A Multidisciplinary Approach in Head and Neck Malignancies

A Multidisciplinary Approach in Head and Neck Malignancies

Editors

Marco Zeppieri
Tamara Ius
Filippo Flavio Angileri
Antonio Pontoriero
Alessandro Tel

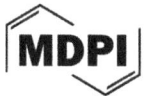

Basel • Beijing • Wuhan • Barcelona • Belgrade • Novi Sad • Cluj • Manchester

Editors

Marco Zeppieri
Department of
Ophthalmology, University
Hospital of Udine
Udine
Italy

Tamara Ius
Neurosurgery Unit,
Head-Neck and
NeuroScience Department,
University Hospital of Udine
Udine
Italy

Filippo Flavio Angileri
Department of Biomedical
and Dental Sciences and
Morphofunctional Imaging,
Neurosurgery Unit,
University of Messina
Messina
Italy

Antonio Pontoriero
Radiotherapy Unit,
University of Messina
Messina
Italy

Alessandro Tel
Department of Maxillofacial
Surgery, University of Udine
Udine
Italy

Editorial Office
MDPI
St. Alban-Anlage 66
4052 Basel, Switzerland

This is a reprint of articles from the Special Issue published online in the open access journal *Journal of Clinical Medicine* (ISSN 2077-0383) (available at: https://www.mdpi.com/journal/jcm/special_issues/6K256X4CM8).

For citation purposes, cite each article independently as indicated on the article page online and as indicated below:

Lastname, A.A.; Lastname, B.B. Article Title. *Journal Name* **Year**, *Volume Number*, Page Range.

ISBN 978-3-7258-0987-5 (Hbk)
ISBN 978-3-7258-0988-2 (PDF)
doi.org/10.3390/books978-3-7258-0988-2

© 2024 by the authors. Articles in this book are Open Access and distributed under the Creative Commons Attribution (CC BY) license. The book as a whole is distributed by MDPI under the terms and conditions of the Creative Commons Attribution-NonCommercial-NoDerivs (CC BY-NC-ND) license.

Contents

About the Editors vii

Denis Aiudi, Alessio Iacoangeli, Mauro Dobran, Gabriele Polonara, Mario Chiapponi, Andrea Mattioli, Maurizio Gladi and Maurizio Iacoangeli
The Prognostic Role of Volumetric MRI Evaluation in the Surgical Treatment of Glioblastoma
Reprinted from: *J. Clin. Med.* **2024**, *13*, 849, doi:10.3390/jcm13030849 1

Luca Zanin, Edoardo Agosti, Florian Ebner, Lucio de Maria, Francesco Belotti, Barbara Buffoli, Rita Rezzani, et al.
Quantitative Anatomical Comparison of Surgical Approaches to Meckel's Cave
Reprinted from: *J. Clin. Med.* **2023**, *12*, 6847, doi:10.3390/jcm12216847 16

Matteo de Notaris, Matteo Sacco, Francesco Corrivetti, Michele Grasso, Sergio Corvino, Amedeo Piazza, Doo-Sik Kong, et al.
The Transorbital Approach, A Game-Changer in Neurosurgery: A Guide to Safe and Reliable Surgery Based on Anatomical Principles
Reprinted from: *J. Clin. Med.* **2023**, *12*, 6484, doi:10.3390/jcm12206484 36

Alberto D'Amico, Giulia Melinda Furlanis, Valentina Baro, Luca Sartori, Andrea Landi, Domenico d'Avella, Francesco Sala, et al.
Thalamopeduncular Tumors in Pediatric Age: Advanced Preoperative Imaging to Define Safe Surgical Planning: A Multicentric Experience
Reprinted from: *J. Clin. Med.* **2023**, *12*, 5521, doi:10.3390/jcm12175521 51

Aniek T. Zwart, Laurence M. C. Kok, Julius de Vries, Marloes S. van Kester, Rudi A. J. O. Dierckx, Geertruida H. de Bock, Anouk van der Hoorn, et al.
Radiologically Defined Sarcopenia as a Biomarker for Frailty and Malnutrition in Head and Neck Skin Cancer Patients
Reprinted from: *J. Clin. Med.* **2023**, *12*, 3445, doi:10.3390/jcm12103445 61

Daniele Armocida, Alessandro Pesce, Mauro Palmieri, Fabio Cofano, Giuseppe Palmieri, Paola Cassoni, Carla Letizia Busceti, et al.
EGFR-Driven Mutation in Non-Small-Cell Lung Cancer (NSCLC) Influences the Features and Outcome of Brain Metastases
Reprinted from: *J. Clin. Med.* **2023**, *12*, 3372, doi:10.3390/jcm12103372 75

Yu-Hsuan Lai, Chien-Chou Su, Shang-Yin Wu, Wei-Ting Hsueh, Yuan-Hua Wu, Helen H. W. Chen, Jenn-Ren Hsiao, et al.
Impact of Alcohol and Smoking on Outcomes of HPV-Related Oropharyngeal Cancer
Reprinted from: *J. Clin. Med.* **2022**, *11*, 6510, doi:10.3390/jcm11216510 88

Andrea Bianconi, Flavio Panico, Bruna Lo Zito, Andrea Do Trinh, Paola Cassoni, Umberto Ricardi, Diego Garbossa, et al.
Understanding and Managing Pineal Parenchymal Tumors of Intermediate Differentiation: An In-Depth Exploration from Pathology to Adjuvant Therapies
Reprinted from: *J. Clin. Med.* **2024**, *13*, 1266, doi:10.3390/jcm13051266 101

Domenico La Torre, Attilio Della Torre, Erica Lo Turco, Prospero Longo, Dorotea Pugliese, Paola Lacroce, Giuseppe Raudino, et al.
Primary Intracranial Gliosarcoma: Is It Really a Variant of Glioblastoma? An Update of the Clinical, Radiological, and Biomolecular Characteristics
Reprinted from: *J. Clin. Med.* **2024**, *13*, 83, doi:10.3390/jcm13010083 113

Antonio Colamaria, Augusto Leone, Francesco Carbone, Yasser Andres Dallos Laguado, Nicola Pio Fochi, Matteo Sacco, Cinzia Fesce, et al.
Primary Anaplastic-Lymphoma-Kinase-Positive Large-Cell Lymphoma of the Central Nervous System: Comprehensive Review of the Literature
Reprinted from: *J. Clin. Med.* **2023**, *12*, 7516, doi:10.3390/jcm12247516 . . . . **130**

Grazia D'Onofrio, Nadia Icolaro, Elena Fazzari, Domenico Catapano, Antonello Curcio, Antonio Izzi, Aldo Manuali, et al.
Real-Time Neuropsychological Testing (RTNT) and Music Listening during Glioblastoma Excision in Awake Surgery: A Case Report
Reprinted from: *J. Clin. Med.* **2023**, *12*, 6086, doi:10.3390/jcm12186086 . . . . **142**

Edoardo Agosti, Marco Zeppieri, Lucio De Maria, Marcello Mangili, Alessandro Rapisarda, Tamara Ius, Leopoldo Spadea, et al.
Surgical Treatment of Spheno-Orbital Meningiomas: A Systematic Review and Meta-Analysis of Surgical Techniques and Outcomes
Reprinted from: *J. Clin. Med.* **2023**, *12*, 5840, doi:10.3390/jcm12185840 . . . . **154**

Tobias Moest, Marco Rainer Kesting, Maximilian Rohde, Werner Lang, Alexander Meyer, Manuel Weber and Rainer Lutz
A Treatment Approach for Carotid Blowout Syndrome and Soft Tissue Reconstruction after Radiotherapy in Patients with Oral Cancer: A Report of 2 Cases
Reprinted from: *J. Clin. Med.* **2023**, *12*, 3221, doi:10.3390/jcm12093221 . . . . **182**

About the Editors

Marco Zeppieri

Marco Zeppieri obtained a degree in biology from the University of Toronto in 1992, his medical degree from the University of Milano-Bicocca, Italy, in 2003, and his specialization in ophthalmology from the University of Udine in 2007. In 2012, he completed his Ph.D. at the University of Udine. He also completed a post-doctoral glaucoma research fellowship at the Discoveries in Sight, Devers Eye Institute in Portland, Oregon, USA, in 2006. He obtained his national qualifications as a second-level university professor in 2018. Since January 2008, he has worked as an ophthalmologist at the Department of Ophthalmology at Santa Maria Della Misericordia Hospital in Udine, Italy. His scientific interests include new techniques for the morphological and functional diagnosis of ocular hypertension and glaucoma, the utilization of stem cells for corneal wound lesions, ocular surface and lid diagnostics and treatments, and community-based screening procedures. He has participated at numerous national and international ophthalmology conferences as an invited speaker. He is a reviewer for numerous international peer-reviewed journals, as well as the author of over 100 book chapters and indexed scientific publications in international scientific journals.

Tamara Ius

Tamara Ius graduated from the University of Trieste Medical School (2004) and trained in neurosurgery at Udine Medical Center (2005–2010). She obtained her Ph.D. degree in Robotics, Brain, and Cognitive Function at the Italian Institute of Technology in 2014. She is a member of SINch, EANS, AINO, and EANO. She has been a member of the AINO board since November 2017 and a coordinator of the SINch Neuro-Oncology Section since 2020. She is involved in research in the field of neuro-oncology (brain mapping and awake surgery, skull base surgery, DTI fiber-tracking, glioma, brain tumor-associated stem cell research, molecular markers in glioma, new nanotechnology frontiers in brain mapping, NGS in glioma, and the application of artificial intelligence and machine learning in glioma and meningiomas).

Filippo Flavio Angileri

Filippo Flavio Angileri, a distinguished figure in the field of neurosurgery, holds the esteemed position of Full Professor at the University of Messina, Italy. Graduating with honors from the Catholic University of Rome Medical School in 1993, Dr. Angileri embarked on a journey of specialization, completing his residency in Neurosurgery at the University of Messina before undertaking a Fellowship in Neuro-oncology at the same institution. Over the years, he has contributed significantly to academia, holding positions ranging from Assistant Professor to his current role as Full Professor. Dr. Angileri's expertise extends beyond the confines of academia; he has chaired prominent programs and departments, notably serving as Chairman of the Department of Neurosurgery at AOU Policlinico "G. Martino", University of Messina. Actively engaged in scientific societies, he is a member of several esteemed organizations, including the Italian Society of Neurosurgery, Congress of Neurological Surgeons, and European Association of Neurosurgical Societies, among others. Dr. Angileri's leadership is further exemplified through his roles as Chairman of the Neuro-oncology Section of the Italian Society of Neurosurgery and as the Italian Delegate of the Young Neurosurgical Forum of the World Federation of Neurosurgical Societies.

Antonio Pontoriero

Antonio Pontoriero graduated from the University of Messina Medical School (2000) and trained in Radiotherapy at the University of Messina Medical School (2002–2005). Roles have included the following: Assistant Researcher in the Department of Radiological Science, Operative Unit of Radiation Oncology University of Messina (2006–2011); Associate Medical Director Department of Radiological Science, Operative Unit of Radiation Oncology Messina University School of Medicine (2011–2024); Researcher (RTD-A, Assistant Professor), Department of Biomedical Sciences and Morphological and Functional Images, Section of Radiological Science, Operative Unit of Radiation Oncology (2012–2015); Senior Researcher (RTD-B), Department of Biomedical Sciences and Morphological and Functional Images, Section of Radiological Science, Operative Unit of Radiation Oncology Messina (2021-2024). Since 2024, Prof. Antonio has acted as an Associate Professor in Radiation Oncology at the Department of Biomedical Sciences and Morphological and Functional Images. He is a reviewer for numerous international peer-reviewed journals and is the author of over 86 book chapters and indexed scientific publications in international scientific journals.

Alessandro Tel

Alessandro Tel graduated from the University of Udine Medical School (2017) with honors and completed his residency in CMF Surgery at the University of Verona with honors. Currently, he is a consultant in CMF surgery at the University Hospital of Udine. Dr. Tel's career mainly focuses on the application of high technology in CMF surgery, with special attention paid to innovative technologies, including AR and AI. Moreover, he is active in the fields of reconstructive surgery and surgical and molecular oncology, with a special interest in the topic of liquid biopsy. Currently, Dr. Tel's scientific activity includes more than 70 publications registered in ORCID. Moreover, Dr. Tel's editorial project of the first Atlas for VSP in CMF surgery, in collaboration with highly renowned international partners, was accepted by Springer and will be released in 2025.

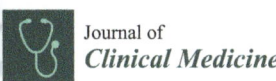

Article

The Prognostic Role of Volumetric MRI Evaluation in the Surgical Treatment of Glioblastoma

Denis Aiudi [1,*], Alessio Iacoangeli [1], Mauro Dobran [1], Gabriele Polonara [2], Mario Chiapponi [1], Andrea Mattioli [1], Maurizio Gladi [1] and Maurizio Iacoangeli [1]

1. Department of Neurosurgery, Università Politecnica delle Marche, Azienda Ospedaliero Universitaria delle Marche, 60121 Ancona, Italy; alessio.iacoangeli95@gmail.com (A.I.); dobran@libero.it (M.D.); mario.chiapponi.med@gmail.com (M.C.); andrea.mattioli.92@gmail.com (A.M.); mauriziogladi@gmail.com (M.G.); neurotra@gmail.com (M.I.)
2. Department of Neuroradiology, Università Politecnica delle Marche, Azienda Ospedaliero Universitaria delle Marche, 60121 Ancona, Italy; gabriele.polonara@ospedaliriuniti.marche.it
* Correspondence: denis.aiudi@gmail.com; Tel.: +39-0715964567

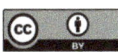

Citation: Aiudi, D.; Iacoangeli, A.; Dobran, M.; Polonara, G.; Chiapponi, M.; Mattioli, A.; Gladi, M.; Iacoangeli, M. The Prognostic Role of Volumetric MRI Evaluation in the Surgical Treatment of Glioblastoma. *J. Clin. Med.* **2024**, *13*, 849. https://doi.org/10.3390/jcm13030849

Academic Editor: Mario Ganau

Received: 25 September 2023
Revised: 26 January 2024
Accepted: 30 January 2024
Published: 1 February 2024

Copyright: © 2024 by the authors. Licensee MDPI, Basel, Switzerland. This article is an open access article distributed under the terms and conditions of the Creative Commons Attribution (CC BY) license (https://creativecommons.org/licenses/by/4.0/).

Abstract: Background: Glioblastoma is the most common primary brain neoplasm in adults, with a poor prognosis despite a constant effort to improve patient survival. Some neuroradiological volumetric parameters seem to play a predictive role in overall survival (OS) and progression-free survival (PFS). The aim of this study was to analyze the impact of the volumetric areas of contrast-enhancing tumors and perineoplastic edema on the survival of patients treated for glioblastoma. **Methods**: A series of 87 patients who underwent surgery was retrospectively analyzed; OS and PFS were considered the end points of the study. For each patient, a multidisciplinary revision was conducted in collaboration with the Neuroradiology and Neuro-Oncology Board. Manual and semiautomatic measurements were adopted to perform the radiological evaluation, and the following quantitative parameters were retrospectively analyzed: contrast enhancement preoperative tumor volume (CE-PTV), contrast enhancement postoperative tumor volume (CE-RTV), edema/infiltration preoperative volume (T2/FLAIR-PV), edema/infiltration postoperative volume (T2/FLAIR-RV), necrosis volume inside the tumor (NV), and total tumor volume including necrosis (TV). **Results**: The median OS value was 9 months, and the median PFS value was 4 months; the mean values were 12.3 and 6.9 months, respectively. Multivariate analysis showed that the OS-related factors were adjuvant chemoradiotherapy ($p < 0.0001$), CE-PTV < 15 cm^3 ($p = 0.03$), surgical resection $> 95\%$ ($p = 0.004$), and the presence of a "pseudocapsulated" radiological morphology ($p = 0.04$). **Conclusions**: Maximal safe resection is one of the most relevant predictive factors for patient survival. Semiautomatic preoperative MRI evaluation could play a key role in prognostically categorizing these tumors.

Keywords: FLAIR infiltration; brain tumors; extent of surgical resection; glioblastoma; overall survival; progression-free survival; pseudocapsule; neuro-oncology; tumor volume

1. Introduction

Glioblastoma (GB) is the most common primary brain neoplasm in adults and the most common malignancy of the CNS (approximately 49% of malignant brain tumors are glioblastomas) [1], It is described by the WHO as grade 4 according to the most recent updates to the WHO classification (2021) [2,3].

Age, sex, and race/ethnicity influence the incidence rate, which exponentially increases beyond 40 years of age. The mean age of diagnosis is 65 years, and it peaks between 75 and 84 years. GB is more common in males and Caucasians compared to African-American patients [4].

Adult-type diffuse gliomas now consist of only three categories: astrocytoma, IDH-mutant; oligodendroglioma, IDH-mutant and 1p/19-codeleted; and glioblastoma, IDH-wildtype. Thus, astrocytic tumors are grouped as those with and without IDH mutations;

those without IDH mutations (wildtype) are named glioblastomas IDH-wildtype. The term "glioblastoma multiforme" should not be used [1,2].

Despite decades of advances in surgery and discoveries in molecular research, encouraging outcomes are not typically observed; patients diagnosed with this tumor generally have a dismal prognosis and poor quality of life as the disease progresses. The median survival time has been reported to be less than 15 months on average. Survival longer than 3–5 years has been reported for approximately 0.5% of GB patients [5].

These data have led to an increasing number of studies focused on acquiring knowledge about GB prognostic factors. According to the literature, the most relevant prognostic factors are age, sex, Karnofsky Performance Status (KPS), surgical resection rate, adjuvant therapies performed, and tumor molecular biology [6]. This last characteristic has grown in importance because several genetic mutations have been shown to have a prognostic role, such as MGMT promoter methylation, loss of 10q heterozygosity, miRNA dysregulation, EGFR mutation, PTEN mutation, P53 mutation, and especially IDH1 mutation.

Positive GB prognostic elements:

MGMT promoter methylation: Methylation of the MGMT (O6-methylguanine-DNA methyltransferase) promoter is associated with an improved response to temozolomide chemotherapy, leading to a more favorable prognosis in glioblastoma patients.

ATRX mutations: ATRX mutations, particularly in the context of the IDH-mutant, 1p/19q non-codeleted subtype, are generally associated with a more favorable prognosis and longer overall survival rates.

IDH1 R132H and IDH2 R173 mutations: In the rare instances of glioblastoma harboring these specific IDH mutations, patients tend to have a better prognosis compared to IDH wildtype glioblastomas. However, it is important to note that these mutations are relatively rare in glioblastoma.

Negative GB prognostic elements:

EGFR amplification: Amplification of the EGFR (epidermal growth factor receptor) gene is associated with increased tumor aggressiveness and a poorer prognosis in glioblastoma patients.

TERTp mutations: Mutations in the TERT (telomerase reverse transcriptase) promoter are often associated with increased telomerase activity and contribute to the aggressiveness of glioblastoma, resulting in a poorer prognosis.

Gain of Chr.7 and loss of Chr.10: Chromosomal alterations involving the gain of chromosome 7 and the loss of chromosome 10 are commonly observed in glioblastoma and are associated with more aggressive tumor behavior and a worse prognosis [1].

Recent studies have also shown increasing interest in some neuroradiological parameters, evaluated both prior and after surgery, that seem to play a predictive role in overall survival (OS) and progression-free survival (PFS) [7–10].

Glioblastomas are typically large tumors at diagnosis. They often have thick, irregularly enhancing margins and a central necrotic core, which may also have a hemorrhagic component. They are characterized by their ability to invade surrounding parenchyma and are usually surrounded by vasogenic-type edema, which, in fact, usually contains infiltration by neoplastic cells, making curative resection difficult.

Contrast-enhanced brain magnetic resonance imaging is the gold standard for diagnosis and presurgical planning. T1-weighted (T1) and T2-weighted/fluid-attenuated inversion recovery (T2/FLAIR) sequences are commonly used in the study of glioblastoma.

T1-weighted images provide good anatomical detail and are excellent for visualizing the brain's anatomy, and GB typically appear hypointense (dark) due to their high cellularity and increased protein content, making them distinguishable from surrounding normal brain tissues. Enhancement patterns on T1 postcontrast images are often present and are typically peripheral and irregular with nodular components. They are usually indicative of increased vascularity and blood–brain barrier disruption surrounding a necrotic core, which may also have a hemorrhagic component.

T2-weighted images are sensitive to variations in water content and are useful for highlighting vasogenic-type edema, which usually contains infiltration by neoplastic cells and typically appears hyperintense (bright) in GB. FLAIR sequences suppress cerebrospinal fluid (CSF) signals, enhancing the visibility of abnormalities near CSF-filled spaces and making it easier to identify tumor borders.

The extent of edema seen on T2/FLAIR images can provide information about the tumor's infiltrative nature and its impact on the surrounding brain tissues. The absence of a T2/FLAIR mismatch may also help with differential diagnosis.

The aim of our study was to analyze clinical, radiological, and histologic characteristics as predictive factors for OS and PFS in patients affected by GB who underwent surgery and were monitored at our institute; in particular, the impact of the volumetric areas of contrast-enhancing tumor and perineoplastic edema on the outcome of patients was analyzed.

2. Materials and Methods

A series of 87 patients diagnosed with GB (glioblastoma, IDH-wildtype, CNS WHO grade 4) who underwent surgery at our institution between 2020 and 2022 was retrospectively analyzed.

Overall survival (OS, defined as the time from first surgery until death) and progression-free survival (PFS, defined as the time from first surgery and the radiological evidence of disease relapse/progression on MRI) were considered the end points of the study. For each patient, demographic, clinical, radiological, and histological characteristics were studied as predictive factors, and a multidisciplinary revision of medical records was conducted in collaboration with the Neuroradiology and Neuro-Oncology Board.

Manual and semiautomatic measurements were adopted to perform the radiological evaluation, and the following quantitative parameters were retrospectively analyzed: contrast enhancement preoperative tumor volume (CE-PTV), contrast enhancement postoperative tumor volume (CE-RTV), edema/infiltration preoperative volume (T2/FLAIR-PV), edema/infiltration postoperative volume (T2/FLAIR-RV), necrosis volume inside the tumor (NV), and total tumor volume including necrosis (TV). Quantitative volumetric assessment was carried out using the Advantage Workstation Server 3.2 (AW Server 3.2, General Electric®, 2009–2015, Boston, MA, USA).

A presurgery MRI was available for all patients; 37 (42.5%) of them also underwent a postoperative MRI within the first 48 h after surgery. All exams were performed on 1.5 T scanners.

CE-PTV was evaluated on 2D axial contrast-enhanced T1 weighted (CE-T1w) images (slice thickness: 5 mm; slice spacing: 5.5–6 mm) by contouring manually enhanced tumor areas on every single axial slice, excluding necrosis; the same analysis was subsequently performed with the semiautomatic method using the specific tool of the AW Server 3.2 (Figures 1 and 2).

CE-RTV was assessed on 2D axial CE-T1w images (slice thickness: 5 mm; slice spacing: 5.5–6 mm) with the subtraction imaging technique to minimize errors due to the spontaneous hyperintensity of degradation products of hemoglobin or those related to the presence of hemostatic/chemotherapeutic agents in the surgical area. As for CE-PTV, the analysis was performed both manually and semiautomatically (Figures 3 and 4).

T2/FLAIR-PV and T2/FLAIR-RV were both evaluated manually on axial hybrid sequences resulting from FLAIR (slice thickness: 5 mm; slice spacing: 5.5 mm) and CE-T1w (slice thickness: 5 mm; slice spacing: 5.5–6 mm) fusion in order to exclusively measure the edema/infiltration component, excluding the tumor (enhancing mass) previously assessed with CE-PTV and CE-RTV measurements (Figures 5 and 6).

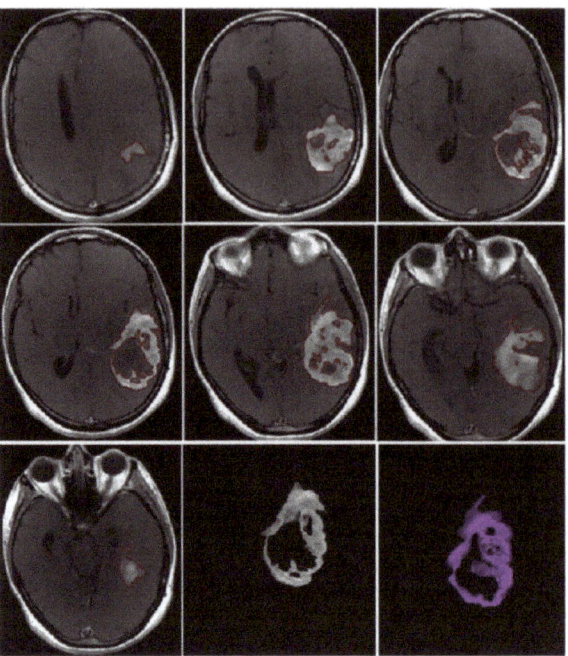

Figure 1. CE-PTV, contrast-enhanced T1 weighted (CE-T1w) images by contouring manually enhanced tumor areas on every single axial slice, excluding necrosis.

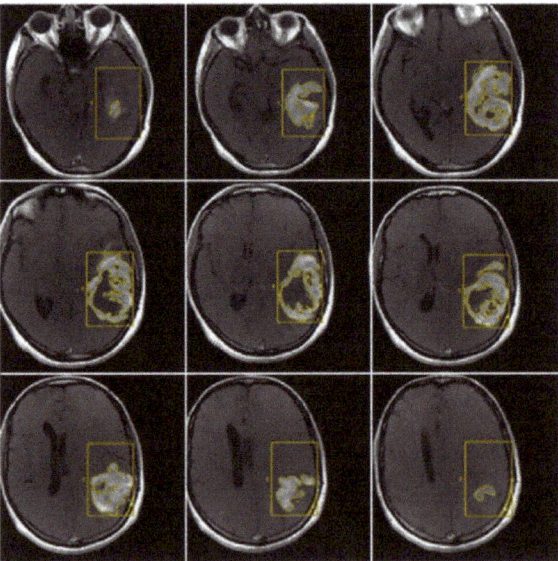

Figure 2. CE-PTV, contrast-enhanced T1 weighted (CE-T1w) images performed with the semiautomatic method using the specific tool of the AW Server 3.2. The yellow box represents the area selected by the radiologist that the software analyzes (semi-automatic method).

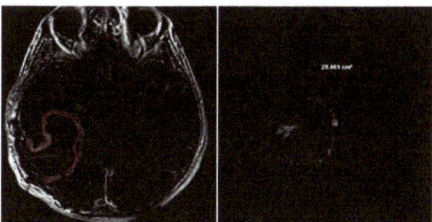

Figure 3. Contrast enhancement postoperative tumor volume (CE-RTV) manual evaluation, achieved with subtraction imaging technique to minimize errors due to the spontaneous hyperintensity of degradation products of hemoglobin.

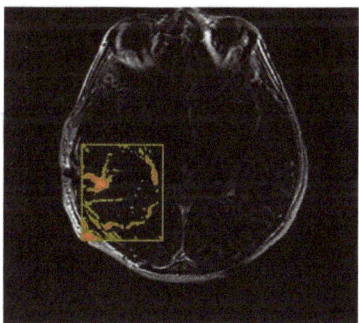

Figure 4. Contrast enhancement postoperative tumor volume (CE-RTV) semiautomatic evaluation, assessed on 2D axial CE-T1w images (slice thickness: 5 mm; slice spacing: 5.5–6 mm), achieved with the semiautomatic subtraction imaging technique.

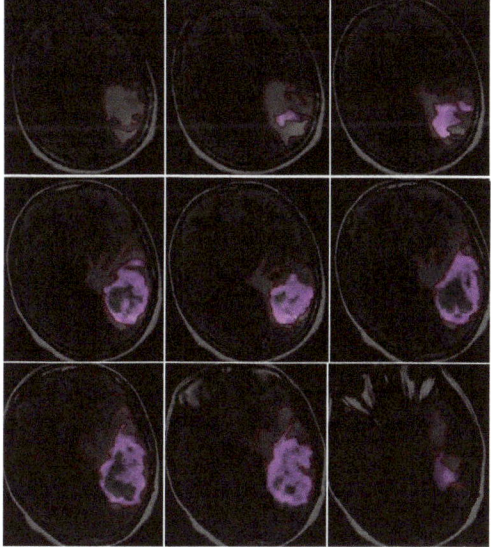

Figure 5. Edema/infiltration preoperative volume (T2/FLAIR-PV), evaluated manually on axial hybrid sequences resulting from FLAIR (slice thickness: 5 mm; slice spacing: 5.5 mm) and CE-T1w in order to exclusively measure the edema/infiltration component, excluding the tumor (enhancing mass) previously assessed with CE-PTV and CE-RTV measurements.

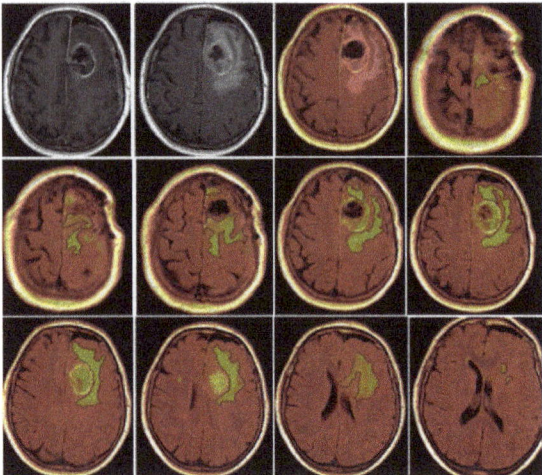

Figure 6. Edema/infiltration postoperative volume (T2/FLAIR-RV), evaluated manually on axial hybrid sequences resulting from FLAIR and CE-T1w fusion in order to exclusively measure the edema/infiltration component, excluding the tumor (enhancing mass).

NV was evaluated manually on preoperative 2D axial CE-T1w images, including only the necrotic area inside the tumor (Figure 7).

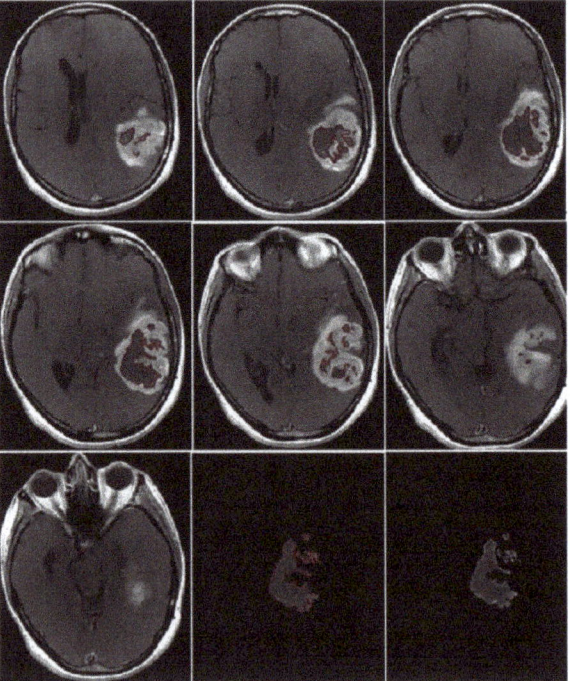

Figure 7. Necrosis volume inside the tumor, evaluated manually on preoperative 2D axial CE-T1w images, including only the necrotic area inside the tumor.

TV was calculated as the sum of NV and CE-PTV, both assessed on 2D axial CE-T1w images (slice thickness: 5 mm; slice spacing: 5.5–6 mm).

In the case of tumor localization near eloquent brain areas, the extent of surgical resection was modulated based on neurophysiological monitoring techniques such as sensorimotor evoked potentials and electrocorticography.

Furthermore, we investigated the following relevant qualitative characteristics of GB: tumor localization (the lobe containing the enhancing mass or, in case of radiological multifocality, the lobe corresponding to the main tumor mass was considered as the tumor site); eloquent area involvement (defined as neoplastic infiltration of the cortex or iuxta-cortical white matter of eloquent areas, such as motor, visual, Wernicke's area, or Broca's area); and radiological appearance (distinguished by three different patterns based on the enhancing wall thickness on CE-T1w sequences: thin, with enhancing wall thickness < 3 mm; thin-nodular, with enhancing wall showing focal thickening > 3 mm; and nodular, with solid appearance predominant and intratumoral necrosis absent or less than 1.5 cm^3) (Figure 8). Similarly, we identified two morphological categories: "pseudocapsulated" and non-pseudo-capsulated masses, depending on the macroscopic appearance of a pseudocleavage plane at the time of neurosurgery. Furthermore, we analyzed the presence of ependymal involvement (defined as visible signal alteration on FLAIR images or tumor mass joining the ependymal interface) and focal or multifocal disease (focal if only a single mass was observed; multifocal if multiple tumor foci were visible, contiguous to FLAIR signal alterations or not, with no difference between the terms "multifocal" and "multicenter").

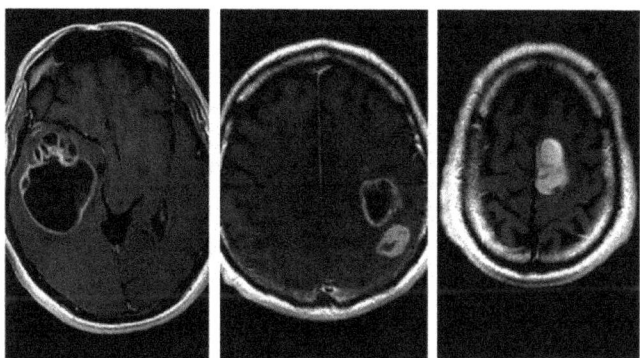

Figure 8. Thin, with enhancing wall thickness < 3 mm (**left**); thin-nodular, with enhancing wall focal thickenings > 3 mm (**center**); and nodular, with solid appearance predominant and intratumoral necrosis absent or less than 1.5 cm^3 (**right**).

Patients with incomplete data sets were not included in the study sample.

Statistical analysis was performed using the MedCalc 15.8 Portable software.

Univariate analysis was carried out using the Kaplan–Meier method, and patient subgroups were compared employing the log-rank test. Both univariate and multivariate analyses were based on the Cox proportional hazard regression stepwise method to identify predictive factors for OS and PFS.

A p-value < 0.05 was considered statistically significant.

All procedures performed in the study were conducted in accordance with the ethics standards given in the 1964 Declaration of Helsinki, as revised in 2013. The study protocol was approved by the Institutional Ethics Review Board at our institution. All participants provided written informed consent for their participation in the study, and patient consent was obtained for the purpose of the study with due care to maintain their privacy.

3. Results

Our sample included 87 patients; 45 (51.7%) were males and 42 (48.3%) were females, and the mean age was 67 years (range: 25–85 years). At the time of our study, 22 (25.3%) patients were still alive, and 65 (74.7%) were deceased.

All patients underwent neurosurgical intervention; 68 (78.1%) of them received adjuvant therapy as follows: 4 (4.6%) patients received only chemotherapy, 7 (8%) patients received only radiotherapy, and 57 (65.5%) received both chemo- and radiotherapy. A total of 19 (21.9%) patients did not receive any adjuvant treatment.

The median OS was 9 months, and the median PFS was 4 months; the mean values were 12.3 months for OS and 6.9 months for PFS.

The KPS was evaluated before and after surgery: 74 (85%) patients showed a preoperative KPS > 80 and 13 (15%) had a preoperative KPS < 80; two months after surgery, there were 49 (59%) patients with a postoperative KPS < 80, while there were 34 (41%) patients who had a postoperative KPS > 80. Four patients died within the first month after surgery.

3.1. Qualitative Analysis

- Localization: All tumors had a supratentorial localization; 31 (36%) were in the frontal lobe, 18 (21%) were in the parietal lobe, 36 (41%) in the temporal lobe, and 2 (2%) in the occipital lobe.
- Eloquent areas: 35 of the 87 lesions (40%) were in eloquent areas.
- Ependymal involvement: Ependymal involvement was observed in 52 (60%) patients; 35 (40%) lesions had no connection with the periventricular zone.
- Morphological appearance: We divided GB lesions into three categories based on the enhancing wall thickness: thin, <3 mm; thin-nodular, when the enhancing wall showed focal thickenings > 3 mm; and nodular, when solid appearance was predominant and intratumoral necrosis was absent or <1.5 cm^3. A total of 11 (13%) masses showed a thin pattern, 51 (58%) showed a thin-nodular pattern, and 25 (29%) showed a nodular pattern.
- Multifocal disease: Multifocal disease was found in 20 (23.3%) patients (Table 1).

Table 1. Qualitative analysis.

Localization	n (%)	Morphology	n (%)
Frontal lobe	31 (36%)	Multifocal	20 (23.3%)
Parietal lobe	18 (21%)	Thin (d < 3 mm)	11 (13%)
Temporal lobe	36 (41%)	Thin-nodular (d > 3 mm)	51 (58%)
Occipital lobe	2 (2%)	Nodular	25 (29%)
Eloquent areas	35 (40%)	Pseudocapsulated	62 (71%)
Ependymal involvment	52 (60%)		

3.2. Quantitative Analysis

Median CE-PTV values obtained by manual and semiautomatic methods were 24.8 and 22.6 cm^3, respectively. A good concordance value (R^2: 0.86) between manual and semiautomatic measurements was observed; a greater dispersion rate was noticeable for volume values > 25 cm^3.

We also calculated the percent deviation between manual and semiautomatic volumes, and the resulting deviation mean value was 4%, despite a mean squared deviation value of 34%. This result is probably due to the high values of the mean squared deviation corresponding to mass volumes > 40 cm^3. Similar results were observed for the CE-RTV manual and semiautomatic volume correlation; the CE-RTV median values obtained by manual and semiautomatic methods were 5.8 and 6.8 cm^3, respectively.

The TV median value was 37.7 cm^3, and the surgical resection median value was 78%.

T2/FLAIR-PV and T2/FLAIR-RV were 59.2 and 42.3 cm^3, respectively; the preoperative necrosis volume median value was 6.6 cm^3.

3.3. Overall Survival—Univariate Analysis

The univariate analysis showed that adjuvant therapies (chemotherapy, radiotherapy, and chemoradiotherapy) and CE-RTV < 5.8 cm^3 were the only variables connected with OS.

- Chemotherapy: The median OS values were 15 months for patients who received adjuvant chemotherapy (n = 61) and 3 months for patients who did not (n = 26); the difference between the two groups was statistically significant ($p < 0.0001$).
- Radiotherapy: The median OS values were 14 months for patients who received adjuvant radiotherapy (n = 64) and 3 months for patients who did not (n = 23); the difference between the two groups was statistically significant ($p < 0.0001$).
- Chemoradiotherapy: The median OS values were 16 months for patients who received chemoradiotherapy (n = 57), 6 months for patients who received radiotherapy alone (n = 7), and 5 months for patients who received chemotherapy alone (n = 4); the median OS value was 2 months for patients who did not receive any adjuvant treatment (n = 19). The difference was statistically significant ($p < 0.0001$).
- CE-RTV: The median OS value was 19 months for patients with CE-RTV < 5.8 cm^3 and 9 months for patients with CE-RTV > 5.8 cm^3. The difference was statistically significant ($p < 0.004$) (Table 2).

Table 2. Overall survival.

	Median OS Treated (n)	Median OS Not Treated (n)	p-Value
AC	15 (n = 61)	3 (n = 26)	<0.0001
ART	14 (n = 64)	3 (n = 23)	<0.0001
CRT	16 (n = 57)	2 (n = 19)	<0.0001
CT	5 (n = 4)		
RT	6 (n = 7)		
NT	2 (n = 19)		
CE-RTV	<5.8 cm^3: 19	>5.8 cm^3: 9	<0.004

OS, overall survival; AC, adjuvant chemotherapy; ART, adjuvant radiotherapy; CRT, chemoradiotherapy; CT, chemotherapy; RT, radiotherapy; NT, not treated.

3.4. Overall Survival—Multivariate Analysis

Similar to univariate analysis, multivariate analysis showed that adjuvant chemo- and radiotherapy were OS-related prognostic factors ($p < 0.0001$). Furthermore, multivariate analysis proved that the only OS-related radiological prognostic factor was CE-PTV < 15 cm^3 ($p = 0.03$).

3.5. Progression-Free Survival—Univariate Analysis

During follow-up, 70 patients showed disease relapse or progression; the median PFS value was 4 months, while the mean PFS value was 6.9 months.

Univariate analysis demonstrated that PFS-related variables were gender, adjuvant chemo- and radiotherapy, postoperative KPS, and CE-RTV.

- Gender: The median PFS value was 4 months for men and 5 months for women. The difference was statistically significant ($p = 0.02$).
- Chemotherapy: The median PFS value was 6 months for patients who underwent chemotherapy and 1 month for patients who did not. The difference was statistically significant ($p < 0.0001$).

- Radiotherapy: The median PFS value was 5 months for patients who received radiotherapy and 1 month for patients who did not. The difference was statistically significant ($p < 0.0001$).
- Postoperative KPS: The median PFS value was 3 months in patients with postoperative KPS < 80 and 7 months in patients with postoperative KPS > 80. The difference was statistically significant ($p < 0.0001$).
- CE-RTV: The median PFS value was 5 months in patients with CE-RTV < 5.8 cm^3 and 4 months in patients with CE-RTV > 5.8 cm^3. The difference was statistically significant ($p = 0.04$).
- Surgical resection: The median PFS value was 6 months in patients with a surgical resection percentage > 95% and 4 months if the surgical resection percentage was <95%. The difference was statistically significant ($p = 0.02$).

3.6. Progression-Free Survival—Multivariate Analysis

PFS-related variables in multivariate analysis were adjuvant radiotherapy ($p = 0.01$), surgical resection percentage > 95% ($p = 0.004$), and the presence of "pseudocapsulated" morphologic gross appearance ($p = 0.04$).

The preliminary analysis, performed with the McNemar test for qualitative dichotomous nominal variables to find a correlation between "pseudocapsulated" appearance and other parameters, showed a strong match between the macroscopic presence of pseudocapsule and the nodular pattern observed in preoperative MRI ($p < 0.0001$) (Table 3).

Table 3. Progression-free survival.

	Median PFS (Months)		p-Value
Sex (M/F)	Male 4	Female 5	$p = 0.02$
Chemotherapy	With: 6 /	Without: 1	$p < 0.0001$
Radiotherapy	With: 5 /	Without: 1	$p < 0.0001$
Postoperative KPS	<80: 3	>80: 7	$p < 0.0001$
CE-RTV	<5.8 cm^3: 5	>5.8 cm^3: 4	$p = 0.04$
Surgical resection (%)	>95%: 6	>95%: 4	$p = 0.02$
Pseudocapsulated	with: 6	Without: 3	$p < 0.0001$

All quantitative data for CE-PTV and CE-RTV evaluations are shown in Table 4.

Table 4. Quantitative data for CE-PTV and CE-RTV evaluations.

Patient	Semiautomatic CE-PTV (cm^3)	Manual CE-PTV (cm^3)	CE-RTV (cm^3)
1	34.89	31.14	
2	30.00	33.51	16.37
3	27.32	33.33	0.00
4	17.53	15.46	
5	12.21	5.24	
6	5.21	4.70	0.00
7	21.99	24.04	10.71
8	59.10	38.78	5.82
9	20.15	21.31	6.98
10	64.52	72.11	
11	11.83	10.58	10.12
12	49.81	49.72	
13	11.01	10.17	
14	20.87	17.97	
15	32.55	39.27	
16	46.11	42.10	

Table 4. Cont.

Patient	Semiautomatic CE-PTV (cm³)	Manual CE-PTV (cm³)	CE-RTV (cm³)
17	35.88	36.29	
18	23.65	39.15	
19	5.87	5.21	4.65
20	25.75	24.16	10.49
21	17.78	14.68	
22	20.43	21.26	
23	1.18	0.39	0.00
24	10.93	11.26	
25	16.06	14.84	0.00
26	20.11	18.65	13.28
27	25.89	25.40	0.00
28	19.49	13.90	0.00
29	39.34	42.64	16.67
30	38.90	42.41	
31	20.24	22.89	
32	43.90	42.09	4.17
33	14.30	13.22	8.44
34	24.87	23.45	6.85
35	4.51	5.29	2.85
36	28.13	24.56	
37	68.11	61.67	
38	51.79	54.13	
39	59.65	64.19	
40	83.58	65.28	
41	18.34	13.45	
42	8.03	10.69	
43	49.64	28.78	5.27
44	62.41	51.74	
45	22.34	12.37	
46	5.69	9.09	
47	20.00	17.02	0.00
48	47.05	44.89	
49	2.12	1.60	
50	31.19	34.89	
51	6.73	5.93	
52	28.91	34.66	
53	8.54	8.50	3.30
54	50.48	60.56	
55	12.72	11.05	7.75
56	28.14	27.22	12.23
57	37.39	32.12	
58	37.98	31.05	0.00
59	36.26	51.17	
60	22.56	27.87	5.32
61	28.90	44.36	
62	16.00	15.98	14.46
63	5.97	17.10	
64	17.40	17.61	7.38
65	14.28	15.88	5.78
66	8.80	10.30	
67	46.00	49.34	28.97
68	0.79	0.97	
69	15.53	12.24	0.73
70	29.56	41.62	
71	10.79	11.25	
72	37.61	51.02	
73	21.61	29.19	
74	24.86	33.77	

Table 4. Cont.

Patient	Semiautomatic CE-PTV (cm³)	Manual CE-PTV (cm³)	CE-RTV (cm³)
75	18.46	20.99	
76	42.89	46.64	42.96
77	42.32	54.07	
78	24.09	24.08	0.58
79	83.44	84.80	29.46
80	12.51	11.59	
81	14.12	10.71	1.30
82	37.00	54.50	
83	47.58	37.95	
84	2.35	2.98	0.00
85	12.98	12.60	11.45
86	15.53	21.01	
87	39.18	42.70	8.17

4. Discussion

According to the most recent literature, OS median values in patients with GB ranges from 6 to 14 months [11], while the PFS median value is 6 months [12]. Our data (OS median value: 9 months; PFS median value: 4 months) seems to be consistent with this evidence. CE-PTV and TV median values of our sample were 24 and 39 cm³, respectively, compared to other studies such as Wangaryattawanich et al.'s series that reported a median CE-PTV = 21 cm³ and Ellingson et al.'s work with a median TV = 15 cm³; this difference may depend on the fact that larger masses were resected in our series, and this could explain our lower survival rate [13,14]. CE-PTV < 15 cm³ was an independent predictive factor for OS together with adjuvant radio and chemotherapy in multivariate analysis; especially when combined, it significantly increased the OS. Total tumor volume including necrosis (TV), with a 15 cm³ cut-off, represented a relevant independent prognostic factor in multivariate analysis, in accordance with the aforementioned studies. Additionally, these findings underscore the importance of accurate tumor volume assessment for optimizing treatment strategies and predicting outcomes in GB patients.

Chaichana et al. established thresholds for the extent of resection and residual volume that impact the survival and recurrence rates in patients with newly diagnosed intracranial glioblastoma. Our analysis confirmed these findings by analyzing postoperative enhancing mass volume (CE-RTV), resulting in a significance cut-off value of 5.8 cm³. This parameter emerged as an important independent prognostic factor in univariate analysis. Notably, patients with CE-RTV < 5.8 cm³ demonstrated superior OS and PFS values, emphasizing the pivotal role of surgical mass removal rates [15]. Univariate analysis concerning PFS revealed that factors such as female gender, adjuvant chemo- and radiotherapy, absence of postoperative neurological deficits, CE-RTV < 5.8 cm³, and surgical resection rate > 95% of TV significantly increased its median value. Multivariate analysis pointed towards adjuvant radiotherapy and surgical resection rate > 95% of TV as independent predictive prognostic factors. The absence of postoperative neurological deficits was a noteworthy parameter influencing PFS, leading to higher values in patients without deficiencies. This condition strongly correlated with Karnofsky Performance Status (KPS) values > 80, emphasizing the crucial role of KPS as a prognostic factor, a notion well-supported in the existing literature [16–18]. A reduction in KPS value postsurgery emerged as a negative prognostic factor. In our experience, a surgical resection rate > 95% proved to be a relevant independent prognostic factor for PFS in multivariate analysis, further affirming its significance alongside adjuvant chemo- and radiotherapy. These factors, which are well documented in the literature, played a decisive role in our series, significantly associating with both OS and PFS [6,19–23].

In our investigation, we identified an additional independent prognostic factor for progression-free survival (PFS): the presence of a morphological "pseudocapsulated" gross appearance in the tumoral mass. This phenomenon is characterized by a lesion displaying an apparent "pseudocapsule" at the superficial aspect, possibly attributed to regions of necrosis and hemorrhage, as suggested by Khadijeh Abdal et al. [24]. Our preliminary experience indicates that this more compact mass, with evidence of a pseudocleavage plan, is correlated with the nodular preoperative MRI pattern. To our knowledge, this specific association has not been widely documented in the existing literature. The identification of this aspect by the neurosurgeon, coupled with neuroradiological findings, may be related to the anatomopathological characterization.

Some tumors exhibit a type of "pseudoplane" surrounding the nodule, facilitating easier and more effective removal. Al-Holou et al. [8] demonstrated that circumferential perilesional resection of glioblastoma (GB) was linked to significantly higher rates of complete resection and lower rates of neurological complications, even for tumors in eloquent locations. Perilesional resection, when feasible, should be considered a preferred option.

Our analysis did not identify them as significant in our T2/FLAIR-PV and T2/FLAIR-RV cohorts as significant prognostic factors, even though some studies have suggested these volumetric parameters as important OS (T2/FLAIR-PV = 85 cm^3) and PFS (T2/FLAIR-RV = 24.85 cm^3) predictive factors. Grossman R. et al. [25] noticed that OS was related to CE-RTV assessed immediately after surgery and that a FLAIR alteration signal volume reduction of at least 46% of preoperative volume (or a postoperative FLAIR alteration signal volume < 19.3 cm^3) evaluated 3 months after surgery represented a favorable prognostic factor for OS, suggesting that surgical resection beyond contrast-enhancing boundaries could represent a promising strategy to improve outcomes in GB patients. In relation to the amount of FLAIR abnormality removal (defined as the rate of resection of the infiltrative tumor component), Pessina et al. recorded a cut-off value for conditioning survival of 45% [9].

While these data necessitate correlation with main predictive factors such as KPS and adjuvant therapies, quantitative imaging emerges as a reliable and valuable tool in predicting overall and progression-free survival in glioblastoma patients undergoing surgery. Notably, the removal of the surrounding perinodular area stands out as a significant prognostic factor. Tumors exhibiting a nodular pattern, in our experience, correlate with enhanced surgical removal, leading to maximal safe asportation and an improved prognosis. This, however, needs to be carefully balanced with the goal of minimizing neurological deficits. Glioblastoma is not merely a surgical disease but a complex condition demanding multimodal treatment and multidisciplinary management. It remains crucial to acknowledge that increasing resection volume, at the cost of inducing new or permanent neurological deficits, may nullify the survival benefit conferred to patients. Therefore, a judicious approach is essential to optimizing both surgical outcomes and overall patient well-being.

5. Conclusions

In conclusion, despite the incorporation of diverse therapies, the prognosis for GB patients remains bleak. A radical, yet safe, maximal surgical resection still retains its role as a crucial predictive factor for patient survival. The integration of quantitative MRI volumetric imaging, particularly semiautomatic preoperative evaluation, emerges as pivotal in stratifying the prognostic categories of these tumors and shows the intricate interplay between surgical precision, imaging technologies, and overall patient outcomes. Therefore, advancing our understanding of these dynamics holds promise for refining treatment strategies and ultimately improving the challenging prognosis faced by GB patients.

Author Contributions: Conceptualization: D.A., A.I. and G.P.; methodology: M.D. and D.A.; formal analysis: D.A., M.C. and A.M.; investigation: D.A., M.I., G.P., A.I., A.M., M.G., M.D. and M.C.; data curation: D.A.; writing—original draft preparation: D.A., A.I., A.M. and M.C.; writing—review and editing: M.G. and M.I. All authors have read and agreed to the published version of the manuscript.

Funding: This research received no external funding.

Institutional Review Board Statement: The study was conducted in accordance with the Declaration of Helsinki, and ethical review and approval were waived for this study due to the retrospective nature of the study and the fact that all the procedures being performed were part of routine care.

Informed Consent Statement: Informed consent was obtained from the patients to publish this paper.

Data Availability Statement: The data presented in this study are available on request from the corresponding author. The data are not publicly available due to privacy reasons.

Conflicts of Interest: The authors declare no conflicts of interest.

References

1. Schaff, L.R.; Mellinghoff, I.K. Glioblastoma and Other Primary Brain Malignancies in Adults: A Review. *JAMA* **2023**, *329*, 574–587. [CrossRef]
2. Torp, S.H.; Solheim, O.; Skjulsvik, A.J. The WHO 2021 Classification of Central Nervous System tumours: A practical update on what neurosurgeons need to know—A minireview. *Acta Neurochir.* **2022**, *164*, 2453–2464. [CrossRef]
3. Stoyanov, G.S.; Lyutfi, E.; Georgieva, R.; Georgiev, R.; Dzhenkov, D.L.; Petkova, L.; Ivanov, B.D.; Kaprelyan, A.; Ghenev, P. Reclassification of Glioblastoma Multiforme According to the 2021 World Health Organization Classification of Central Nervous System Tumors: A Single Institution Report and Practical Significance. *Cureus* **2022**, *14*, e21822. [CrossRef] [PubMed]
4. Melhem, J.M.; Detsky, J.; Lim-Fat, M.J.; Perry, J.R. Updates in IDH-Wildtype Glioblastoma. *Neurotherapeutics* **2022**, *19*, 1705–1723. [CrossRef] [PubMed]
5. Lakomy, R.; Kazda, T.; Selingerova, I.; Poprach, A.; Pospisil, P.; Belanova, R.; Fadrus, P.; Vybihal, V.; Smrcka, M.; Jancalek, R.; et al. Real-World Evidence in Glioblastoma: Stupp's Regimen after a Decade. *Front. Oncol.* **2020**, *10*, 840. [CrossRef]
6. Delgado-López, P.D.; Corrales-García, E.M. Survival in glioblastoma: A review on the impact of treatment modalities. *Clin. Transl. Oncol.* **2016**, *18*, 1062–1071. [CrossRef] [PubMed]
7. Polonara, G.; Aiudi, D.; Iacoangeli, A.; Raggi, A.; Ottaviani, M.M.; Antonini, R.; Iacoangeli, M.; Dobran, M. Glioblastoma: A Retrospective Analysis of the Role of the Maximal Surgical Resection on Overall Survival and Progression Free Survival. *Biomedicines* **2023**, *11*, 739. [CrossRef]
8. Al-Holou, W.N.; Hodges, T.R.; Everson, R.G.; Freeman, J.; Zhou, S.; Suki, D.; Rao, G.; Ferguson, S.D.; Heimberger, A.B.; McCutcheon, I.E.; et al. Perilesional Resection of Glioblastoma Is Independently Associated with Improved Outcomes. *Neurosurgery* **2020**, *86*, 112–121. [CrossRef]
9. Pessina, F.; Navarria, P.; Cozzi, L.; Ascolese, A.M.; Simonelli, M.; Santoro, A.; Clerici, E.; Rossi, M.; Scorsetti, M.; Bello, L. Maximize surgical resection beyond contrast-enhancing boundaries in newly diagnosed glioblastoma multiforme: Is it useful and safe? A single institution retrospective experience. *J. Neurooncol.* **2017**, *135*, 129–139. [CrossRef]
10. Hooper, G.W.; Ansari, S.; Johnson, J.M.; Ginat, D.T. Advances in the Radiological Evaluation of and Theranostics for Glioblastoma. *Cancers* **2023**, *15*, 4162. [CrossRef]
11. Brown, N.F.; Ottaviani, D.; Tazare, J.; Gregson, J.; Kitchen, N.; Brandner, S.; Fersht, N.; Mulholland, P. Survival Outcomes and Prognostic Factors in Glioblastoma. *Cancers* **2022**, *14*, 3161. [CrossRef] [PubMed]
12. Soffietti, R.; Trevisan, E.; Bertero, L.; Cassoni, P.; Morra, I.; Fabrini, M.G.; Pasqualetti, F.; Lolli, I.; Castiglione, A.; Ciccone, G.; et al. Bevacizumab and fotemustine for recurrent glioblastoma: A phase II study of AINO (Italian Association of Neuro-Oncology). *J. Neurooncol.* **2014**, *116*, 533–541. [CrossRef] [PubMed]
13. Wangaryattawanich, P.; Hatami, M.; Wang, J.; Thomas, G.; Flanders, A.; Kirby, J.; Wintermark, M.; Huang, E.S.; Bakhtiari, A.S.; Luedi, M.M.; et al. Multicenter imaging outcomes study of the Cancer Genome Atlas glioblastoma patient cohort: Imaging predictors of overall and progression-free survival. *Neuro Oncol.* **2015**, *17*, 1525–1537. [CrossRef]
14. Ellingson, B.M.; Harris, R.J.; Woodworth, D.C.; Leu, K.; Zaw, O.; Mason, W.P.; Sahebjam, S.; Abrey, L.E.; Aftab, D.T.; Schwab, G.M.; et al. Baseline pretreatment contrast enhancing tumor volume including central necrosis as a prognostic factor in recurrent glioblastoma: Evidence from single and multicenter trials. *Neuro Oncol.* **2017**, *19*, 89–98. [CrossRef] [PubMed]
15. Chaichana, K.L.; Jusue-Torres, I.; Navarro-Ramirez, R.; Raza, S.M.; Pascual-Gallego, M.; Ibrahim, A.; Hernandez-Hermann, M.; Gomez, L.; Ye, X.; Weingart, J.D.; et al. Establishing percent resection and residual volume thresholds affecting survival and recurrence for patients with newly diagnosed intracranial glioblastoma. *Neuro Oncol.* **2014**, *16*, 113–122. [CrossRef] [PubMed]
16. Ostrom, Q.T.; Gittleman, H.; Farah, P.; Ondracek, A.; Chen, Y.; Wolinsky, Y.; Stroup, N.E.; Kruchko, C.; Barnholtz-Sloan, J.S. CBTRUS statistical report: Primary brain and central nervous system tumors diagnosed in the United States in 2006–2010. *Neuro Oncol.* **2013**, *15* (Suppl. S2), ii1–ii56, Erratum in: *Neuro Oncol.* **2014**, *16*, 760. [CrossRef] [PubMed]
17. Stepp, H.; Beck, T.; Pongratz, T.; Meinel, T.; Kreth, F.W.; Tonn, J.C.; Stummer, W. ALA and malignant glioma: Fluorescence-guided resection and photodynamic treatment. *J. Environ. Pathol. Toxicol. Oncol.* **2007**, *26*, 157–164. [CrossRef]
18. Lacroix, M.; Abi-Said, D.; Fourney, D.R.; Gokaslan, Z.L.; Shi, W.; DeMonte, F.; Lang, F.F.; McCutcheon, I.E.; Hassenbusch, S.J.; Holland, E.; et al. A multivariate analysis of 416 patients with glioblastoma multiforme: Prognosis, extent of resection, and survival. *J. Neurosurg.* **2001**, *95*, 190–198. [CrossRef]

19. deSouza, R.M.; Shaweis, H.; Han, C.; Sivasubramaniam, V.; Brazil, L.; Beaney, R.; Sadler, G.; Al-Sarraj, S.; Hampton, T.; Logan, J.; et al. Has the survival of patients with glioblastoma changed over the years? *Br. J. Cancer* **2016**, *114*, 146–150, Erratum in: *Br. J. Cancer* **2016**, *114*, e20. [CrossRef]
20. Stewart, L.A. Chemotherapy in adult high-grade glioma: A systematic review and meta-analysis of individual patient data from 12 randomised trials. *Lancet* **2002**, *359*, 1011–1018. [CrossRef]
21. Stupp, R.; Hegi, M.E.; Mason, W.P.; van den Bent, M.J.; Taphoorn, M.J.; Janzer, R.C.; Ludwin, S.K.; Allgeier, A.; Fisher, B.; Belanger, K.; et al. Effects of radiotherapy with concomitant and adjuvant temozolomide versus radiotherapy alone on survival in glioblastoma in a randomised phase III study: 5-year analysis of the EORTC-NCIC trial. *Lancet Oncol.* **2009**, *10*, 459–466. [CrossRef] [PubMed]
22. Walid, M.S. Prognostic factors for long-term survival after glioblastoma. *Perm. J.* **2008**, *12*, 45–48. [CrossRef] [PubMed]
23. Karschnia, P.; Young, J.S.; Dono, A.; Häni, L.; Sciortino, T.; Bruno, F.; Juenger, S.T.; Teske, N.; Morshed, R.A.; Haddad, A.F.; et al. Prognostic validation of a new classification system for extent of resection in glioblastoma: A report of the RANO resect group. *Neuro Oncol.* **2023**, *25*, 940–954. [CrossRef] [PubMed]
24. Abdal, K.; Darvish, M.; Ahmadi, M.H. Rapid Progression of Primary Glioblastoma to the Maxillofacial Area in a 29-year-old Woman. *World J. Dent.* **2016**, *9*, 122–125. [CrossRef]
25. Grossman, R.; Shimony, N.; Shir, D.; Gonen, T.; Sitt, R.; Kimchi, T.J.; Harosh, C.B.; Ram, Z. Dynamics of FLAIR Volume Changes in Glioblastoma and Prediction of Survival. *Ann. Surg. Oncol.* **2017**, *24*, 794–800. [CrossRef]

Disclaimer/Publisher's Note: The statements, opinions and data contained in all publications are solely those of the individual author(s) and contributor(s) and not of MDPI and/or the editor(s). MDPI and/or the editor(s) disclaim responsibility for any injury to people or property resulting from any ideas, methods, instructions or products referred to in the content.

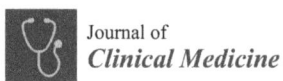

Article

Quantitative Anatomical Comparison of Surgical Approaches to Meckel's Cave

Luca Zanin [1,†], Edoardo Agosti [1,†], Florian Ebner [2], Lucio de Maria [1], Francesco Belotti [1], Barbara Buffoli [3], Rita Rezzani [3], Bernard Hirt [4], Marco Ravanelli [5], Tamara Ius [6], Marco Zeppieri [7,*], Marcos Soares Tatagiba [2], Marco Maria Fontanella [1] and Francesco Doglietto [8,9]

[1] Neurosurgery Unit, Department of Medical and Surgical Specialties, Radiological Sciences and Public Health, University of Brescia, 25123 Brescia, Italy; edoardo_agosti@libero.it (E.A.)
[2] Department of Neurological Surgery, Eberhard-Karls University, Tübingen University Hospital, D-72076 Tübingen, Germany
[3] Section of Anatomy and Physiopathology, Department of Clinical and Experimental Sciences, University of Brescia, 25123 Brescia, Italy
[4] Department of Clinical Anatomy, Eberhard-Karls-University, Tübingen University Hospital, D-72076 Tübingen, Germany
[5] Radiology Unit, Department of Medical and Surgical Specialties, Radiological Sciences and Public Health, University of Brescia, 25123 Brescia, Italy
[6] Neurosurgery Unit, Head-Neck and NeuroScience Department, University Hospital of Udine, p.le S. Maria della Misericordia 15, 33100 Udine, Italy
[7] Department of Ophthalmology, University Hospital of Udine, p.le S. Maria della Misericordia 15, 33100 Udine, Italy
[8] Neurosurgery, Fondazione Policlinico Universitario A. Gemelli IRCSS, 00168 Rome, Italy
[9] Neurosurgery, Università Cattolica del Sacro Cuore, 20123 Rome, Italy
* Correspondence: markzeppieri@hotmail.com
† These authors contributed equally to this work.

Citation: Zanin, L.; Agosti, E.; Ebner, F.; de Maria, L.; Belotti, F.; Buffoli, B.; Rezzani, R.; Hirt, B.; Ravanelli, M.; Ius, T.; et al. Quantitative Anatomical Comparison of Surgical Approaches to Meckel's Cave. *J. Clin. Med.* **2023**, *12*, 6847. https://doi.org/10.3390/jcm12216847

Academic Editor: Petra Klinge

Received: 8 October 2023
Revised: 27 October 2023
Accepted: 28 October 2023
Published: 30 October 2023

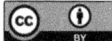

Copyright: © 2023 by the authors. Licensee MDPI, Basel, Switzerland. This article is an open access article distributed under the terms and conditions of the Creative Commons Attribution (CC BY) license (https://creativecommons.org/licenses/by/4.0/).

Abstract: Background: Meckel's cave is a challenging surgical target due to its deep location and proximity to vital neurovascular structures. Surgeons have developed various microsurgical transcranial approaches (MTAs) to access it, but there is no consensus on the best method. Newer endoscopic approaches have also emerged. This study seeks to quantitatively compare these surgical approaches to Meckel's cave, offering insights into surgical volumes and exposure areas. Methods: Fifteen surgical approaches were performed bilaterally in six specimens, including the pterional approach (PTA), fronto-temporal-orbito-zygomatic approach (FTOZA), subtemporal approach (STA), Kawase approach (KWA), retrosigmoid approach (RSA), retrosigmoid approach with suprameatal extension (RSAS), endoscopic endonasal transpterygoid approach (EETPA), inferolateral transorbital approach (ILTEA) and superior eyelid approach (SEYA). All the MTAs were performed both with 10 mm and 15 mm of brain retraction, to consider different percentages of surface exposure. A dedicated navigation system was used to quantify the surgical working volumes and exposure of different areas of Meckel's cave (ApproachViewer, part of GTx-Eyes II, University Health Network, Toronto, Canada). Microsurgical transcranial approaches were quantified with two different degrees of brain retraction (10 mm and 15 mm). Statistical analysis was performed using a mixed linear model with bootstrap resampling. Results: The RSAS with 15 mm of retraction offered the maximum exposure of the trigeminal stem (TS). If compared to the KWA, the RSA exposed more of the TS (69% vs. 46%; $p = 0.01$). The EETPA and ILTEA exposed the Gasserian ganglion (GG) mainly in the anteromedial portion, but with a significant 20% gain in exposure provided by the EETPA compared to ILTEA (42% vs. 22%; $p = 0.06$). The STA with 15 mm of retraction offered the maximum exposure of the GG, with a significant gain in exposure compared to the STA with 10 mm of retraction (50% vs. 35%; $p = 0.03$). The medial part of the three trigeminal branches was mainly exposed by the EETPA, particularly for the ophthalmic (66%) and maxillary (83%) nerves. The EETPA offered the maximum exposure of the medial part of the mandibular nerve, with a significant gain in exposure compared to the ILTEA (42% vs. 11%; $p = 0.01$) and the SEY (42% vs. 2%; $p = 0.01$). The FTOZA offered the maximum exposure of the lateral part of the ophthalmic nerve, with a significant gain of 67% ($p = 0.03$) and 48% ($p = 0.04$)

in exposure compared to the PTA and STA, respectively. The STA with 15 mm of retraction offered the maximum exposure of the lateral part of the maxillary nerve, with a significant gain in exposure compared to the STA with 10 mm of retraction (58% vs. 45%; $p = 0.04$). The STA with 15 mm of retraction provided a significant exposure gain of 23% for the lateral part of the mandibular nerve compared to FTOZA with 15 mm of retraction ($p = 0.03$). Conclusions: The endoscopic approaches, through the endonasal and transorbital routes, can provide adequate exposure of Meckel's cave, especially for its more medial portions, bypassing the impediment of major neurovascular structures and significant brain retraction. As far as the most lateral portion of Meckel's cave, MTA approaches still seem to be the gold standard in obtaining optimal exposure and adequate surgical volumes.

Keywords: Meckel's cave; quantitative comparison; skull base surgery; endoscopy; microsurgery; anatomy

1. Introduction

The trigeminal cave, or Meckel's cave, originally described by Johann Friedrich Meckel the Elder in 1748, is a cerebrospinal-fluid-containing dural pouch in the medial portion of the middle cranial fossa and adjacent to the cavernous sinus [1]. It opens to the posterior cranial fossa and houses the trigeminal ganglion (TG). Its deep location, the presence of the temporal lobe, and the anatomical proximity to vital neurovascular structures make its surgical access challenging [2].

Several microsurgical transcranial approaches (MTAs) to Meckel's cave have been described over time, but a common opinion among authors is still lacking as to which approach can quantitatively offer the best exposure. Conversely, the choice of a surgical approach often relies on personal preference, the level of comfort of the surgeon, and the overall goals of the procedure (e.g., simple debulking for mass effect release, radical resection, etc.). Moreover, with the recent introduction of endoscopic endonasal approaches and endoscopic transorbital approaches (ETOAs), new surgical trajectories to Meckel's cave have been proposed.

Although clinical comparative analyses of different surgical approaches to Meckel's cave are available [3,4], they often include a small number of patients of single-center case series or do not consider all the commonly used surgical approaches to Meckel's cave. Therefore, the aim of this study is to perform a quantitative anatomical comparison of the most used surgical approaches to Meckel's cave, describing surgical volumes and areas of exposure.

2. Materials and Methods

Cadavers were obtained from the body donation program of the Institute of Anatomy at the University of Brescia. Prior to death, the donors had all given written consent to the use of the body for educational and research purposes. The general use of cadavers for teaching purposes is a common practice and has been widely approved by the University Ethics Board. Formal ethics committee approval for this type of research on cadavers was not required by our University. The research was conducted in full compliance with the ethical guidelines established by our Institutional Review Board. All investigations involving human cadavers were carried out in strict adherence to the ethical principles outlined in the 1964 Declaration of Helsinki and its subsequent revisions.

Of note, the methods of this study were replicated from previous peer-reviewed anatomical studies both from our group and in the literature [5–8].

2.1. Preparation of Specimens and Neuronavigation

A total of 6 alcohol-fixed specimens (12 sides) were dissected. Intracranial arteries were injected with red silicone rubber.

Each specimen underwent a 128-multidetector computed tomography scan (Somatom® Definition Flash, Siemens, Forcheim, Germany). Subsequently, the Digital Imaging and Communications in Medicine (DICOM) records of the CT scans were transferred to a specialized neuronavigation software program (v. 1, GTx-Eyes II Approach Viewer, University Health Network, University of Toronto, Toronto, ON, Canada) [8].

2.2. Surgical Approaches to Dissection

The dissections were conducted at the Anatomy Laboratory of the University of Brescia (Italy) and the Anatomy Laboratory of the University of Tubingen (Germany) with the utilization of conventional microsurgical and endoscopic tools from Karl Storz® (Tüttlingen, Germany). To capture and record the intricate details of the microsurgical and endoscopic anatomy, a Leica M320® surgical microscope (Leica Microsystems Srl, Buccinasco, Italy) and a 4 K camera head from Olympus® (Segrate, Italy) were employed, respectively.

Fifteen surgical approaches were performed on each specimen. A schematic representation of these approaches is shown in Figure 1.

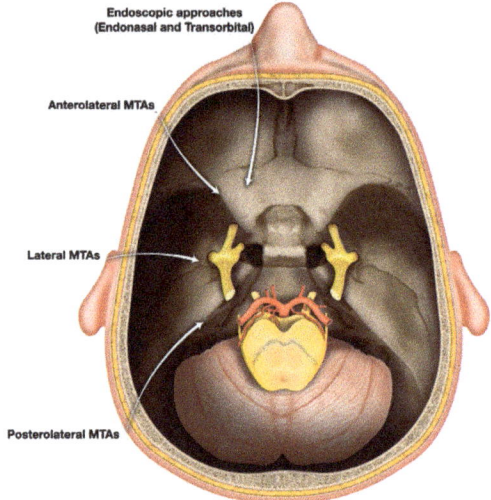

Figure 1. Schematic representation of the surgical approaches performed on each specimen.

The following anterolateral MTAs were investigated:

1. Pterional approach (PTA), according to Yasargil et al. [9], with 10 and 15 mm of retraction;
2. Fronto-temporal-orbito-zygomatic approach (FTOZA) according to Van Furth et al. [10], with 10 and 15 mm of retraction.

The following lateral MTAs were investigated:

1. Kawase approach (KWA), according to Kawase et al. [11], with 10 and 15 mm of retraction;
2. Subtemporal approach (STA), according to Dolenc et al. [12], with 10 and 15 mm of retraction.

The following posterolateral MTAs were investigated:

1. Retrosigmoid approach (RSA) according to Samii et al. [13], with 10 and 15 mm of retraction;
2. Retrosigmoid approach with suprameatal extension (RSAS) according to Samii et al. [5], with 10 and 15 mm of retraction.

The following endoscopic approaches were investigated:

1. Endoscopic endonasal transpterygoid approach (EETPA), according to Agosti et al. [7];
2. Inferolateral transorbital endoscopic approach (ILTEA), according to Ferrari et al. [7];
3. Superior eyelid approach (SEYA), according to Locatelli et al. [14].

As for MTAs, the surgical volumes were quantified with two different retraction degrees (i.e., 10 and 15 mm), to evaluate the exposure advantage as cerebral retraction increases. Brain retraction was kept constant during the quantification with the use of a Greenberg® Retractor System, parallelly positioned at 10 and 15 mm from the sphenoid ridge, middle cranial fossa, and posterior surface of the petrous bone for the anterolateral, lateral, and posterolateral MTAs, respectively [7].

2.3. Quantification of the Surgical Corridor

We employed an optical neuronavigation system (Polaris Vicra®; NDI, Waterloo, ON, Canada) in conjunction with GTx-Eyes II for the assessment of the maximum surgical volume with optimal maneuverability, termed the "crossing" modality, and the largest exposure achievable with straight instruments, referred to as the "non-crossing" modality [7]. Each modality was evaluated through three data collection iterations.

For MTAs, the height of the surgical corridor was established at the level of the craniotomy, while, for ETOAs, it was set at the orbital rim. In the case of EETPA, the surgical corridor height was aligned with the nasal pyriform aperture.

2.4. Surface Rendering and Quantification of the Exposed Area

Meckel's cave was considered as an open-ended three-fingered glove, enveloping the trigeminal ganglion, the ophthalmic nerve (V1), maxillary nerve (V2), and mandibular nerve (V3) divisions until they reach the correspondent skull base foramina [1,2].

Meckel's cave was divided into 8 surfaces, rendered with the ITK-SNAP software v. 4.0.2 from each CT scan (Figure 2). Dedicated software (Autodesk Meshmixer v. 3.5® and ApproachViewer v. 1), part of GTX-Eyes-II) quantified the percentage value of the exposed area by all approaches for each of the 8 surfaces [7].

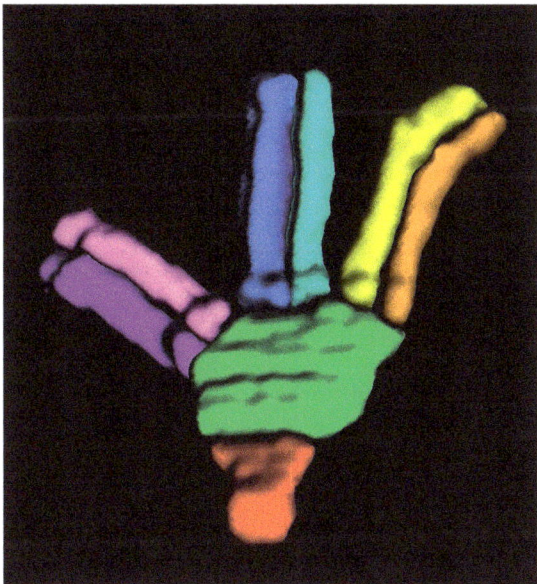

Figure 2. The 8 surfaces of Meckel's cave that were rendered with ITK-SNAP software from CT scans. Red: trigeminal stem; green: Gasserian ganglion; orange: V1 medial; yellow: V1 lateral; light-blue: V2 medial; blue: V2 lateral; purple: V3 medial; violet: V3 lateral.

2.5. Statistical Analysis

The Meckel's cave exposure and surgical volume of the different approaches were compared using linear mixed models with random intercepts for specimens. The final estimate was expressed as the β coefficient and 95% CI and was calculated using the bootstrap resampling method with 1000-fold replications. Statistical significance was set at $p < 0.05$. All analyses were performed using the STATA® software v. 16.1 (StataCorp® LLC., College Station, TX, USA).

3. Results

A grand total of 720 intersection data points were gathered through the execution of surgical procedures involving MTAs, EETPA, and ETOAs, all directed towards Meckel's cave. Detailed breakdowns of the average percentages of the exposed area on each surface of Meckel's cave, facilitated by each respective surgical approach, can be found in Tables 1–8. A visual representation of these findings is depicted in Figure 3. Additionally, Figures 4–7 provide illustrative screen captures from the Approach Viewer for each of the distinct surgical approaches.

Table 1. Comparison of surgical exposure for GG.

	Gasserian Ganglion (GG)	
	% (95% CI)	
	Non-crossing	Crossing
EETPA	41.8 (39.3, 45.8)	47.4 (42.6, 50.6)
FTOZA (10 mm)	0	0
FTOZA (15 mm)	18.6 (4.6, 12.5)	24.5 (15.4, 31.6)
ILTEA	22.4 (17.8, 25.9)	27.1 (18.3, 32.5)
KWA (10 mm)	2.1 (1.2, 4.5)	4.8 (3.2, 5.1)
KWA (15 mm)	3.2 (1.8, 4.8)	6.3 (3.2, 7.8)
PTA (10 mm)	0	0
PTA (15 mm)	0	0
RSA (10 mm)	0	0
RSA (15 mm)	0	0
RSAS (10 mm)	0	0
RSAS (15 mm)	0	0
SEYA	5.6 (4.6, 6.0)	6.7 (5.8, 7.5)
STA (10 mm)	35.3 (29.5, 39.4)	43.9 (33.4, 47.9)
STA (15 mm)	49.7 (42.5, 53.6)	64.2 (51.5, 70.4)

Abbreviations: CI, confidential interval; EETPA, endoscopic endonasal transpterygoid approach; FTOZA, fronto-temporal-orbito-zygomatic approach; ILTEA, infero-lateral transorbital endoscopic approach; RSA, retrosigmoid approach; RSAS, retrosigmoid approach with suprameatal extension; PTA, pterional approach; SEYA, superior eyelid approach; KWA, Kawase approach; STA, subtemporal approach.

Table 2. Comparison of surgical exposure for TS.

	Trigeminal Stem (TS)	
	% (95% CI)	
	Non-crossing	Crossing
EETPA	8.0 (1.2, 12.9)	11.5 (3.4, 17.3)
FTOZA (10 mm)	0	0
FTOZA (15 mm)	0	0

Table 2. Cont.

	Trigeminal Stem (TS)	
ILTEA	0	0
KWA (10 mm)	33.0 (28.2, 35.7)	36.5 (31.2, 42.8)
KWA (15 mm)	46.3 (42.3, 52.1)	55.2 (39.2, 65.6)
PTA (10 mm)	0	0
PTA (15 mm)	0	0
RSA (10 mm)	58.1 (55.3, 62.7)	61.4 (60.3, 63.5)
RSA (15 mm)	68.6 (65.9, 71.9)	73.2 (69.8, 78.8)
RSAS (10 mm)	74.5 (68.2, 78.5)	78.0 (64.1, 82.0)
RSAS (15 mm)	78.2 (67.6, 81.7)	82.3 (78.6, 85.4)
SEYA	0	0
STA (10 mm)	0	0
STA (15 mm)	0	0

Abbreviations: CI, confidential interval; EETPA, endoscopic endonasal transpterygoid approach; FTOZA, fronto-temporal-orbito-zygomatic approach; ILTEA, infero-lateral transorbital endoscopic approach; RSA, retrosigmoid approach; RSAS, retrosigmoid approach with suprameatal extension; PTA, pterional approach; SEYA, superior eyelid approach; KWA, Kawase approach; STA, subtemporal approach.

Table 3. Comparison of surgical exposure for V1m.

	V1 Medial (V1m)	
	% (95% CI)	
	Non-crossing	Crossing
EETPA	66.3 (52.1, 74.2)	73.9 (61.6, 88.5)
FTOZA (10 mm)	0	0
FTOZA (15 mm)	0	0
ILTEA	0	0
KWA (10 mm)	0	0
KWA (15 mm)	0	0
PTA (10 mm)	0	0
PTA (15 mm)	0	0
RSA (10 mm)	0	0
RSA (15 mm)	0	0
RSAS (10 mm)	0	0
RSAS (15 mm)	0	0
SEYA	0	0
STA (10 mm)	0	0
STA (15 mm)	0	0

Abbreviations: CI, confidential interval; EETPA, endoscopic endonasal transpterygoid approach; FTOZA, fronto-temporal-orbito-zygomatic approach; ILTEA, infero-lateral transorbital endoscopic approach; RSA, retrosigmoid approach; RSAS, retrosigmoid approach with suprameatal extension; PTA, pterional approach; SEYA, superior eyelid approach; KWA, Kawase approach; STA, subtemporal approach.

Table 4. Comparison of surgical exposure for V1l.

	V1 Lateral (V1l)	
	% (95% CI)	
	Non-crossing	Crossing
EETPA	5.3 (2.1, 6.2)	6.1 (3.6, 8.5)
FTOZA (10 mm)	89.4 (84.5, 93.1)	93.4 (88.5, 98.4)
FTOZA (15 mm)	93.8 (81.8, 95.9)	96.2 (91.3, 98.4)
ILTEA	60.7 (48.5, 72.4)	68.2 (56.3, 76.8)
KWA (10 mm)	0	0
KWA (15 mm)	0	0
PTA (10 mm)	23.5 (44.6, 57.1)	36.1 (49.0, 59.9)
PTA (15 mm)	27.1 (47.8, 58.3)	39.2 (53.2, 61.3)
RSA (10 mm)	0	0
RSA (15 mm)	0	0
RSAS (10 mm)	0	0
RSAS (15 mm)	0	0
SEYA	2.3 (1.2, 3.4)	2.9 (1.2, 3.5)
STA (10 mm)	40.3 (34.2, 48.9)	51.9 (41.0, 63.8)
STA (15 mm)	45.9 (35.8, 54.1)	57.6 (44.2, 69.2)

Abbreviations: CI, confidential interval; EETPA, endoscopic endonasal transpterygoid approach; FTOZA, fronto-temporal-orbito-zygomatic approach; ILTEA, infero-lateral transorbital endoscopic approach; RSA, retrosigmoid approach; RSAS, retrosigmoid approach with suprameatal extension; PTA, pterional approach; SEYA, superior eyelid approach; KWA, Kawase approach; STA, subtemporal approach.

Table 5. Comparison of surgical exposure for V2m.

	V2 Medial (V2m)	
	% (95% CI)	
	Non-crossing	Crossing
EETPA	83.1 (75.3, 92.6)	91.3 (82.7, 96.0)
FTOZA (10 mm)	0	0
FTOZA (15 mm)	0	0
ILTEA	1.6 (1.0, 2.5)	5.3 (2.4, 6.8)
KWA (10 mm)	0	0
KWA (15 mm)	0	0
PTA (10 mm)	0	0
PTA (15 mm)	0	0
RSA (10 mm)	0	0
RSA (15 mm)	0	0
RSAS (10 mm)	0	0
RSAS (15 mm)	0	0
SEYA	0	0
STA (10 mm)	0	0
STA (15 mm)	0	0

Abbreviations: CI, confidential interval; EETPA, endoscopic endonasal transpterygoid approach; FTOZA, fronto-temporal-orbito-zygomatic approach; ILTEA, infero-lateral transorbital endoscopic approach; RSA, retrosigmoid approach; RSAS, retrosigmoid approach with suprameatal extension; PTA, pterional approach; SEYA, superior eyelid approach; KWA, Kawase approach; STA, subtemporal approach.

Table 6. Comparison of surgical exposure for V2l.

	V2 Lateral (V2l)	
	% (95% CI)	
	Non-crossing	Crossing
EETPA	8.1 (2.9, 15.4)	13.5 (12.0, 21.8)
FTOZA (10 mm)	19.1 (14.4, 26.0)	23.7 (18.5, 30.9)
FTOZA (15 mm)	30.6 (21.8, 38.5)	39.8 (31.6, 44.5)
ILTEA	28.6 (21.0, 34.6)	35.3 (26.4, 46.1)
KWA (10 mm)	0	0
KWA (15 mm)	0	0
PTA (10 mm)	3.1 (1.5, 5.6)	5.0 (3.8, 9.5)
PTA (15 mm)	5.4 (3.8, 8.3)	9.2 (6.6, 11.9)
RSA (10 mm)	0	0
RSA (15 mm)	0	0
RSAS (10 mm)	0	0
RSAS (15 mm)	0	0
SEYA	0	0
STA (10 mm)	44.7 (35.6, 52.9)	60.1 (51.8, 71.0)
STA (15 mm)	57.9 (49.1, 64.3)	72.4 (58.2, 79.3)

Abbreviations: CI, confidential interval; EETPA, endoscopic endonasal transpterygoid approach; FTOZA, fronto-temporal-orbito-zygomatic approach; ILTEA, infero-lateral transorbital endoscopic approach; RSA, retrosigmoid approach; RSAS, retrosigmoid approach with suprameatal extension; PTA, pterional approach; SEYA, superior eyelid approach; KWA, Kawase approach; STA, subtemporal approach.

Table 7. Comparison of surgical exposure for V3m.

	V3 Medial (V3m)	
	% (95% CI)	
	Non-crossing	Crossing
EETPA	41.9 (35.7, 52.6)	50.3 (46.5, 63.0)
FTOZA (10 mm)	0	0
FTOZA (15 mm)	0	0
ILTEA	11.2 (9.0, 16.4)	15.8 (11.1, 20.6)
KWA (10 mm)	0	0
KWA (15 mm)	0	0
PTA (10 mm)	0	0
PTA (15 mm)	0	0
RSA (10 mm)	0	0
RSA (15 mm)	0	0
RSAS (10 mm)	0	0
RSAS (15 mm)	0	0
SEYA	2.3 (1.9, 5.5)	7.1 (4.4, 10.9)
STA (10 mm)	0	0
STA (15 mm)	0	0

Abbreviations: CI, confidential interval; EETPA, endoscopic endonasal transpterygoid approach; FTOZA, fronto-temporal-orbito-zygomatic approach; ILTEA, infero-lateral transorbital endoscopic approach; RSA, retrosigmoid approach; RSAS, retrosigmoid approach with suprameatal extension; PTA, pterional approach; SEYA, superior eyelid approach; KWA, Kawase approach; STA, subtemporal approach.

Table 8. Comparison of surgical exposure for V3l.

	V3 Lateral (V3l)	
	% (95% CI)	
	Non-crossing	Crossing
EETPA	0.5 (0, 1.3)	3.6 (2.2, 6.3)
FTOZA (10 mm)	29.6 (24.5, 36.9)	37.3 (28.9, 48.2)
FTOZA (15 mm)	42.4 (30.0, 47.4)	49.1 (35.6, 56.0)
ILTEA	44.9 (31.8, 53.7)	53.7 (42.1, 58.5)
KWA (10 mm)	0	0
KWA (15 mm)	0	0
PTA (10 mm)	13.6 (8.2, 17.9)	15.3 (10.1, 21.5)
PTA (15 mm)	25.7 (13.6, 31.4)	31.8 (26.8, 42.3)
RSA (10 mm)	0	0
RSA (15 mm)	0	0
RSAS (10 mm)	0	0
RSAS (15 mm)	0	0
SEYA	17.0 (11.8, 23.6)	25.8 (12.4, 31.9)
STA (10 mm)	56.5 (41.3, 62.7)	65.6 (60.9, 77.4)
STA (15 mm)	64.6 (54.2, 76.9)	73.6 (64.8, 81.9)

Abbreviations: CI, confidential interval; EETPA, endoscopic endonasal transpterygoid approach; FTOZA, fronto-temporal-orbito-zygomatic approach; ILTEA, infero-lateral transorbital endoscopic approach; RSA, retrosigmoid approach; RSAS, retrosigmoid approach with suprameatal extension; PTA, pterional approach; SEYA, superior eyelid approach; KWA, Kawase approach; STA, subtemporal approach.

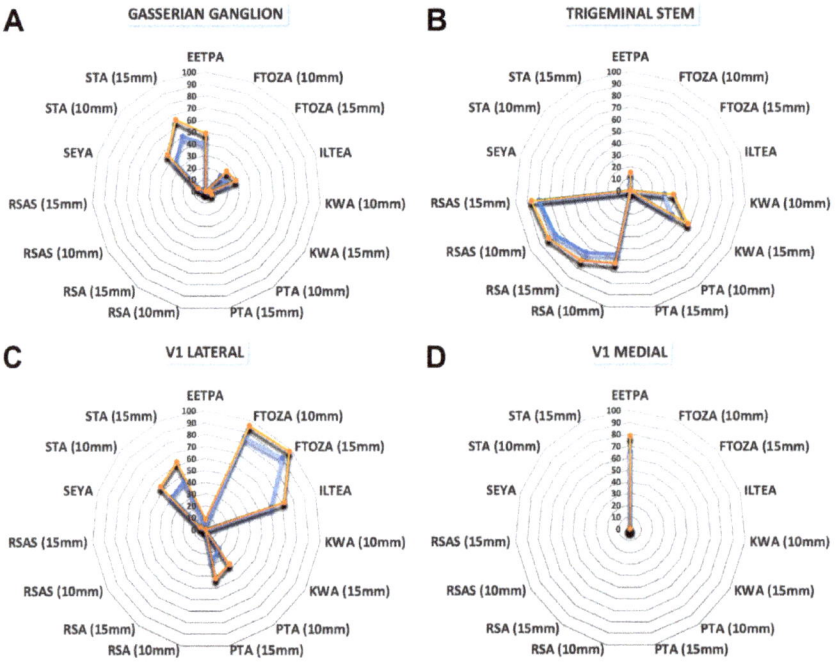

Figure 3. *Cont.*

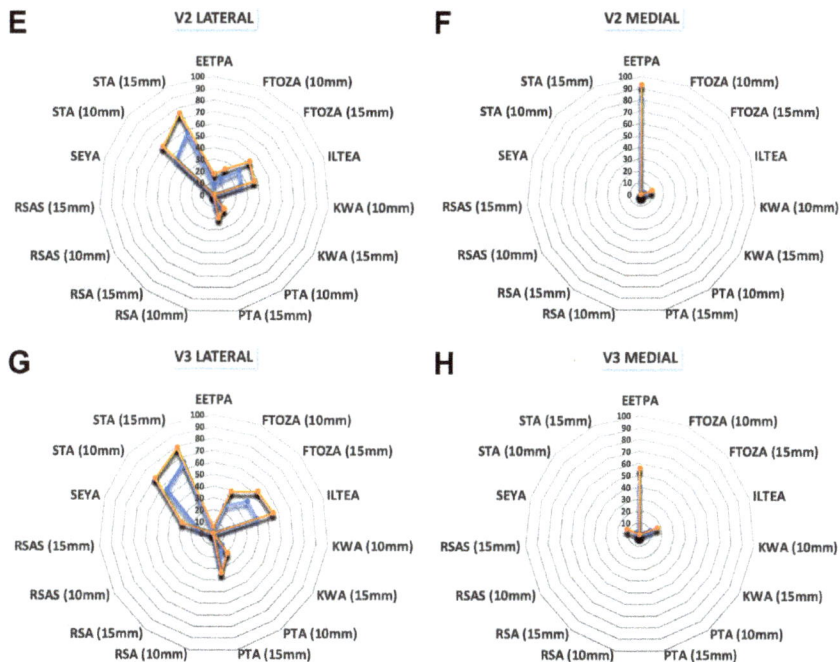

Figure 3. Visual depiction of the average exposed surface area percentages for each surgical approach in relation to Meckel's cave. Orange line: crossing measurements; blue line: non-crossing measurements. Abbreviations: EETPA, endoscopic endonasal transpterygoid approach; FTOZA, fronto-temporal-orbito-zygomatic approach; ILTEA, infero-lateral transorbital endoscopic approach; RSA, retrosigmoid approach; RSAS, retrosigmoid approach with suprameatal extension; PTA, pterional approach; SEYA, superior eyelid approach; KWA, Kawase approach; STA, subtemporal approach.

3.1. Areas of Exposure

3.1.1. Gasserian Ganglion (GG)

The STA with 15 mm of retraction offered the maximum exposure of the GG, with a significant gain in exposure compared to the STA with 10 mm of retraction (50% vs. 35%; $p = 0.03$). The EETPA and ILTEA exposed the GG mainly in the anteromedial portion, but with a significant 20% gain in exposure provided by the EETPA compared to ILTEA (42% vs. 22%; $p = 0.06$). The lowest exposure of the GG was provided by the KWA (2%).

3.1.2. Trigeminal Stem (TS)

The RSAS with 15 mm of retraction offered the maximum exposure of the TS, without any significant gain in exposure compared to the RSAS with 10 mm of retraction (78% vs. 75%; $p = 0.73$). If compared to the KWA, the RSA exposed more of the TS (69% vs. 46%; $p = 0.01$). Neither the anterolateral MTAs nor the ETOAs provided any exposure to this region.

3.1.3. Ophthalmic Nerve (V1): Medial (V1m) and Lateral (V1l) Portions

The V1m is mainly exposed by the EETPA (66%). The FTOZA offered the maximum exposure of the V1l, with a significant gain of 67% ($p = 0.03$) and 48% ($p = 0.04$) in exposure compared to the PTA and STA, respectively. The ILTEA is the endoscopic approach that offers the major exposure (61%) of the V1l. Neither the anterolateral EETPA nor the SEYA provided any significant exposure to this region.

3.1.4. Maxillary Nerve (V2): Medial (V2m) and Lateral (V2l) Portions

The EETPA offered the greatest exposure of the V2m (83%). The STA with 15 mm of retraction offered the maximum exposure of the V2l, with a significant gain in exposure compared to the STA with 10 mm of retraction (58% vs. 45%; $p = 0.04$). The STA with 15 mm of retraction provided a significant exposure gain of 27% and 53% compared to FTOZA and PTA with parity of retraction, respectively. The ILTEA is the endoscopic approach that offers the greatest exposure (29%) of the V2l.

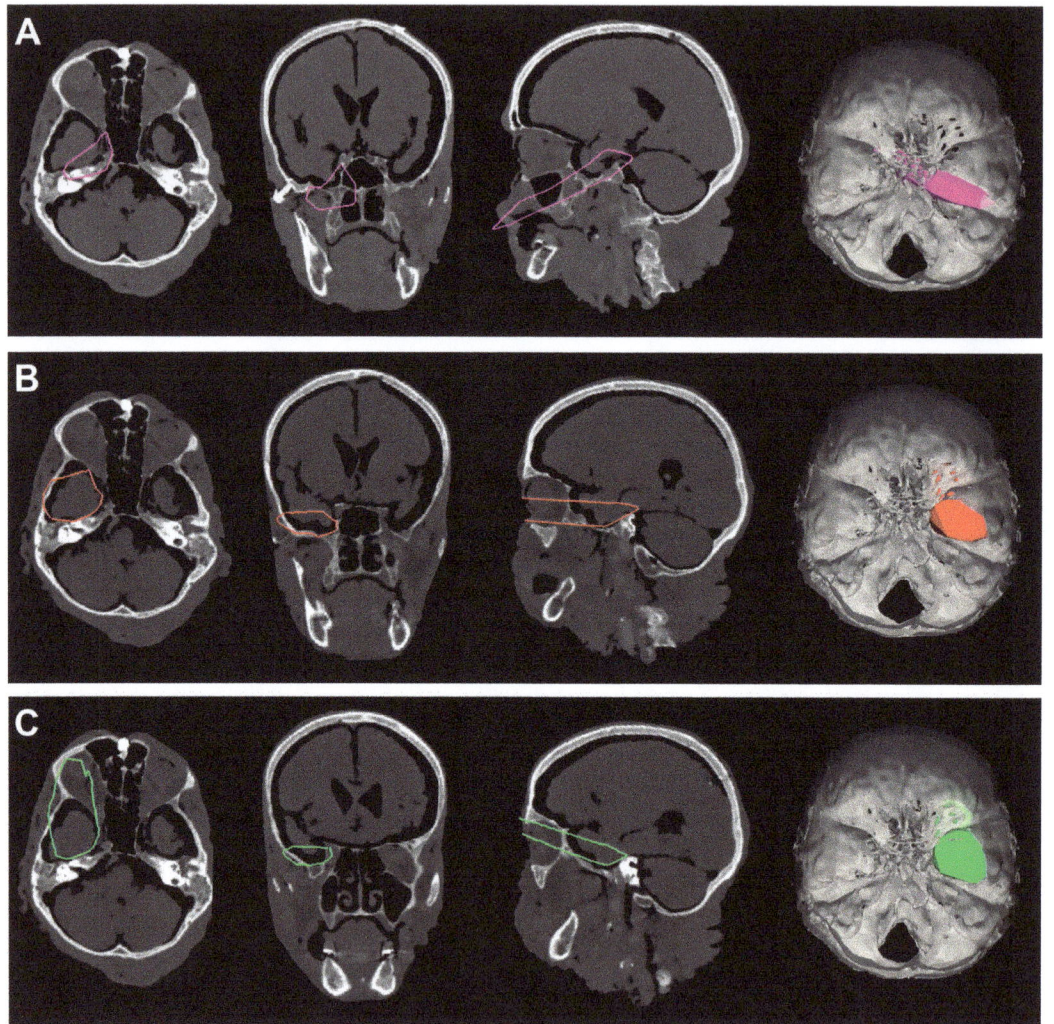

Figure 4. (**A**). Exemplificative screenshot from Approach Viewer of the EETPA. (**B**). Exemplificative screenshot from Approach Viewer of the ILTEA. (**C**). Exemplificative screenshot from Approach Viewer of the SEYA.

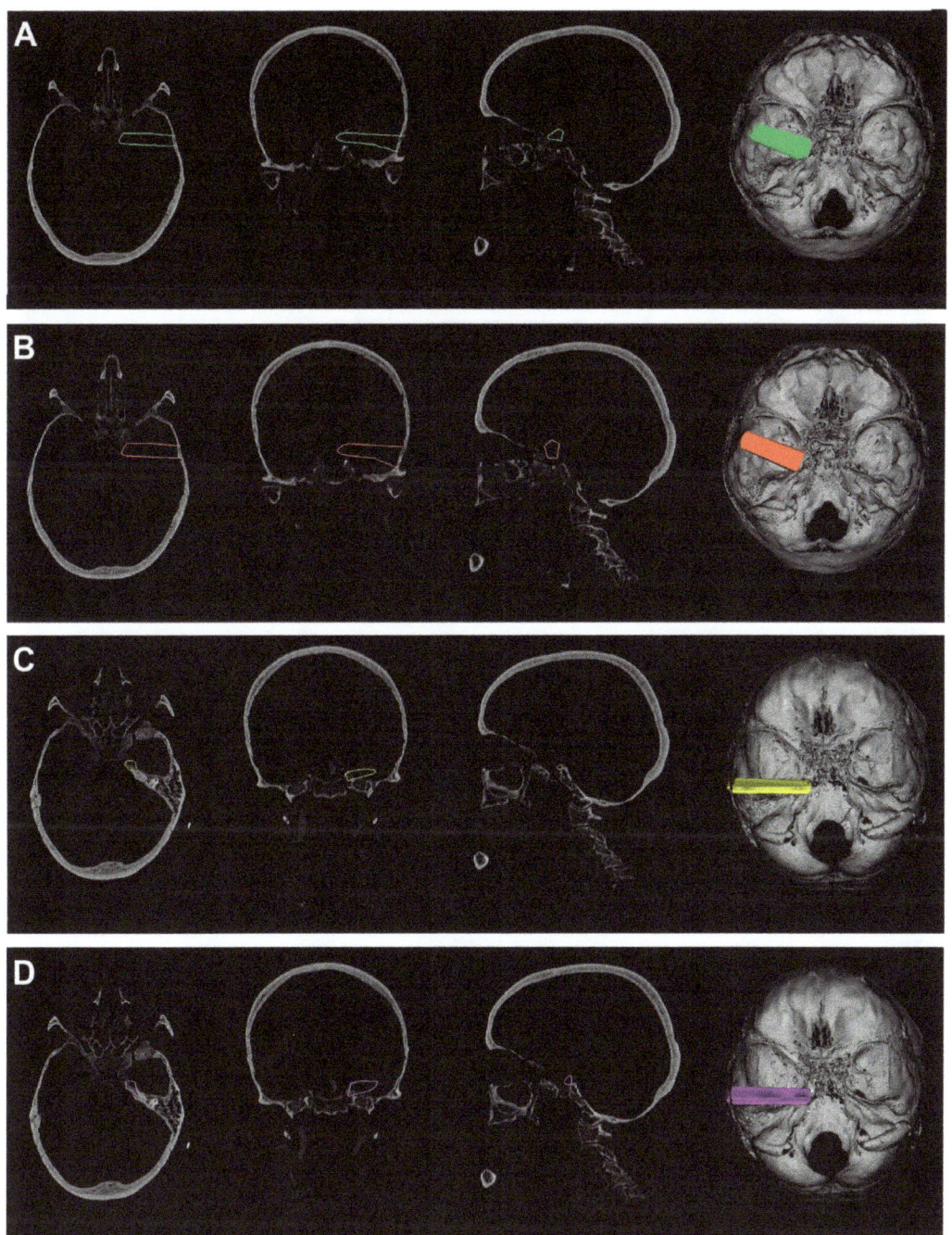

Figure 5. (**A**). Exemplificative screenshot from Approach Viewer of the STA with 10 mm of retraction. (**B**). Exemplificative screenshot from Approach Viewer of the STA with 15 mm of retraction. (**C**). Exemplificative screenshot from Approach Viewer of the KWA with 10 mm of retraction. (**D**). Exemplificative screenshot from Approach Viewer of the KWA with 15 mm of retraction.

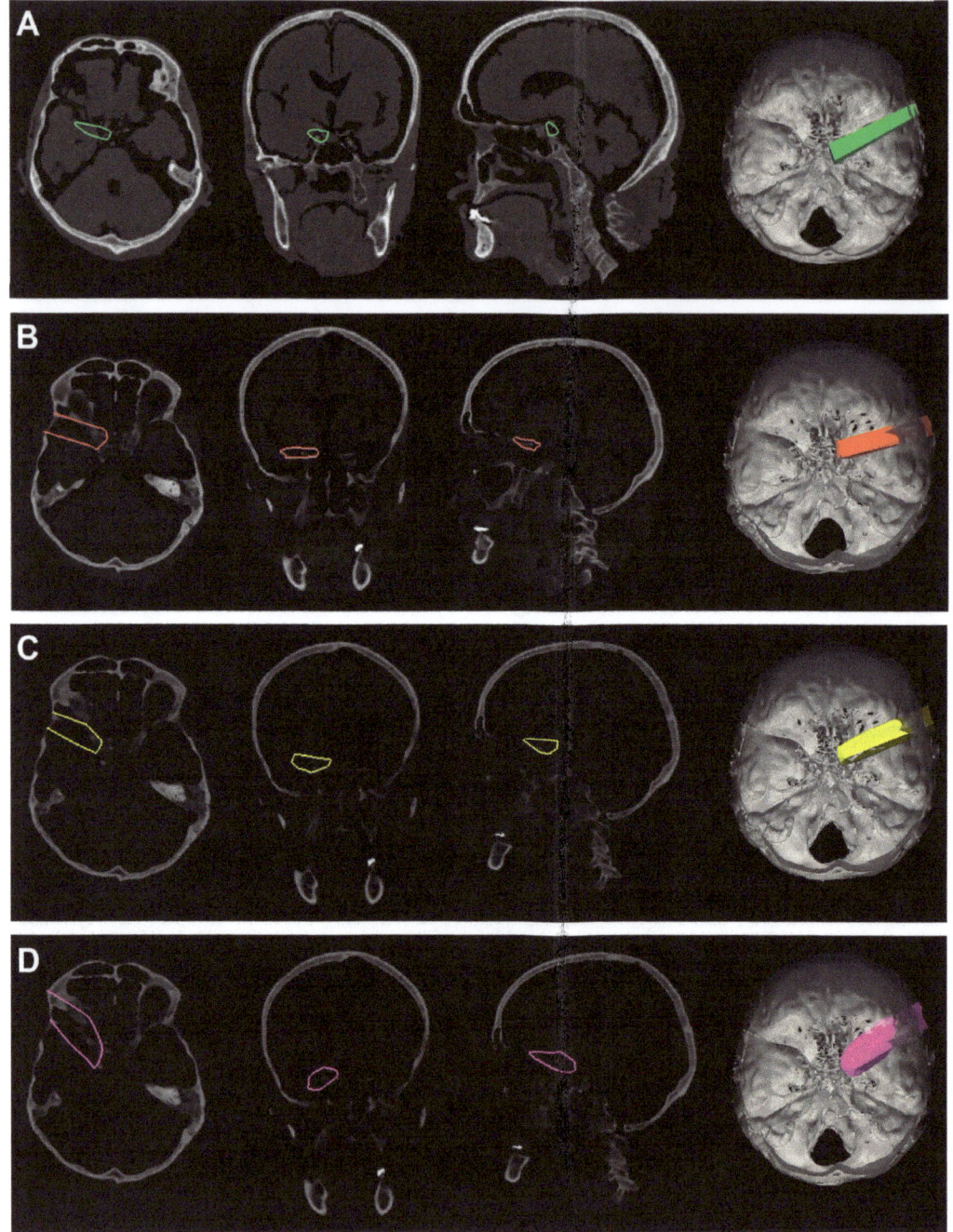

Figure 6. (**A**). Exemplificative screenshot from Approach Viewer of the PTA with 10 mm of retraction. (**B**). Exemplificative screenshot from Approach Viewer of the PTA with 15 mm of retraction. (**C**). Exemplificative screenshot from Approach Viewer of the FTOZ with 10 mm of retraction. (**D**). Exemplificative screenshot from Approach Viewer of the FTOZ with 15 mm of retraction.

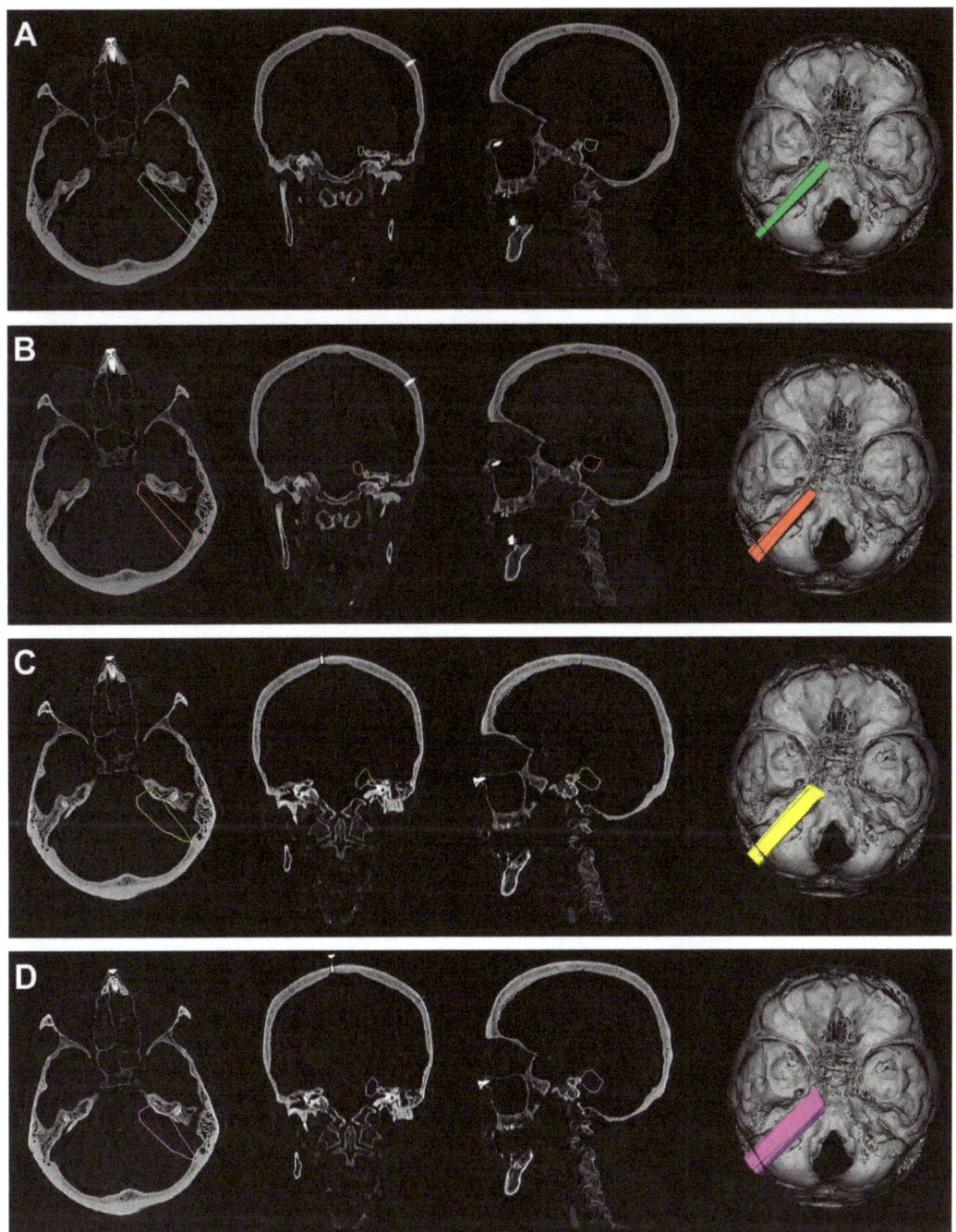

Figure 7. (**A**). Exemplificative screenshot from Approach Viewer of the RSA with 10 mm of retraction. (**B**). Exemplificative screenshot from Approach Viewer of the RSA with 10 mm of retraction. (**C**). Exemplificative screenshot from Approach Viewer of the RSAS with 10 mm of retraction. (**D**). Exemplificative screenshot from Approach Viewer of the RSAS with 15 mm of retraction.

3.1.5. Mandibular Nerve (V3): Medial (V3m) and Lateral (V3l) Portions

The EETPA is the endoscopic approach that offers the maximum exposure of the V3m, with a significant gain in exposure compared to the ILTEA (42% vs. 11%; $p = 0.01$) and the SEY (42% vs. 2%; $p = 0.01$). The STA with 15 mm of retraction offered the maximum exposure of the V3l, without any significant gain in exposure compared to the STA with 10 mm of retraction (65% vs. 57%; $p = 0.23$). The STA with 15 mm of retraction provided a significant exposure gain of 23% compared to FTOZA with 15 mm of retraction ($p = 0.03$). The FTOZA with 15 mm of retraction is the anterolateral MTA that offers the maximum exposure of the V3l, with a significant gain in exposure compared to the PTA with 15 mm of retraction (42% vs. 26%; $p = 0.04$).

3.2. Surgical Volumes

The endoscopic methods demonstrated comparable working volumes (EETPA: 84 cm^3; ETOAs: 66–75 cm^3), albeit with varying distances from the target (EETPA: 12 cm; ETOAs: 11 cm). In contrast, the working volume for MTAs expanded in proportion to the craniotomy size (FTOZAA: 63 cm^3; RSA: 25 cm^3). The average distance from the target was shorter than that of the endoscopic approaches (9 cm). Refer to Table 9 for a summary of the minimum, mean, maximum, and standard deviation values pertaining to the non-crossing volume of each simulated approach, with a visual representation provided in Figure 8.

Table 9. Table featuring the minimum, mean, maximum, and standard deviation values, measured in cubic centimeters (cm^3), for the non-crossing volume in each simulated approach.

Approach	Average	Minimum	Maximum	Standard Deviation
EETPA	84.7	68.1	95.3	9.6
FTOZA	62.9	56.4	77.2	5.4
ILTEA	75.4	66.2	86.8	8.2
KWA	35.6	26.9	44.3	4.2
PTA	35.5	29.2	46.7	4.0
RSA	25.1	20.7	33.9	3.7
RSAS	30.4	21.0	38.5	3.9
SEYA	66.3	46.0	75.5	7.3
STA	33.1	27.4	41.8	3.9

Abbreviations: EETPA, endoscopic endonasal transpterygoid approach; FTOZA, fronto-temporal-orbito-zygomatic approach; ILTEA, infero-lateral transorbital endoscopic approach; RSA, retrosigmoid approach; RSAS, retrosigmoid approach with suprameatal extension; PTA, pterional approach; SEYA, superior eyelid approach; KWA, Kawase approach; STA, subtemporal approach.

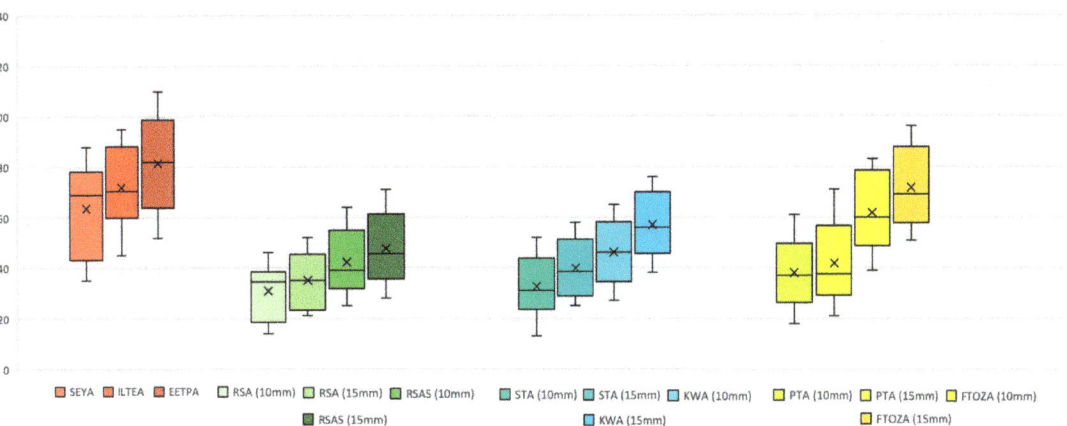

Figure 8. Graphical representation of the minimum, average, maximum, and standard deviation values of the non-crossing volume of each simulated approach. Abbreviations: EETPA, endoscopic endonasal transpterygoid approach; FTOZA, fronto-temporal-orbito-zygomatic approach; ILTEA, infero-lateral transorbital endoscopic approach; RSA, retrosigmoid approach; RSAS, retrosigmoid approach with suprameatal extension; PTA, pterional approach; SEYA, superior eyelid approach; KWA, Kawase approach; STA, subtemporal approach.

4. Discussion

In this anatomical pre-clinical study, we quantitatively compared the percentages of exposure of eight different surfaces of Meckel's cave by 15 surgical approaches. The experimental findings can be summarized into three main results: (1) the TS is mainly exposed by the RSA; (2) the STA and EETPA can both efficiently expose the GG but the need for major parenchymal retraction must be considered in the microsurgical approach; (3) the EETPA and ETOAs can provide adequate exposure of the most medial compartments of Meckel's cave, especially for the trigeminal branches, while the MTAs seem to offer the greatest surgical exposure of the lateral compartment of Meckel's cave. Our data furthermore show clearly how moving anteriorly along the petrous part of the temporal bone posterior approaches causes a loss of exposure power, while that for anterior ones increases.

The existing literature contains a scarcity of quantitative anatomical investigations. These studies have primarily focused on comparing a small selection of surgical approaches to Meckel's cave, often neglecting the full spectrum of available options and occasionally failing to comprehensively analyze the extent of exposure within the surgical field [15–17].

Beyond the anatomical factors, when translating these preclinical findings into a clinical context, it is imperative to remain cognizant of the inherent advantages and disadvantages associated with each surgical approach. Our results are useful for the management of tumors involving Meckel's cave. These closely related anatomical regions remain a formidable challenge for today's skull base surgeons due to the intricate bone structures and the presence of critical neurovascular elements that converge within these areas [18–20].

Trigeminal schwannomas can present in three different anatomical situations [19,21–23]. (1) Schwannomas that involve the trigeminal branches and extend to the pterygopalatine or infratemporal fossae. In this case, the best surgical approach seems to be the EETPA with surface exposure of the medial part of V1, V2, and V3 of 73.9%, 91.3%, and 50.3%; the GG is also well reached by this approach, with surface exposure of 47.4%. This approach is a minimally invasive technique that provides direct access to the pterygopalatine and infratemporal fossae. It has gained popularity in recent years due to its reduced morbidity and faster recovery times [24]. (2) Schwannomas involving only the middle cranial fossa. These tumors grow laterally and medially, pressing Meckel's cave. In this case, the best surgical approach seems to be the STA with surface exposure of 43.9%. It is interesting to note the gain of exposed surface with brain retraction of 15 mm instead of 10 mm (64.2% vs. 43.9%). This allows the surgeon to carefully evaluate the balance between the benefits and risks of parenchymal retraction, knowing that he will obtain a significant gain in terms of surgical exposure. (3) Trigeminal schwannomas with extension to the TS and/or invasion of the posterior fossa. In this case, the best surgical approaches are KWA or RSAS. KWA is a highly complex but essential middle fossa approach, able to serve a wide array of pathologies together with its extensions. It is very accurate in performing hearing preservation surgery, but not without caveats and an inherent risk of complications [25]. RSAS provides greater exposure of the brainstem and petroclival areas, according to our findings (82.3%) but also according to the literature [15,16].

The KWA is ideally suited for lesions around Meckel's cave involving the TS but with a main extension into the middle fossa. The KWA exposes significantly less ventral brainstem area than RSAS, as previous studies have confirmed [15]. The mean petroclival area of exposure through the KWA was significantly smaller than that obtained through the RSAS. However, these approaches can be used in conjunction with one another to access petroclival tumors [25]. While trigeminal schwannomas are quite rare, meningiomas are the most frequent Meckel's cave tumors [26].

Traditionally, three surgical approaches have been described to remove Meckel's cave meningioma: the STA, the RSA, and the KWA [27]. Still, endoscopic approaches are increasingly used [28], above all when tumors are located anteriorly at the cavernous sinus apex. Biopsy can be performed with EETPA when the percutaneous approach fails, but it also allows tumor removal during the same procedure if indicated. According to our results, EETPA can expose a wide portion of the GG and most of the medial portions of the three trigeminal branches, being particularly useful for small tumors that are located in the anterior portion of Meckel's cave and that are not associated with significant compression of the trigeminal nerve or other adjacent structures, as Kassam [29] and Jouanneau [28] previously described. For meningiomas located posteriorly in the petrous apex extending to the cerebellopontine angle, without expanding the upper and lower quadrangular spaces of the sphenoid, as described by Cavallo [30], the KWA or RSA is more appropriate.

We found particularly interesting also the trans-orbital approaches, recently described in clinical practice, both as single approaches and combined with EETPA [31,32]. Previous studies have proposed ILTEA as a minimally invasive surgical approach that provides access to the anterior and middle cranial fossae, the cavernous sinus, and the petrous apex [32–34]. According to our results, ILTEA can expose wide portions of the lateral parts of V1 and V3 (68.2% and 53.7%) but can reach also the GG with 27.1% of exposure. ILTEAs should be considered as an additional tool rather than a replacement for EETPA or external approaches, to optimize visualization and maneuverability, especially for multicompartmental lesions with extension to the cavernous sinus and petrous apex. SEYA can be used to target lesions involving the anterolateral skull base, as previously described [31].

As far as lesions with parasellar extension are concerned, however, the approach to be preferred is undoubtedly EETPA, given that it allows a wide range of exposure of all the sellar and parasellar regions, as already reported in the literature [35–41]. To obtain a general overview from the analysis of our anatomical results, it is possible to state that for lesions that grow medially and displace Meckel's cave laterally, it appears more convenient to perform EETPA, while, for lesions that grow lateral to Meckel's cave and cause therefore medial compression, it is more appropriate to perform one of the MTAs; if the lesions develop laterally but also present medial involvement, then it may be appropriate to add ILTEA to EETPA.

Our study has several limitations. This was an experimental preclinical investigation, and, as such, it did not consider any distortions in intracranial anatomy, such as the mass effect of the tumor or CSF diversion, when conducting measurements. Additionally, it is important to note that fixation tends to make tissues less flexible and more rigid, potentially resulting in a decreased area of surgical exposure for both endoscopic and transcranial approaches.

5. Conclusions

The endoscopic approaches, through the endonasal and transorbital routes, can provide adequate exposure of Meckel's cave, especially for its more medial portions, bypassing the impediment of major neurovascular structures and significant brain retraction. As far as the most lateral portion of Meckel's cave, MTAs still seem to be the gold standard in obtaining optimal exposure and adequate surgical volumes. Although limited to a preclinical setting, these findings can provide a valuable contribution to everyday neurosurgical practice and aid in the selection of the most accurate surgical approach to Meckel's cave.

Author Contributions: Conceptualization, E.A., M.Z., L.d.M., M.M.F., T.I., M.M.F. and F.D.; methodology, E.A., M.Z., L.d.M., M.M.F., T.I., M.M.F. and F.D.; validation, L.Z., E.A., F.E., L.d.M., F.B., B.B., R.R., B.H., M.R., T.I., M.Z., M.S.T., M.M.F. and F.D.; formal analysis, E.A. and L.D; investigation, E.A. and L.d.M.; resources, M.M.F. and F.D.; data curation, E.A. and L.d.M.; writing—original draft preparation, E.A. and L.d.M.; writing—review and editing, E.A., M.Z. and L.d.M.; visualization, L.Z., E.A., F.E., L.d.M., F.B., B.B., R.R., B.H., M.R., T.I., M.Z., M.S.T., M.M.F. and F.D.; supervision, M.Z.; project administration, M.M.F. and F.D. All authors have read and agreed to the published version of the manuscript.

Funding: This research received no external funding.

Institutional Review Board Statement: Cadavers were obtained from the body donation program of the Institute of Anatomy at the University of Brescia. Prior to death, the donors had all given written consent to the use of the body for educational and research purposes. The general use of cadavers for teaching purposes is a common practice and has been widely approved by the University Ethics Board. Formal ethics committee approval for this type of research on cadavers was not required by our University. This study was performed according to the ethical standards of our Institutional Review Board. All human cadaveric studies were performed in accordance with the ethical standards laid down in the 1964 Declaration of Helsinki and its later amendments.

Informed Consent Statement: Not applicable.

Data Availability Statement: Data available in a publicly accessible repository.

Conflicts of Interest: The authors declare no conflict of interest.

Abbreviations

CI = confidential interval; EETPA = endoscopic endonasal transpterygoid approach; ETOA = endoscopic transorbital approach; FTOZA = fronto-temporal-orbito-zygomatic approach; GG = Gasserian ganglion; ILTEA = infero-lateral transorbital endoscopic approach; KWA = Kawase approach; MTA = microsurgical transcranial approach; RSA = retrosigmoid approach; RSAS = retrosigmoid approach with suprameatal extension; PTA = pterional approach; SEYA = superior eyelid approach; TS = trigeminal stem; STA = subtemporal approach; V1l = lateral ophthalmic nerve; V1m = medial ophthalmic nerve; V2m = medial maxillary nerve; V2l = lateral maxillary nerve; V3m = medial mandibular nerve; V3l = lateral mandibular nerve.

References

1. Sabancı, P.A.; Batay, F.; Civelek, E.; Al Mefty, O.; Husain, M.; Abdulrauf, S.I.; Karasu, A. Meckel's Cave. *World Neurosurg.* **2011**, *76*, 335–341, discussion 266–267. [CrossRef] [PubMed]
2. Bond, J.D.; Xu, Z.; Zhang, H.; Zhang, M. Meckel's Cave and Somatotopy of the Trigeminal Ganglion. *World Neurosurg.* **2021**, *148*, 178–187. [CrossRef] [PubMed]
3. Van Rompaey, J.; Suruliraj, A.; Carrau, R.; Panizza, B.; Solares, C.A. Meckel's Cave Access: Anatomic Study Comparing the Endoscopic Transantral and Endonasal Approaches. *Eur. Arch. Otorhinolaryngol.* **2014**, *271*, 787–794. [CrossRef] [PubMed]
4. Van Rompaey, J.; Bush, C.; Khabbaz, E.; Vender, J.; Panizza, B.; Solares, C.A. What Is the Best Route to the Meckel Cave? Anatomical Comparison between the Endoscopic Endonasal Approach and a Lateral Approach. *J. Neurol. Surg. B Skull Base* **2013**, *74*, 331–336. [CrossRef]
5. Agosti, E.; Saraceno, G.; Rampinelli, V.; Raffetti, E.; Veiceschi, P.; Buffoli, B.; Rezzani, R.; Giorgianni, A.; Hirtler, L.; Alexander, A.Y.; et al. Quantitative Anatomic Comparison of Endoscopic Transnasal and Microsurgical Transcranial Approaches to the Anterior Cranial Fossa. *Oper. Neurosurg.* **2022**, *23*, e256–e266. [CrossRef]

6. Rampinelli, V.; Agosti, E.; Saraceno, G.; Ferrari, M.; Taboni, S.; Mattavelli, D.; Schreiber, A.; Tomasoni, M.; Gualtieri, T.; Ravanelli, M.; et al. Endoscopic Subtemporal Epidural Key-Hole Approach: Quantitative Anatomic Analysis of Three Surgical Corridors. *World Neurosurg.* **2021**, *152*, e128–e137. [CrossRef]
7. Agosti, E.; Turri-Zanoni, M.; Saraceno, G.; Belotti, F.; Karligkiotis, A.; Rocca, G.; Buffoli, B.; Raffetti, E.; Hirtler, L.; Rezzani, R.; et al. Quantitative Anatomic Comparison of Microsurgical Transcranial, Endoscopic Endonasal, and Transorbital Approaches to the Spheno-Orbital Region. *Oper. Neurosurg.* **2021**, *21*, E494–E505. [CrossRef]
8. Agosti, E.; Saraceno, G.; Qiu, J.; Buffoli, B.; Ferrari, M.; Raffetti, E.; Belotti, F.; Ravanelli, M.; Mattavelli, D.; Schreiber, A.; et al. Quantitative Anatomical Comparison of Transnasal and Transcranial Approaches to the Clivus. *Acta Neurochir.* **2020**, *162*, 649–660. [CrossRef]
9. Yasargil, M.G.; Antic, J.; Laciga, R.; Jain, K.K.; Hodosh, R.M.; Smith, R.D. Microsurgical Pterional Approach to Aneurysms of the Basilar Bifurcation. *Surg. Neurol.* **1976**, *6*, 83–91.
10. van Furth, W.R.; Agur, A.M.R.; Woolridge, N.; Cusimano, M.D. The Orbitozygomatic Approach. *Neurosurgery* **2006**, *58*, ONS103–ONS107, discussion ONS103–ONS107. [CrossRef]
11. Kawase, T.; Toya, S.; Shiobara, R.; Mine, T. Transpetrosal Approach for Aneurysms of the Lower Basilar Artery. *J. Neurosurg.* **1985**, *63*, 857–861. [CrossRef]
12. Dolenc, V. Direct Microsurgical Repair of Intracavernous Vascular Lesions. *J. Neurosurg.* **1983**, *58*, 824–831. [CrossRef]
13. Samii, M.; Metwali, H.; Samii, A.; Gerganov, V. Retrosigmoid Intradural Inframeatal Approach: Indications and Technique. *Neurosurgery* **2013**, *73*, ons53–ons59, discussion ons60. [CrossRef]
14. Locatelli, D.; Restelli, F.; Alfiero, T.; Campione, A.; Pozzi, F.; Balbi, S.; Arosio, A.; Castelnuovo, P. The Role of the Transorbital Superior Eyelid Approach in the Management of Selected Spheno-Orbital Meningiomas: In-Depth Analysis of Indications, Technique, and Outcomes from the Study of a Cohort of 35 Patients. *J. Neurol. Surg. B Skull Base* **2022**, *83*, 145–158. [CrossRef] [PubMed]
15. Chang, S.W.; Wu, A.; Gore, P.A.; Beres, E.J.; Porter, R.W.; Preul, M.C.; Spetzler, R.F.; Bambakidis, N.C. Quantitative Comparison of Kawase's Approach versus the Retrosigmoid Approach: Implications for Tumors Involving Both Middle and Posterior Fossae. *Neurosurgery* **2009**, *64*, ons44–ons52. [CrossRef] [PubMed]
16. Sharma, M.; Ambekar, S.; Guthikonda, B.; Nanda, A. A Comparison between the Kawase and Extended Retrosigmoid Approaches (Retrosigmoid Transtentorial and Retrosigmoid Intradural Suprameatal Approaches) for Accessing the Petroclival Tumors. A Cadaveric Study. *Skull Base Surg.* **2014**, *75*, 171–176. [CrossRef] [PubMed]
17. Meling, T.R. Letter: How I Do It: Retrosigmoid Intradural Inframeatal Petrosectomy. *Acta Neurochir.* **2021**, *163*, 2191. [CrossRef] [PubMed]
18. Sun, D.Q.; Menezes, A.H.; Howard, M.A.; Gantz, B.J.; Hasan, D.M.; Hansen, M.R. Surgical Management of Tumors Involving Meckel's Cave and Cavernous Sinus: Role of an Extended Middle Fossa and Lateral Sphenoidectomy Approach. *Otol. Neurotol.* **2018**, *39*, 82–91. [CrossRef]
19. Li, M.; Wang, X.; Chen, G.; Liang, J.; Guo, H.; Song, G.; Bao, Y. Trigeminal Schwannoma: A Single-Center Experience with 43 Cases and Review of Literature. *Br. J. Neurosurg.* **2021**, *35*, 49–56. [CrossRef]
20. Zhang, Q.; Feng, K.; Ge, C.; Hongchuan, G.; Mingchu, L. Endoscopic Endonasal Management of Trigeminal Schwannomas Extending into the Infratemporal Fossa. *J. Clin. Neurosci.* **2012**, *19*, 862–865. [CrossRef]
21. An, K.; Spallone, A.; Mukhamedjanov, D.J.; Tcherekajev, V.A.; Makhmudov, U.B. Trigeminal Neurinomas a Series of 111 Surgical Cases from a Single Institution. *Acta Neurochir.* **1996**, *138*, 1027–1035. [CrossRef]
22. Dabas, S.K.; Menon, N.N.; Ranjan, R.; Gurung, B.; Tiwari, S.; Shukla, H.; Sharma, A.; Sinha, A.; Singh, J.; Singal, R.; et al. Trigeminal Schwannoma—Case Report of a Rare Tumour. *Indian J. Otolaryngol. Head Neck Surg.* **2023**, *75*, 1–6. [CrossRef] [PubMed]
23. Evans, L.K.; Peraza, L.R.; Zamboni, A. A Trigeminal Schwannoma Masked by Solely Vestibulocochlear Symptoms. *J. Am. Acad. Audiol.* **2019**, *31*, 449–454. [CrossRef]
24. Nguyen, D.-A.; Nguyen, T.-H.; Vo, H.-L. Successful Endoscopic Endonasal Surgery for Very Huge Trigeminal Schwannomas in Nasopharynx. *Br. J. Neurosurg.* **2021**, *35*, 73–76. [CrossRef] [PubMed]
25. Lin, Y.; Gao, Q.; Jin, H.; Wang, N.; Xu, D.; Wang, F.; Guo, A.B.; Zang, W.; Li, Z.; Guo, F. Analysis of Approaches in the Microsurgical Treatment of 102 Cases of Petroclival Meningioma in a Single Center. *Front. Neurol.* **2021**, *12*, 627736. [CrossRef] [PubMed]
26. Malhotra, A.; Tu, L.; Kalra, V.B.; Wu, X.; Mian, A.; Mangla, R.; Michaelides, E.; Sanelli, P.; Gandhi, D. Neuroimaging of Meckel's Cave in Normal and Disease Conditions. *Insights Imaging* **2018**, *9*, 499–510. [CrossRef]
27. Muto, J.; Kawase, T.; Yoshida, K. Meckel's Cave Tumors: Relation to the Meninges and Minimally Invasive Approaches for Surgery: Anatomic and Clinical Studies. *Neurosurgery* **2010**, *67*, ons291–ons298, discussion ons298–ons299. [CrossRef]
28. Jouanneau, E.; Simon, E.; Jacquesson, T.; Sindou, M.; Tringali, S.; Messerer, M.; Berhouma, M. The Endoscopic Endonasal Approach to the Meckel's Cave Tumors: Surgical Technique and Indications. *World Neurosurg.* **2014**, *82*, S155–S161. [CrossRef]
29. Kassam, A.B.; Prevedello, D.M.; Carrau, R.L.; Snyderman, C.H.; Gardner, P.; Osawa, S.; Seker, A.; Rhoton, A.L. The Front Door to Meckel's Cave: An Anteromedial Corridor via Expanded Endoscopic Endonasal Approach- Technical Considerations and Clinical Series. *Neurosurgery* **2009**, *64*, ons71–ons82, discussion ons82–ons83. [CrossRef]
30. Mastantuoni, C.; Cavallo, L.M.; Esposito, F.; d'Avella, E.; de Divitiis, O.; Somma, T.; Bocchino, A.; Fabozzi, G.L.; Cappabianca, P.; Solari, D. Midline Skull Base Meningiomas: Transcranial and Endonasal Perspectives. *Cancers* **2022**, *14*, 2878. [CrossRef]

1. Di Somma, A.; Langdon, C.; de Notaris, M.; Reyes, L.; Ortiz-Perez, S.; Alobid, I.; Enseñat, J. Combined and Simultaneous Endoscopic Endonasal and Transorbital Surgery for a Meckel's Cave Schwannoma: Technical Nuances of a Mini-Invasive, Multiportal Approach. *J. Neurosurg.* **2020**, *134*, 1836–1845. [CrossRef] [PubMed]
2. Lee, M.H.; Hong, S.D.; Woo, K.I.; Kim, Y.-D.; Choi, J.W.; Seol, H.J.; Lee, J.-I.; Shin, H.J.; Nam, D.-H.; Kong, D.-S. Endoscopic Endonasal Versus Transorbital Surgery for Middle Cranial Fossa Tumors: Comparison of Clinical Outcomes Based on Surgical Corridors. *World Neurosurg.* **2019**, *122*, e1491–e1504. [CrossRef] [PubMed]
3. Ferrari, M.; Schreiber, A.; Mattavelli, D.; Belotti, F.; Rampinelli, V.; Lancini, D.; Doglietto, F.; Fontanella, M.M.; Tschabitscher, M.; Rodella, L.F.; et al. The Inferolateral Transorbital Endoscopic Approach: A Preclinical Anatomic Study. *World Neurosurg.* **2016**, *90*, 403–413. [CrossRef] [PubMed]
4. Han, X.; Yang, H.; Wang, Z.; Li, L.; Li, C.; Han, S.; Wu, A. Endoscopic Transorbital Approach for Skull Base Lesions: A Report of 16 Clinical Cases. *Neurosurg. Rev.* **2023**, *46*, 74. [CrossRef] [PubMed]
5. Erdogan, U.; Turhal, G.; Kaya, I.; Biceroglu, H.; Midilli, R.; Gode, S.; Karci, B. Cavernous Sinus and Parasellar Region: An Endoscopic Endonasal Anatomic Cadaver Dissection. *J. Craniofacial Surg.* **2018**, *29*, e667–e670. [CrossRef]
6. Bozkurt, G.; Turri-Zanoni, M.; Coden, E.; Russo, F.; Elhassan, H.A.; Gallo, S.; Zocchi, J.; Bignami, M.; Locatelli, D.; Castelnuovo, P. Endoscopic Endonasal Transpterygoid Approach to Sphenoid Sinus Lateral Recess Defects. *J. Neurol. Surg. B Skull Base* **2020**, *81*, 553–561. [CrossRef]
7. Hofstetter, C.P.; Singh, A.; Anand, V.K.; Kacker, A.; Schwartz, T.H. The endoscopic, endonasal, transmaxillary transpterygoid approach to the pterygopalatine fossa, infratemporal fossa, petrous apex, and the Meckel cave. *J. Neurosurg.* **2010**, *113*, 967–974. [CrossRef]
8. de Lara, D.; Ditzel Filho, L.F.; Prevedello, D.M.; Carrau, R.L.; Kasemsiri, P.; Otto, B.A.; Kassam, A.B. Endonasal endoscopic approaches to the paramedian skull base. *World Neurosurg.* **2014**, *82*, S121–S129. [CrossRef]
9. Oyama, K.; Tahara, S.; Hirohata, T.; Ishii, Y.; Prevedello, D.M.; Carrau, R.L.; Froelich, S.; Teramoto, A.; Morita, A.; Matsuno, A. Surgical Anatomy for the Endoscopic Endonasal Approach to the Ventrolateral Skull Base. *Neurol. Med. Chir.* **2017**, *57*, 534–541. [CrossRef]
10. Hardesty, D.A.; Montaser, A.S.; Carrau, R.L.; Prevedello, D.M. Limits of endoscopic endonasal transpterygoid approach to cavernous sinus and Meckel's cave. *J. Neurosurg. Sci.* **2018**, *62*, 332–338. [CrossRef]
11. Martínez-Pérez, R.; Zachariah, M.; Li, R.; Silveira-Bertazzo, G.; Carrau, R.L.; Prevedello, D.M. Expanded endoscopic endonasal transpterygoid transmaxillary approach for a giant trigeminal schwannoma. *Neurosurg. Focus. Video* **2020**, *2*, V15. [CrossRef] [PubMed]

Disclaimer/Publisher's Note: The statements, opinions and data contained in all publications are solely those of the individual author(s) and contributor(s) and not of MDPI and/or the editor(s). MDPI and/or the editor(s) disclaim responsibility for any injury to people or property resulting from any ideas, methods, instructions or products referred to in the content.

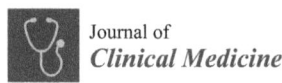

Article

The Transorbital Approach, A Game-Changer in Neurosurgery: A Guide to Safe and Reliable Surgery Based on Anatomical Principles

Matteo de Notaris [1,2], Matteo Sacco [3], Francesco Corrivetti [1,*], Michele Grasso [4], Sergio Corvino [1,5], Amedeo Piazza [1,6], Doo-Sik Kong [7] and Giorgio Iaconetta [8]

1. Laboratory of Neuroanatomy, EBRIS Foundation, European Biomedical Research Institute of Salerno, 84125 Salerno, Italy
2. Department of Neuroscience, Neurosurgery Operative Unit, "San Pio" Hospital, 82100 Benevento, Italy
3. Department of Neurosurgery, University of Foggia, 71122 Foggia, Italy
4. Department of Surgery, Otorhinolaryngology Operative Unit, "San Pio" Hospital, 82100 Benevento, Italy
5. Department of Neurological Sciences, Division of Neurosurgery, Università degli Studi di Napoli Federico II, 80055 Naples, Italy
6. Department of Neurosurgery, Sapienza University, 00185 Rome, Italy
7. Department of Neurosurgery, Samsung Medical Center, School of Medicine, Sungkyunkwan University, Seoul 06531, Republic of Korea
8. Unit of Neurosurgery, University Hospital San Giovanni di Dio e Ruggi d'Aragona, University of Salerno, 84084 Salerno, Italy
* Correspondence: corrivettifrancesco@hotmail.it or f.corrivetti@aslsalerno.it; Tel.: +39-3289185517

Abstract: During the last few years, the superior eyelid endoscopic transorbital approach has been proposed as a new minimally invasive pathway to access skull base lesions, mostly in ophthalmologic, otolaryngologic, and maxillofacial surgeries. However, most neurosurgeons performing minimally invasive endoscopic neurosurgery do not usually employ the orbit as a surgical corridor. The authors undertook this technical and anatomical study to contribute a neurosurgical perspective, exploring the different possibilities of this novel route. Ten dissections were performed on ten formalin-fixed specimens to further refine the transorbital technique. As part of the study, the authors also report an illustrative transorbital surgery case to further detail key surgical landmarks. Herein, we would like to discuss equipment, key anatomical landmarks, and surgical skills and stress the steps and details to ensure a safe and successful procedure. We believe it could be critical to promote and encourage the neurosurgical community to overcome difficulties and ensure a successful surgery by following these key recommendations.

Keywords: transorbital surgery; neuroendoscopy; neuroanatomy; skull base surgery

1. Introduction

During the last few years, neurosurgery has recently been enhanced by a variety of minimally invasive endoscopic procedures to access the ventral skull base. With the advent of transorbital neuroendoscopic surgery (TONES) [1], new modular pathways have been developed for accessing the skull base from the orbit ventrally. This was due to the gradual refinement of endoscopic techniques and anatomical research in minimally invasive skull base surgery. As a matter of fact, anatomic studies have played an important role in the development of transorbital endoscopic approaches, thus providing insights regarding the anatomy [2–6] of the orbit and beyond, such as the paramedian aspect of the anterior and middle cranial fossae and the safest interdural pathway to reach the cavernous sinus laterally to the internal carotid artery (ICA) [7,8] (Figure 1A,B). These studies have allowed surgeons to better understand the relationships between these structures and to identify the safest and most effective approaches for accessing them [4,9–11]. In addition, advances in imaging technology, such as computed tomography (CT) and magnetic resonance imaging (MRI), have enabled surgeons to create detailed 3-D models of the ventral perspective of the skull base, which can be used to plan and guide transorbital endoscopic surgeries [12]. Overall, anatomic studies have been instrumental in the development of transorbital endoscopic approaches, helping to make these procedures safer, more precise, and more effective [13,14].

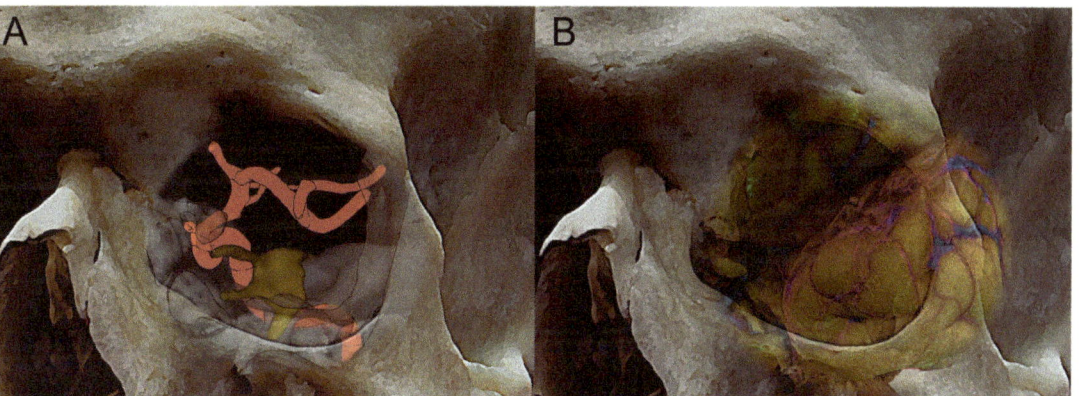

Figure 1. Three-dimensional skull reconstruction of the right orbit with superposition of the course of the internal carotid artey (**A**), the fronto-temporal opercula, and the sylvian fissure (**B**).

Furthermore, transorbital endoscopic approaches have been demonstrated to be feasible for the resection of certain types of tumors, such as trigeminal schwannomas and spheno-orbital meningiomas, with encouraging results [15–17]. However, the decision to use a transorbital endoscopic approach must be made on a case-by-case basis by a multidisciplinary team of specialists involving neurosurgeons, maxillofacial surgeons, ophthalmologists, and ENT surgeons [18,19].

On the other side, transcranial approaches for paramedian skull base lesions often involve extensive surgeries, which can be associated with significant morbidity and prolonged recovery times. Transorbital endoscopic approaches offer a less invasive alternative, with potential advantages such as shorter hospital stays and faster recovery times [20,21].

Another important thing to consider is that, as recently demonstrated, having experience with endonasal techniques can be valuable for the development of transorbital techniques. Indeed, both endonasal and transorbital approaches involve accessing the ventral skull base. As a matter of fact, experience with endonasal techniques may provide valuable insight into navigating the complex anatomy in the skull base region and identifying potential risks and complications associated with accessing this area. The skills and knowledge developed through endonasal techniques, such as using endoscopes and the ergonomy required to manipulate instruments, may also be applicable to transorbital techniques.

In addition, transorbital and endonasal approaches can be used in combination as part of a multiportal approach to access, simultaneously or not, different median and paramedian areas of the skull base [22–24], starting from a key anatomical paradigm: the endonasal approach involves accessing the midline skull base, while the transorbital approach involves accessing the paramedian areas laterally to the parasellar and paraclival segments of the internal carotid artery (Figure 1A) [25]. By combining these approaches in a multiportal approach, surgeons can access a wider range of skull base regions, including areas that may be difficult to reach using a single route [23].

The purpose of this study is to present step-by-step maneuvers that should be observed and accomplished before surgery begins from our 360-degree experience both in anatomy and in clinical settings (endonasal and transorbital surgery). These steps might simplify the often-arduous initial period for beginners, helping them progress more quickly through the steep learning curve. Finally, surgical technique and anatomical studies can provide valuable insights into the potential uses and limitations of the transorbital route.

This specific knowledge can help surgeons plan and perform procedures using reliable landmarks, reducing the risk of complications and improving patient outcomes.

2. Materials and Methods

Anatomical dissections were performed at the Laboratory of Neuroscience, EBRIS, in Salerno (Italy). Ten adult cadaveric embalmed and injected specimens were accessed. Each cadaver head underwent a bilateral superior eyelid transorbital endoscopic approach (TOA). The initial skin and bone step dissections were run under exoscopic visualization for illustrative purposes (Karl Storz) and then continued under endoscopic visualization by means of a rigid 4-mm-diameter endoscope, 18 cm in length, with 0° and 30° rod lenses (Karl Storz GmbH, Tuttlingen, Germany). The common carotid arteries were isolated, cannulated, and injected with red latex. The authors also performed a retrospective review of key and exemplificative transorbital surgery performed by the senior authors to provide specific transorbital techniques applied to an illustrative case.

3. Results

Step-by-Step Paradigm

1. The endoscopic equipment

Endonasal and transorbital approaches share almost the same equipment. While there may be some overlap in the instruments and equipment used in these approaches, they are not identical. Similarly, the endoscopic instrumentation used in the endonasal approach may also include a camera head, instruments such as suction devices, dissectors, and drills, and a neuronavigator.

The endoscopes designed for transorbital surgery are the same as those for endonasal procedures. In our institution, 4-mm-diameter endoscopes, 18 or 30 cm long, with 0 or 30° angled lenses, are used. The 0 degree scope is used at the beginning of the procedure, while 30 degree scopes are usually used at the end of lesion dissection, either for completing the surgical resection or for inspecting the most hidden and lateral aspects of the surgical field. As for the endonasal procedure, a very useful tip is to use the external sheath connected to a manual or automated irrigation system in which the endoscope is inserted to wash the lens when inside the operating field, which renders the procedure clear and dynamic by avoiding frequent in and out movements over the skin incision and keeping the endoscope lens cleaned. In cases where the exoscope is unavailable, the camera head can also be used alone (without the endoscope connected) as a kind of "external eye" at the beginning of the procedure. In such cases, the "external" visual assistance allowed significant increases in maneuverability by eliminating the space occupied by the endoscope. Indeed, at the beginning of the procedure, the space necessary for carrying out the surgical approach is very limited, and the endoscopes, due to their limited field of view and short focal distances, have various limitations during such steps, meaning that they must be placed within the surgical field with the shaft reducing the available working space and thereby reducing maneuverability. To overcome such limitations, the introduction of a 3-D exoscope system offers new possibilities in visualization and ergonomics specifically exploitable for TOA (Figure 2).

Once the dissection proceeds medially and deeply and the great sphenoid wing (GSW) is partially removed, the endoscopic visual assistance showed better surgical exposure with increased magnification and illumination potentials, in our experience.

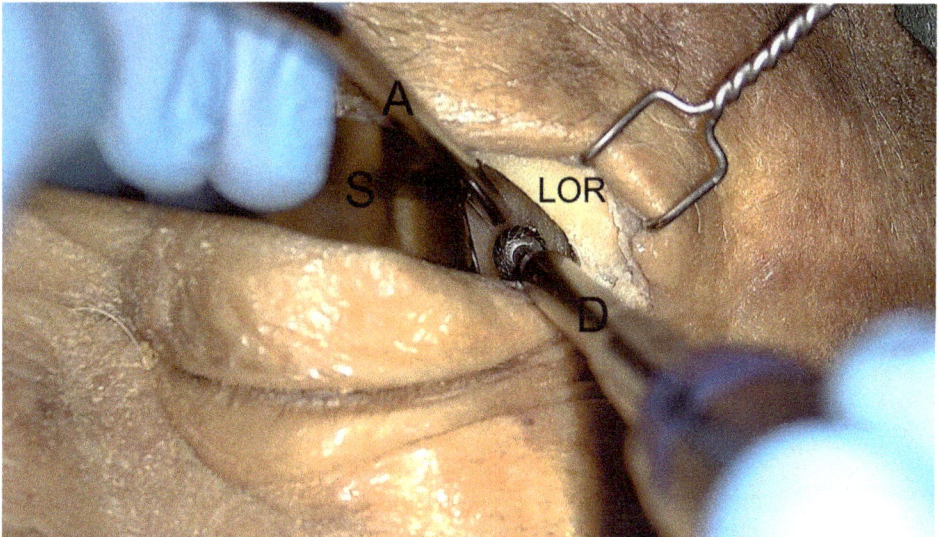

Figure 2. Exoscopic visualization during the first steps of the surgical approach. After superior eyelid incision and subcoutaneous dissection, the lateral orbital rim (LOR) is identified, and a malleable spatula (S) is used to displace medially the orbital content. Two instruments, a low-profile high-speed drill (D) and an aspirator (A), can be inserted inside the surgical corridor along the lateral orbital wall.

2. Drills

The surgical drill used during transorbital procedures should have some specific characteristics to ensure optimal performance and safety. Here are some of the key features:

Low profile: As in the endonasal procedure, the drill should be designed with a low profile to allow easy access to the surgical site without obstructing the surgeon's view.

Cut burr: This type of burr is especially useful in transorbital surgery, where precision and control are crucial, particularly at the beginning of the procedure (4 mm to 5 mm). It can cut through bone with minimal pressure, requiring a large amount of bone to rapidly enlarge the surgical field.

Diamond burr: In addition to the cut burr, the drill may also have a diamond burr (4 mm to 5 mm). Diamond burrs are coated with tiny diamond particles that can grind away bone and other hard tissues with exceptional precision (Figure 2). In addition to their cutting ability, diamond burrs also have the ability to cauterize blood vessels to achieve rapid hemostasis. This can help to reduce bleeding and promote better hemostasis during the final step of the drilling (spongiosum bone) or when the grater sphenoid wing (which represents the first anatomical bony "barrier") is infiltrated by the lesion (i.e., spheno-orbital meningiomas, chordomas). Overall, diamond burrs are a valuable tool for surgeons performing transorbital procedures, as they can help to improve the endoscopic visualization of the surgical field by reducing the bleeding.

3. Navigation system

Neuronavigation is as essential for the transorbital approach as any other skull base surgery. Preoperative imaging, such as CT and MRI scans, allows for the creation of a 3-D roadmap of the patient's anatomy. During surgery, the surgeon uses the navigational probe to track their position in relation to the patient's anatomy in real-time. In addition to improving accuracy and reducing the risk of complications, navigation technology can also help reduce the time required for surgery. Overall, navigation is an important tool for transorbital skull base surgery, especially at the beginning of the procedure to localize the first two main landmarks: the superior (SOF) and inferior orbital fissures (IOF). Other important landmarks to localize at the beginning to check the direction of the approach are the position of the optic canal, the clinoidal process, and the lesser wing of the sphenoid in order to understand the transition of the angle of attack from the middle temporal fossa (caudally) to the anterior cranial fossa (cranially) (Figure 3). In our case series, it met our main goal of significantly limiting device cutaneous displacement near the orbit without invasiveness and postoperative discomfort. Finally, the use of a navigation system seems mandatory when transorbital and endonasal approaches are used in combination as part of a multiportal approach in order to plan and recognize intraoperatively the connection of skull base areas between the two routes.

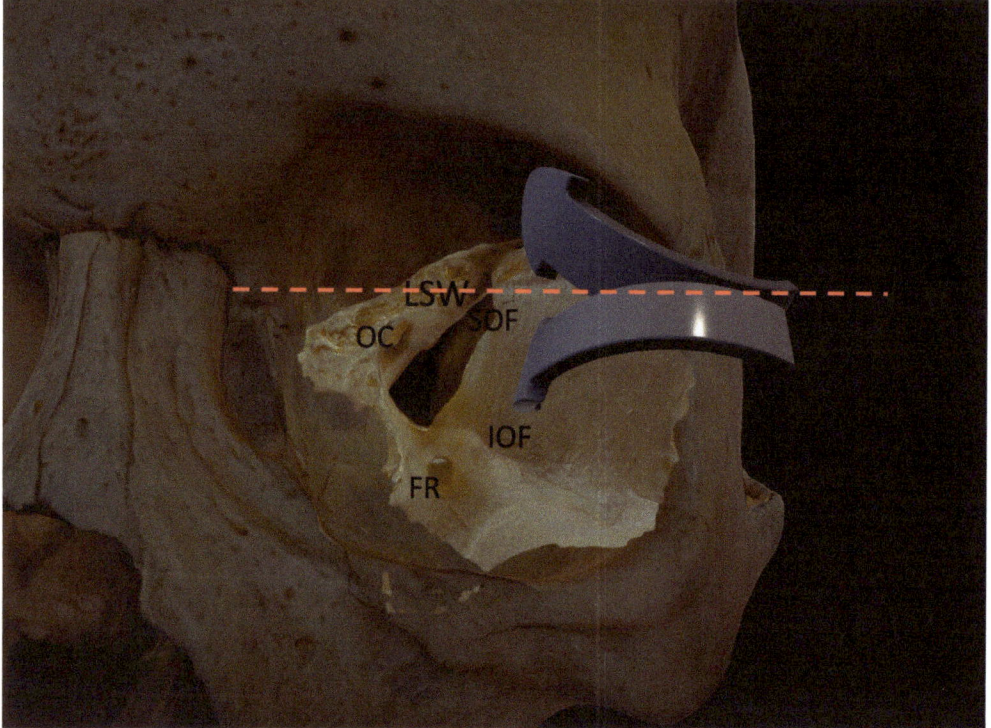

Figure 3. The picture illustrates the two different angles of attack for anterior and middle cranial fossa access. The red dotted line, orthogonal to the fronto-zygomatic suture, represents an imaginary limit between the lateral orbital wall and the orbital roof. FR: foramen rotundum; IOF: inferior orbital fissure; LSW: lesser sphenoid wing; OC: optic canal; SOF: superior orbital fissure.

4. *Operating setup and patient position*

The operating setup and patient position for transorbital surgery are critical to ensuring safety and accuracy during the procedure. The patient is positioned supine on the operating table with their head turned 15 degrees, slightly away from the side of the operation. The head is then secured with a Mayfield skull clamp to provide stability and allow neuronavigation. Regarding the position of the surgical team, in our experience, the first surgeon is positioned at the side of the patient, while the assistant may be positioned ahead of the first surgeon, as in endonasal procedures. This allows for the assistant to provide additional support to hold the endoscope and suction, as well as assist with instruments as needed. The position of the nurse during the procedure may also vary depending on the specific shape of the operating room. However, it is common for the nurse to be positioned in front of the first surgeon, providing additional support and assisting with any needs or requests from the surgical team.

The monitor screens used by the first and second surgeons should ideally be placed in front of them at a comfortable viewing distance and angle. This is important for several reasons: it ensures that they have a clear and unobstructed view of the surgical site; this way, they can maintain a comfortable and ergonomic posture throughout the procedure. This can help to reduce fatigue and improve collaboration between the first and second surgeons, as they can easily communicate and coordinate their actions by referring to the same visual information. The position of the surgical team when a multiportal endonasal and transorbital approach is performed has already been discussed and depicted elsewhere [26] (Figure 4).

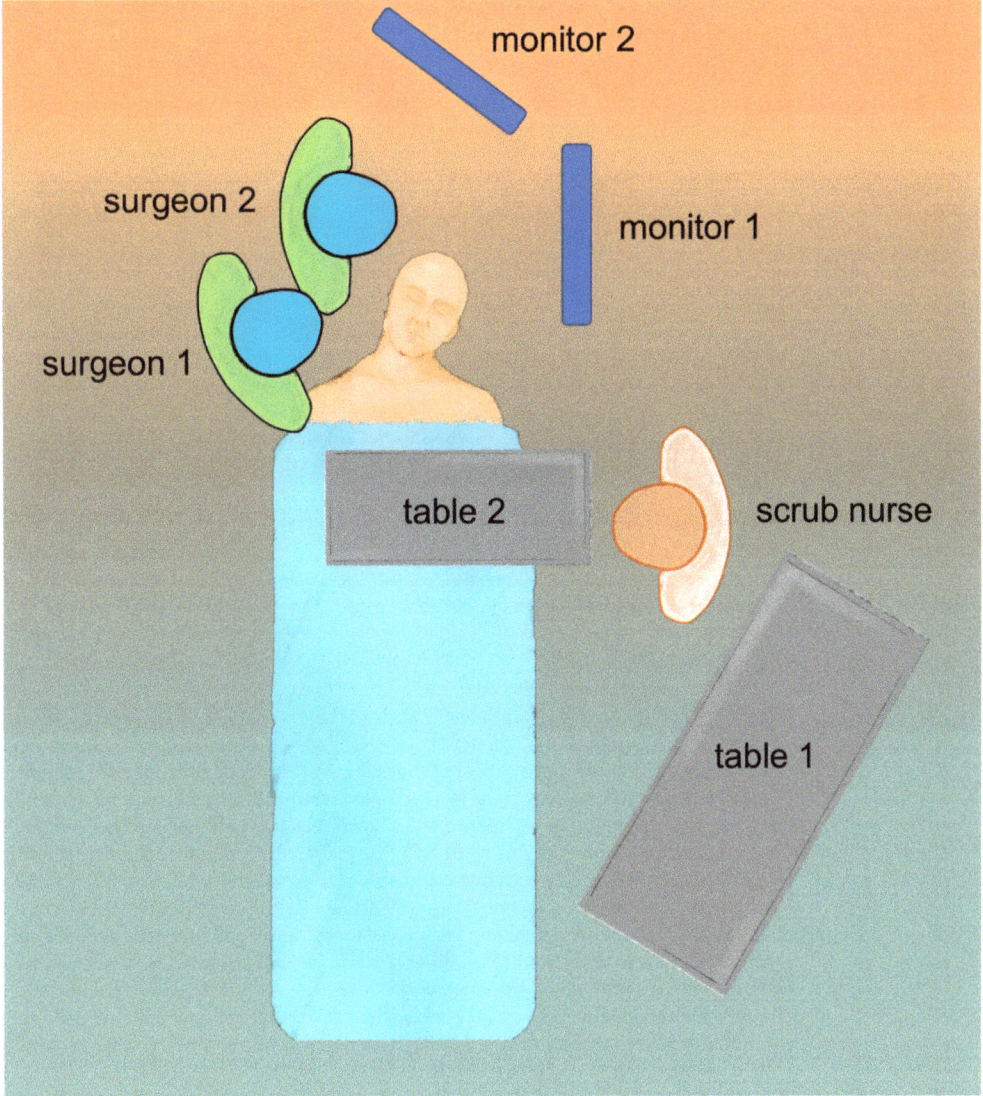

Figure 4. Operative room setup for endoscopic transorbital surgery.

5. *Ergonomics—build up your "triangle"*

In order to perform a successful and safe surgery, degrees of freedom, angles of vision, ergonomics, and instrument positioning are all of paramount importance. The instruments must be positioned correctly during surgery to avoid instrument collisions and obstructing the vision, exactly as during an endonasal procedure. Indeed, the maneuverability of the endoscope itself can be limited by the crowded transorbital entry site, thus increasing the risk of interference between instruments. As a result of these challenges, ergonomics has been taught and practiced in the anatomical lab, as it happened for transsphenoidal approaches, to provide a clear method to ensure the correct position of the instruments during the surgical approach [3]. After the skin incision at the upper eyelid crease and the progressive medial orbital retraction, the endoscope is inserted into a "virtual space" that is gradually enlarged by drilling the GSW. Due to their limited field of view and short focal distances, endoscopes must be placed within the surgical field, with the shaft reducing the available working area and limiting maneuverability. To solve this issue, the surgeon must construct a triangle-shaped operative area as follows: the lateral margin is represented by the lateral orbital rim, the medial margin by the retractor itself, and the base is the lateral aspect of the upper eyelid crease (Figure 5A).

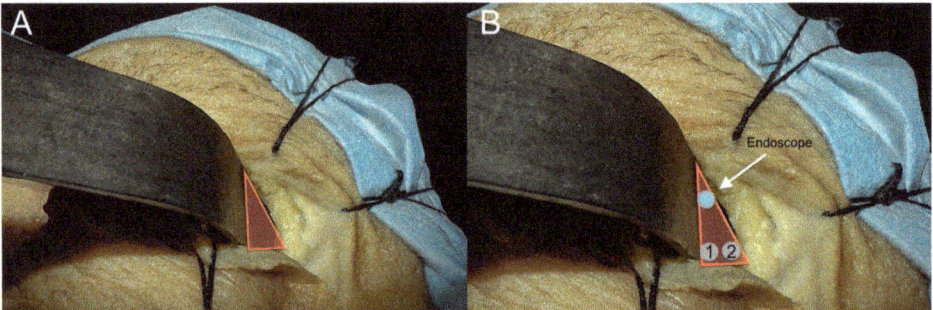

Figure 5. The picture shows the anatomical boundaries of the triangular port. (**A**). The lateral margin is represented by the lateral orbital rim, the medial margin by the retractor itself, and the base is the lateral aspect of the upper eyelid crease. (**B**). The places of insertion of the endoscopic tip are on top, and the two additional instruments are below.

6. *Evolving from endonasal to transorbital*

Neurosurgeons with experience in neuroendoscopy, particularly endoscopic endonasal surgery, may have a solid foundation to expand their expertise to transorbital surgery. They would already possess knowledge of key endoscopic principles, instrument handling, and navigation within complex skull base regions. Indeed, transorbital surgery can be considered a subset of endoscopic neurosurgery. It requires a similar skill set and familiarity with endoscopic techniques, instrumentation, and anatomical knowledge.

As a matter of fact, equipment and ergonomics for the transorbital approach come directly from the EEA, as both procedures involve advanced endoscopic techniques. Concerning the visualization systems, high-definition monitors and HD or 4K camera systems are used in both transorbital and endonasal surgeries. These systems provide surgeons with a clear view of the surgical field and allow for safe surgery. Similar to EEAs, as the corridor is long and narrow, both procedures require an endoscope for visualization. The endoscope can also be held by an external arm or a second surgeon.

While there are similarities in the equipment and ergonomics, it is worth noting that the transorbital approach may require specific instruments and equipment designed for orbital access and manipulation. Indeed, the main difference among surgical instruments for transorbital surgery is the orbital retractor (Figure 5B). There are different types of malleable or rigid orbital retractors that must be used during the initial step of the approach.

For the first cases, we suggest using semi-rigid retractors. These retractors are designed to hold the orbital tissues and maintain the desired exposure without the need for constant manual holding. They come in various sizes and designs that can be adjusted and secured in place. It is important to note that the specific choice of orbital retractors may vary among surgeons and institutions, and there may be other specialized materials utilized for retraction during transorbital procedures, such as protective silastic or silicone sheets. The selection of appropriate retractors depends on the surgeon's experience and preference.

7. Key anatomical transorbital principles to access the middle cranial fossa

According to previously published studies [3,7,25], the skin incision was made through the superior eyelid crease and the orbicularis oculi muscle, and a skin-muscle flap was raised superiorly and inferiorly until the lateral orbital rim was clearly identified.

The periosteal layer was then exposed, and a subperiosteal/subperiorbital dissection plane was found and followed. Dissection proceeded using this plane caudally until the IOF first and then the SOF were reached. This way, it was possible to expose a triangular bony area between both fissures that corresponds to the ventral aspect of the GSW. Afterwards, a malleable retractor was then gently introduced to protect the periorbita, displacing the orbital content infero-medially for about 1 cm from the fronto-zygomatic suture and thus creating room for the next surgical steps (Figure 6).

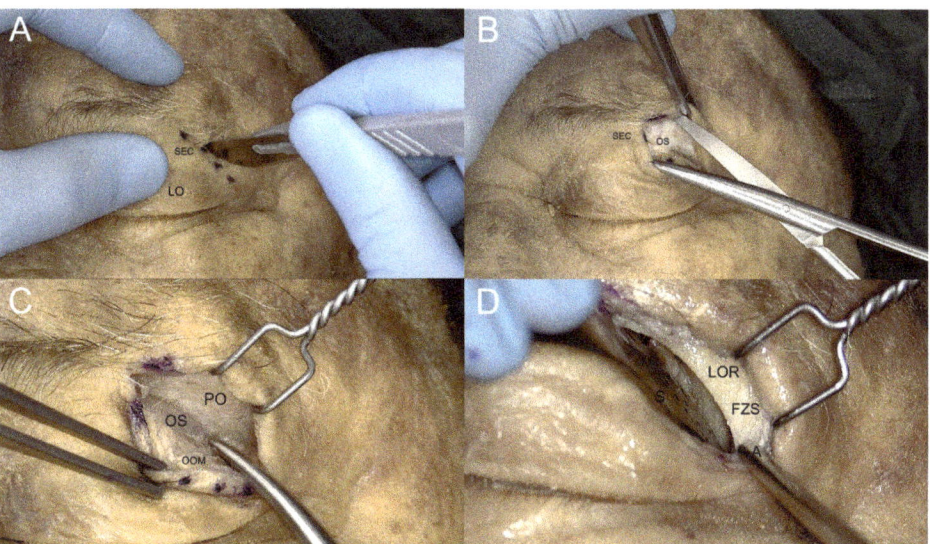

Figure 6. Steps of the superior eyelid transorbital approach. (**A**). Skin incision along the superior eyelid crease (SEC). (**B**). Subcutaneous dissection preserving the optic septum (OS). (**C**). Exposure of the periorbita (PO) of the lateral orbital rim (LOR), with the orbicularis oculi muscle (OOM) separated to preserve the OS underneath. (**D**). Removing the PO and exposing the LOR and the fronto-zygomatic suture (FZS); S: malleable spatula; A: aspirator.

The superior orbital fissure was then protected, and the drilling of the greater sphenoid wing started from laterally to medially. At this point, it was mandatory to first expose the temporal fossa to gain room for further medial progressive dissection. Once the deep temporal muscle fascia is reached, the drilling can turn medially to further remove the medial part of the GSW and gain retrobulbar space.

The "central core" of the transorbital approach is represented by the exposure of the middle cranial fossa; the other possibilities of this very versatile technique are discussed elsewhere [10].

By using this straightforward drilling, it gives access to the middle cranial fossa and exposes the dura mater of the temporal pole. While the bone drilling proceeded caudally until the floor of the middle cranial fossa (MCF), the progressive resection of the lesser sphenoid wing allowed further exposure of the dura mater temporal pole. At this point, the medial limit of bone drilling is represented by the most medial portion of the GSW, where the GSW turns progressively from a coronal to a sagittal plane, forming a triangular bony structure shaping dorsally, named the "sagittal crest" [7]. This crest separates the medial temporal dura from the postero-lateral periorbital layer. The sagittal crest was then meticulously drilled until the anterior aspect of the foramen rotundum was encountered, opening the gate to perform the interdural dissection of the cavernous sinus (CS) through the meningo-orbital band [8,27]. Then, the horizontal part of the MOB was cut, exposing the roof of the SOF corresponding to the base of the anterior clinoidal process (ACP) (Figure 7). At this point, the main landmarks over the middle cranial fossa come into view: the foramen rotundum, the foramen ovale, the foramen spinosum, and the middle meningeal artery. While proceeding with the dissection medially and posteriorly to the FO, direct ventral interdural access to the cavernous sinus is achieved (Figure 8).

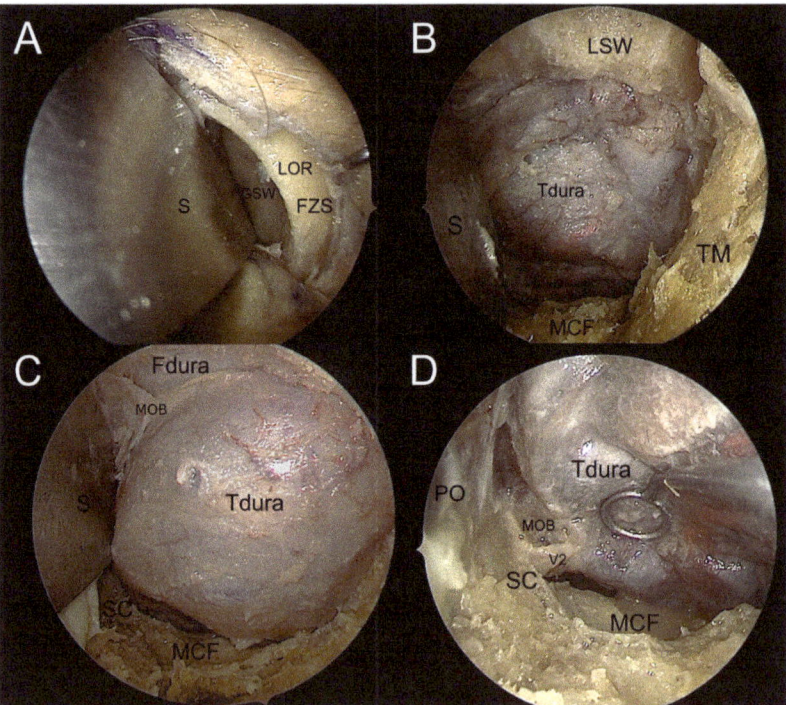

Figure 7. Endoscopic visualization of the transorbital corridor. (**A**). The greater sphenoid wing (GSW) is exposed after identification of the lateral orbital rim (LOR) and frontozygomatic suture (FZS) and subperiosteal dissection of the lateral orbital wall. A malleable spatula (S) is used to retract the orbit. (**B**). Drilling the GSW exposes the dura mater of the temporal lobe (Tdura) in the depth of the surgical field, the temporalis fossa (TF) on the lateral side, the lesser sphenoid wing (LSW) above, and the floor of the middle cranial fossa (MCF) below. (**C**). Drilling the LSW exposes the frontal lobe dura (Fdura) and the meningo-orbital band (MOB) in between; the sagittal crest (SC) is visible in the inferomedial portion of the surgical field. (**D**). Temporal lobe retraction allows for the identification of the maxillary nerve (V2) exiting from the foramen rotundum posterior to the SC; the periorbita (PO) and the MCF can be seen on the medial and inferior sides of the surgical field, respectively.

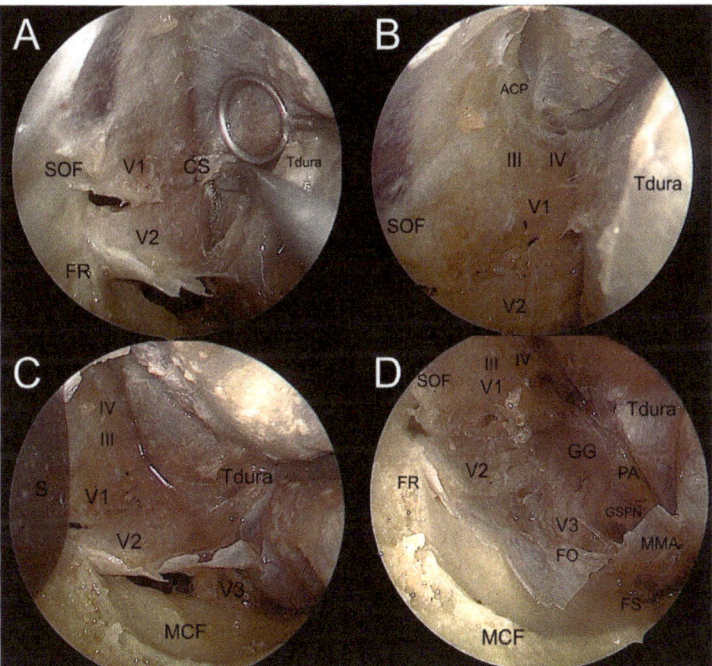

Figure 8. Interdural dissection of the cavernous sinus. (**A**). Exposure of the lateral wall of the cavernous sinus. (**B**). Exposure of the anterior clinoidal process in the upper portion of the surgical field. (**C**). Exposure of the maxillary and mandibulary nerves in the inferior portion of the surgical field. (**D**). Exposure of the entire lateral wall of the cavernous sinus, up to the gasserian ganglion and lateral portion of the middle cranial fossa. ACP: anterior clinoidal process; CS: cavernous sinus; FO: foramen ovale; FR: foramen rotundum; FS: foramen spinosum; III: oculomotor nerve; IV: troclear nerve; GG: gasserian ganglion; GSPN: greater superficial petrosal nerve; MCF: middle cranial fossa; MMA: middle meningeal artery; S: spatula; PA: petrous apex; SOF: superior orbital fissure; Tdura: temporal dura; V1: ophthalmic nerve; V2: maxillary nerve; V3: mandibulary nerve.

8. *Illustrative clinical case (the best case to start)*

The case is represented by a 55-year-old male with a history of tobacco smoking (20 packs/year). He was referred for diagnostic endoscopic endonasal endoscopy by his pneumologist during the follow-up of chronic bronchitis, as the patient complained of weight loss and intermittent difficulty swallowing, with associated dysgeusia (described by the patient as a persistent sensation of sour, bitter, and metal taste in the mouth) and exophthalmos. This was associated with progressive left diplopia and blurred vision in the left eye. On admission to our center, magnetic resonance imaging (MRI) of the nasopharynx (NP) and the whole neck region and chest computed tomography (CT) were performed. A brain and neck MRI and CT scan revealed that the primary pharyngeal tumor infiltrated the left paramedian skull base and temporal pole without metastasizing to the upper neck lymph nodes.

A left endoscopic transorbital decompression and biopsy of the lesion were performed using image guidance by the senior author (MdN) (Figures 9 and 10). The procedure revealed an abnormal appearance of greater sphenoid bone infiltration and meningeal granular tissue, also enhanced by contact endoscopy. A biopsy of the infiltrated bone and dura mater revealed several foci of infiltrating carcinoma consistent with metastatic pharyngeal carcinoma. Pathological examination ultimately confirmed the squamous phenotype of the lesion, as initially suspected.

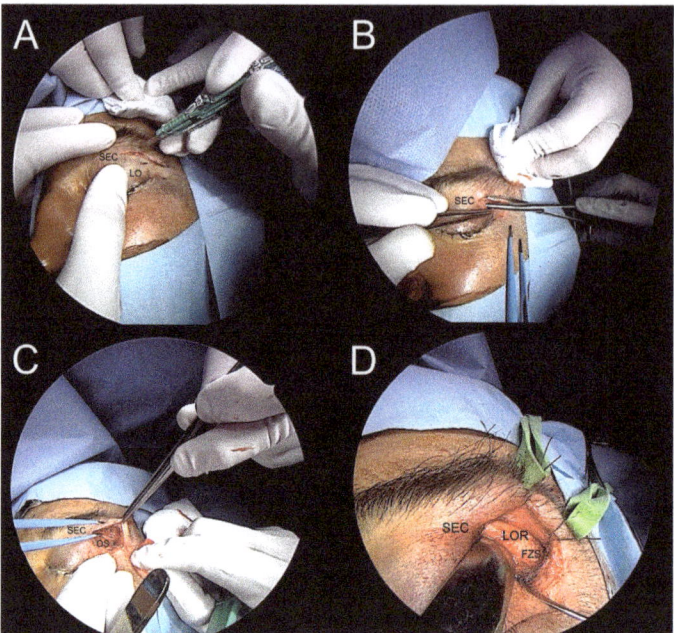

Figure 9. The four steps of transorbital access: (**A**). skin insicion; (**B**,**C**). subcoutaneous dissection; and (**D**). exposure of the lateral orbital rim (LOR). FZS: frontozygomatic suture; LOR: lateral orbital rim; OS: orbital septum; SEC: superior eyelid crease.

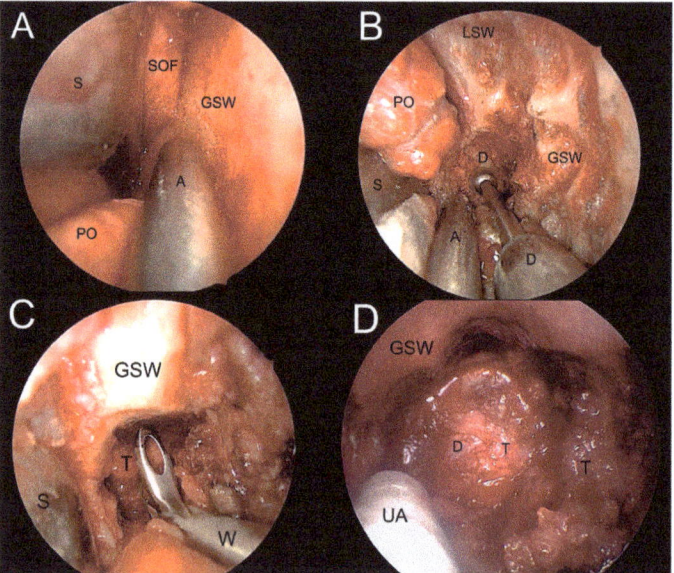

Figure 10. Transorbital corridor and tumor resection. (**A**). Exposure of the lateral orbital wall. (**B**). Drilling the greater sphenoid wing (GSW) to access the middle cranial fossa. (**C**). Tumor biopsy. (**D**). Tumor debulking. A: aspirator; D: dura meter; GSW: greater sphenoid wing; LSW: lesser sphenoid wing; PO: periorbita; T: tumor; S: spatula; UA: ultrasonic aspirator; W: Weil nasal forceps.

A postoperative TC and MRI scan revealed initial orbital decompression without other complications (Figure 11). The patient was dismissed from our department without a new neurological deficit; the exophthalmos improved one week later, and then he was referred urgently to the oncology department for further evaluation and then adjuvant radiotherapy and chemotherapy.

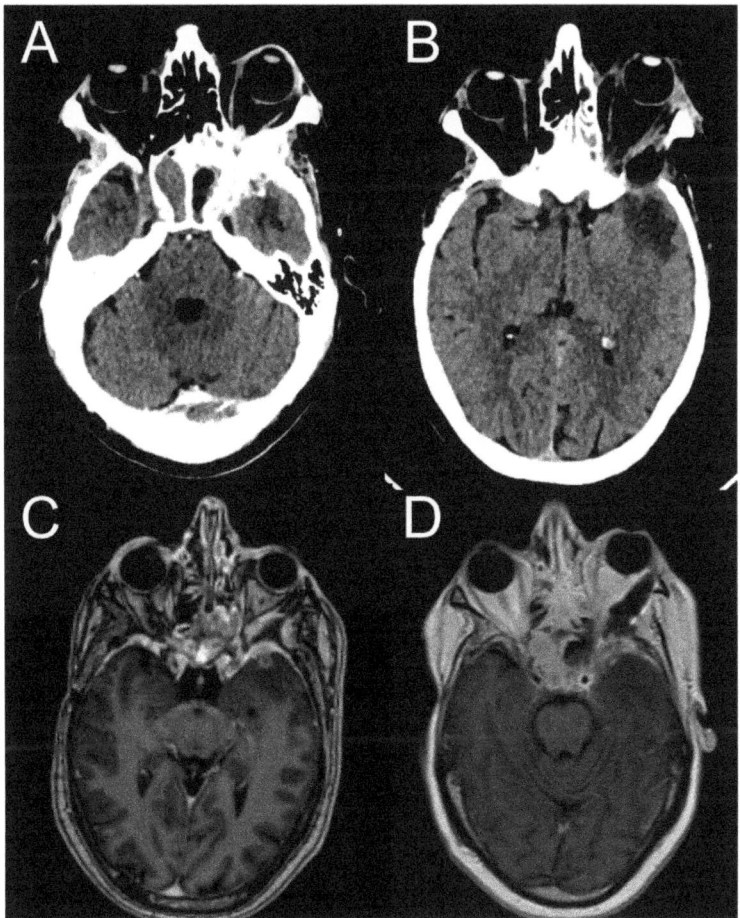

Figure 11. Pre-operative brain CT and MRI (**A,C**)show orbital infiltration by the primary tumor involving the temporal dura and the temporal lobe. Post-operative brain CT and MRI (**B,D**) show orbital decompression and resection of the brain tumor.

4. Discussion

The transorbital approach provides a direct ventral route to the paramedian skull base, which can achieve a favorable ventral angle of attack for several anterior and middle skull base lesions. As a matter of fact, the ventral perspective of most complex skull base paramedian regions (i.e., the lateral wall of the cavernous sinus, the Meckel's cave, and the petroclival synchondrosis) allows the surgeon's eye to be brought close to the target without brain manipulation. Recently, different "extensions" of this ventral paramedian port have been described to reach through a tailored petrous apex drilling in a safe "entry zone" supero-medial to the internal acoustic meatus and without brain retraction or cranial nerve manipulation, the middle tentorial incisura, until the ventral lateral brainstem.

Actually, the transorbital approach is employed for a variety of procedures, including optic nerve decompression [28], biopsy [29], and removal of orbital tumors [30,31], as well as lesions in the anterior and middle skull bases [32] and repair of meningoencephaloceles [33]. It has been shown to be effective and safe in many studies, with low rates of complications and high rates of success [34]. In this context, it can be described as a "game-changer" and revolutionary technique in neurosurgery as a minimally invasive, safe, and reliable technique for multiple reasons: it can lead to reduced morbidity, faster recovery, and shorter hospital stays, avoiding the need for extensive skull base exposure or brain retraction. It provides a direct ventral and paramedian, and intra- and extradural, route to the skull base laterally to the cavernous and clinoidal segments of the internal carotid artery, which can reduce the risk of brain injury, cerebrospinal fluid leak, and infection. This versatility can help surgeons tailor their approach to the specific needs of each patient and surgical target. Furthermore, it can be performed using relatively simple endoscopic equipment, not requiring extensive hospitalization, making it a cost-effective option for many patients.

Finally, this technique is a rapidly evolving field, with ongoing research and development focused on improving surgical techniques and outcomes. New instruments and approaches are being developed to make the transorbital approach even safer and more effective.

5. Conclusions

Overall, the transorbital approach represents a major advance in neurosurgery, providing a safe, minimally invasive, and versatile alternative to traditional open cranial approaches. While the technique is still relatively new, its potential benefits for patients and surgeons are significant, and it is likely to become an increasingly important technique in the neurosurgeon's arsenal.

Author Contributions: Conceptualization, F.C. and M.d.N.; methodology, M.S. and A.P.; validation, G.I., D.-S.K., and M.d.N.; investigation, F.C. and M.S.; resources, M.S. and F.C.; data curation, S.C. and M.G.; writing—original draft preparation, M.d.N. and F.C.; writing—review and editing, M.d.N. and D.-S.K.; visualization, M.G.; supervision, D.-S.K. and M.d.N.; project administration, G.I. and M.d.N. All authors have read and agreed to the published version of the manuscript.

Funding: This research received no external funding.

Institutional Review Board Statement: This study was approved by the Institutional Review Board of the EBRIS Foundation (CS-001131).

Informed Consent Statement: Informed consent was obtained from all subjects involved in the study.

Data Availability Statement: The data used in this study are unavailable due to privacy and ethical restriction.

Conflicts of Interest: The authors declare no conflict of interest.

References

1. Moe, K.S.; Bergeron, C.M.; Ellenbogen, R.G. Transorbital Neuroendoscopic Surgery. *Oper. Neurosurg.* **2010**, *67*, ons16–ons28. [CrossRef] [PubMed]
2. Bly, R.A.; Ramakrishna, R.; Ferreira, M.; Moe, K.S. Lateral Transorbital Neuroendoscopic Approach to the Lateral Cavernous Sinus. *J. Neurol. Surg. B Skull Base* **2014**, *75*, 11–17. [CrossRef]
3. Guizzardi, G.; Di Somma, A.; de Notaris, M.; Corrivetti, F.; Sánchez, J.C.; Alobid, I.; Ferres, A.; Roldan, P.; Reyes, L.; Enseñat, J.; et al. Endoscopic Transorbital Avenue to the Skull Base: Four-Step Conceptual Analysis of the Anatomic Journey. *Front. Oncol.* **2022**, *12*, 988131. [CrossRef] [PubMed]
4. Serioli, S.; Nizzola, M.; Plou, P.; De Bonis, A.; Meyer, J.; Leonel, L.C.P.C.; Tooley, A.A.; Wagner, L.H.; Bradley, E.A.; Van Gompel, J.J.; et al. Surgical Anatomy of the Microscopic and Endoscopic Transorbital Approach to the Middle Fossa and Cavernous Sinus: Anatomo-Radiological Study with Clinical Applications. *Cancers* **2023**, *15*, 4435. [CrossRef]
5. Nannavecchia, B.A.; Ganau, M.; Cebula, H.; Scibilia, A.; Bozzi, M.T.; Zaed, I.; Gallinaro, P.; Boujan, F.; Dietemann, J.-L.; Djennaoui, I.; et al. Endoscopic Transorbital Approaches to Anterior and Middle Cranial Fossa: A Laboratory Investigation on Surgical Anatomy and Potential Routes. *J. Neurol. Surg. B Skull Base* **2021**, *82*, 443–449. [CrossRef]

6. Yanez-Siller, J.C.; Noiphithak, R.; Martinez-Perez, R.; Dallan, I.; Moe, K.S.; Revuelta Barbero, J.M.; Howe, E.; Prevedello, D.M.; Carrau, R.L. The "Crista Ovale": A Reliable Anatomical Landmark in Transorbital Endoscopic Approaches to the Middle Cranial Fossa. *Oper. Neurosurg.* **2023**, *24*, e172–e177. [CrossRef] [PubMed]
7. Corrivetti, F.; de Notaris, M.; Di Somma, A.; Dallan, I.; Enseñat, J.; Topczewski, T.; Solari, D.; Cavallo, L.M.; Cappabianca, P.; Prats-Galino, A. "Sagittal Crest": Definition, Stepwise Dissection, and Clinical Implications From a Transorbital Perspective. *Oper. Neurosurg.* **2022**, *22*, e206–e212. [CrossRef] [PubMed]
8. Dallan, I.; Di Somma, A.; Prats-Galino, A.; Solari, D.; Alobid, I.; Turri-Zanoni, M.; Fiacchini, G.; Castelnuovo, P.; Catapano, G.; de Notaris, M. Endoscopic Transorbital Route to the Cavernous Sinus through the Meningo-Orbital Band: A Descriptive Anatomical Study. *J. Neurosurg.* **2017**, *127*, 622–629. [CrossRef] [PubMed]
9. Houlihan, L.M.; Loymak, T.; Abramov, I.; Jubran, J.H.; Staudinger Knoll, A.J.; Howshar, J.T.; O'Sullivan, M.G.J.; Lawton, M.T.; Preul, M.C. The Biportal Transorbital Approach: Quantitative Comparison of the Anterior Subfrontal Craniotomy, Bilateral Transorbital Endoscopic, and Microscopic Approaches. *J. Neurosurg.* **2023**, 1–10. [CrossRef] [PubMed]
10. Guizzardi, G.; Mosteiro, A.; Hoyos, J.; Ferres, A.; Topczewski, T.; Reyes, L.; Alobid, I.; Matas, J.; Cavallo, L.M.; Cappabianca, P.; et al. Endoscopic Transorbital Approach to the Middle Fossa: Qualitative and Quantitative Anatomic Study. *Oper. Neurosurg.* **2022**, *23*, e267–e275. [CrossRef]
11. Agosti, E.; Turri-Zanoni, M.; Saraceno, G.; Belotti, F.; Karligkiotis, A.; Rocca, G.; Buffoli, B.; Raffetti, E.; Hirtler, L.; Rezzani, R.; et al. Quantitative Anatomic Comparison of Microsurgical Transcranial, Endoscopic Endonasal, and Transorbital Approaches to the Spheno-Orbital Region. *Oper. Neurosurg.* **2021**, *21*, E494–E505. [CrossRef]
12. Lee, W.-J.; Kim, Y.H.; Hong, S.-D.; Rho, T.-H.; Kim, Y.H.; Dho, Y.-S.; Hong, C.-K.; Kong, D.-S. Development of 3-Dimensional Printed Simulation Surgical Training Models for Endoscopic Endonasal and Transorbital Surgery. *Front. Oncol.* **2022**, *12*, 966051. [CrossRef] [PubMed]
13. Park, H.H.; Yoo, J.; Yun, I.-S.; Hong, C.-K. Comparative Analysis of Endoscopic Transorbital Approach and Extended Mini-Pterional Approach for Sphenoid Wing Meningiomas with Osseous Involvement: Preliminary Surgical Results. *World Neurosurg.* **2020**, *139*, e1–e12. [CrossRef]
14. Yoo, J.; Park, H.H.; Yun, I.-S.; Hong, C.-K. Clinical Applications of the Endoscopic Transorbital Approach for Various Lesions. *Acta Neurochir.* **2021**, *163*, 2269–2277. [CrossRef]
15. Almeida, J.P.; Omay, S.B.; Shetty, S.R.; Chen, Y.-N.; Ruiz-Treviño, A.S.; Liang, B.; Anand, V.K.; Levine, B.; Schwartz, T.H. Transorbital Endoscopic Eyelid Approach for Resection of Sphenoorbital Meningiomas with Predominant Hyperostosis: Report of 2 Cases. *J. Neurosurg.* **2018**, *128*, 1885–1895. [CrossRef] [PubMed]
16. Carnevale, J.A.; Ramirez-Loera, C.; Goldberg, J.L.; Godfrey, K.J.; Schwartz, T.H. Transorbital Endoscopic Approach for Middle Fossa Floor/Lateral Cavernous Sinus Meningioma: 2-Dimensional Operative Video. *Oper. Neurosurg.* **2023**, *24*, e201–e202. [CrossRef]
17. Locatelli, D.; Restelli, F.; Alfiero, T.; Campione, A.; Pozzi, F.; Balbi, S.; Arosio, A.; Castelnuovo, P. The Role of the Transorbital Superior Eyelid Approach in the Management of Selected Spheno-Orbital Meningiomas: In-Depth Analysis of Indications, Technique, and Outcomes from the Study of a Cohort of 35 Patients. *J. Neurol. Surg. B Skull Base* **2022**, *83*, 145–158. [CrossRef] [PubMed]
18. Locatelli, D.; Pozzi, F.; Turri-Zanoni, M.; Battaglia, P.; Santi, L.; Dallan, I.; Castelnuovo, P. Transorbital Endoscopic Approaches to the Skull Base: Current Concepts and Future Perspectives. *J. Neurosurg. Sci.* **2016**, *60*, 514–525. [PubMed]
19. Peron, S.; Cividini, A.; Santi, L.; Galante, N.; Castelnuovo, P.; Locatelli, D. Spheno-Orbital Meningiomas: When the Endoscopic Approach Is Better. *Acta Neurochir. Suppl.* **2017**, *124*, 123–128. [CrossRef] [PubMed]
20. Agosti, E.; Zeppieri, M.; De Maria, L.; Mangili, M.; Rapisarda, A.; Ius, T.; Spadea, L.; Salati, C.; Tel, A.; Pontoriero, A.; et al. Surgical Treatment of Spheno-Orbital Meningiomas: A Systematic Review and Meta-Analysis of Surgical Techniques and Outcomes. *J. Clin. Med.* **2023**, *12*, 5840. [CrossRef]
21. Carnevale, J.A.; Pandey, A.; Ramirez-Loera, C.; Goldberg, J.L.; Bander, E.D.; Henderson, F.; Niogi, S.N.; Tabaee, A.; Kacker, A.; Anand, V.K.; et al. Endonasal, Supraorbital, and Transorbital Approaches: Minimal Access Endoscope-Assisted Surgical Approaches for Meningiomas in the Anterior and Middle Cranial Fossae. *J. Neurosurg.* **2023**, 1–9. [CrossRef]
22. Dallan, I.; Castelnuovo, P.; Locatelli, D.; Turri-Zanoni, M.; AlQahtani, A.; Battaglia, P.; Hirt, B.; Sellari-Franceschini, S. Multiportal Combined Transorbital Transnasal Endoscopic Approach for the Management of Selected Skull Base Lesions: Preliminary Experience. *World Neurosurg.* **2015**, *84*, 97–107. [CrossRef] [PubMed]
23. Guizzardi, G.; Prats-Galino, A.; Mosteiro, A.; Santos, C.; Topczewski, T.; Torales, J.; Roldan, P.; Reyes, L.; Di Somma, A.; Enseñat, J. Multiportal Combined Endoscopic Endonasal and Transorbital Pathways: Qualitative and Quantitative Anatomic Studies of the "Connection" Skull Base Areas. *Oper. Neurosurg.* **2023**, *24*, e342–e350. [CrossRef] [PubMed]
24. Ciporen, J.N.; Moe, K.S.; Ramanathan, D.; Lopez, S.; Ledesma, E.; Rostomily, R.; Sekhar, L.N. Multiportal Endoscopic Approaches to the Central Skull Base: A Cadaveric Study. *World Neurosurg.* **2010**, *73*, 705–712. [CrossRef] [PubMed]
25. Corvino, S.; Guizzardi, G.; Sacco, M.; Corrivetti, F.; Bove, I.; Enseñat, J.; Colamaria, A.; Prats-Galino, A.; Solari, D.; Cavallo, L.M.; et al. The Feasibility of Three Port Endonasal, Transorbital, and Sublabial Approach to the Petroclival Region: Neurosurgical Audit and Multiportal Anatomic Quantitative Investigation. *Acta Neurochir.* **2023**, *165*, 1821–1831. [CrossRef]

26. DI Somma, A.; Guizzardi, G.; Valls Cusiné, C.; Hoyos, J.; Ferres, A.; Topczewski, T.E.; Mosteiro, A.; DE Rosa, A.; Solari, D.; Cavallo, L.M.; et al. Combined Endoscopic Endonasal and Transorbital Approach to Skull Base Tumors: A Systematic Literature Review. *J. Neurosurg. Sci.* **2022**, *66*, 406–412. [CrossRef] [PubMed]
27. Froelich, S.C.; Aziz, K.M.A.; Levine, N.B.; Theodosopoulos, P.V.; van Loveren, H.R.; Keller, J.T. Refinement of the Extradural Anterior Clinoidectomy: Surgical Anatomy of the Orbitotemporal Periosteal Fold. *Neurosurgery* **2007**, *61*, 179–185; discussion 185–186. [CrossRef]
28. Ozdogan, S.; Beton, S.; Gungor, Y.; Comert, A.; Bakir, A.; Kahilogullari, G. Alternative Path for Optic Nerve Decompression in Pseudotumor Cerebri With Full Endoscopic Lateral Transorbital Approach. *J. Craniofac Surg.* **2023**, *34*, 1089–1092. [CrossRef] [PubMed]
29. Gerges, M.M.; Godil, S.S.; Younus, I.; Rezk, M.; Schwartz, T.H. Endoscopic Transorbital Approach to the Infratemporal Fossa and Parapharyngeal Space: A Cadaveric Study. *J. Neurosurg.* **2019**, *133*, 1948–1959. [CrossRef]
30. Luzzi, S.; Zoia, C.; Rampini, A.D.; Elia, A.; Del Maestro, M.; Carnevale, S.; Morbini, P.; Galzio, R. Lateral Transorbital Neuroendoscopic Approach for Intraconal Meningioma of the Orbital Apex: Technical Nuances and Literature Review. *World Neurosurg.* **2019**, *131*, 10–17. [CrossRef]
31. Dallan, I.; Castelnuovo, P.; Turri-Zanoni, M.; Fiacchini, G.; Locatelli, D.; Battaglia, P.; Sellari-Franceschini, S. Transorbital Endoscopic Assisted Management of Intraorbital Lesions: Lessons Learned from Our First 9 Cases. *Rhinology* **2016**, *54*, 247–253. [CrossRef]
32. Han, X.; Yang, H.; Wang, Z.; Li, L.; Li, C.; Han, S.; Wu, A. Endoscopic Transorbital Approach for Skull Base Lesions: A Report of 16 Clinical Cases. *Neurosurg. Rev.* **2023**, *46*, 74. [CrossRef]
33. Mathios, D.; Bobeff, E.J.; Longo, D.; Tabaee, A.; Anand, V.K.; Godfrey, K.J.; Schwartz, T.H. Lateral Transorbital Approach for Repair of Lateral Sphenoid Sinus Meningoencephaloceles in Proximity to Foramen Rotundum: Cadaveric Study and Case Report. *Oper. Neurosurg.* **2023**, *25*, 168–175. [CrossRef] [PubMed]
34. Goncalves, N.; Lubbe, D.E. Transorbital Endoscopic Surgery for Sphenoid Wing Meningioma: Long-Term Outcomes and Surgical Technique. *J. Neurol. Surg. B Skull Base* **2020**, *81*, 357–368. [CrossRef]

Disclaimer/Publisher's Note: The statements, opinions and data contained in all publications are solely those of the individual author(s) and contributor(s) and not of MDPI and/or the editor(s). MDPI and/or the editor(s) disclaim responsibility for any injury to people or property resulting from any ideas, methods, instructions or products referred to in the content.

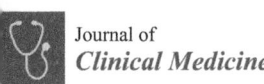

Article

Thalamopeduncular Tumors in Pediatric Age: Advanced Preoperative Imaging to Define Safe Surgical Planning: A Multicentric Experience

Alberto D'Amico [1,*], Giulia Melinda Furlanis [1], Valentina Baro [1], Luca Sartori [1], Andrea Landi [1], Domenico d'Avella [1], Francesco Sala [2] and Luca Denaro [1]

[1] Academic Neurosurgery, Department of Neurosciences, University of Padova, 35122 Padova, Italy
[2] Section of Neurosurgery, Department of Neurological and Movement Sciences, University of Verona, 37100 Verona, Italy
* Correspondence: alberto.damico@unipd.it

Abstract: Background: Thalamopeduncular tumors are challenging lesions arising at the junction between the thalamus and the cerebral peduncle. They represent 1–5% of pediatric brain tumors, are mainly pilocytic astrocytoma and occur within the first two decades of life. To date, the optimal treatment remains unclear. **Methods**: We retrospectively reviewed pediatric patients who underwent surgery for thalamopeduncular tumors in the Academic Pediatric Neurosurgery Unit of Padova and Verona from 2005 to 2022. We collected information on age, sex, symptoms, preoperative and postoperative neuroradiological studies, histological specimens, surgical approaches, and follow-up. **Results**: We identified eight patients with a mean age of 9 years. All lesions were pilocytic astrocytoma. The main symptoms were spastic hemiparesis, cranial nerve palsy, headache, and ataxia. The corticospinal tract was studied in all patients using diffusion-tensor imaging brain MRI and in two patients using navigated transcranial magnetic stimulation. The transsylvian approach was the most frequently used. A gross total resection was achieved in two patients, a subtotal resection in five and a partial resection in one. In three patients, a second treatment was performed due to the regrowth of the tumor, performing an additional surgery in two cases and a second-look surgery followed by adjuvant therapy in one. After the surgery, four patients maintained stability in their postoperative neurological exam, two patients improved, and two worsened but in one of them, an improvement during recovery occurred. At the last follow-up available, three patients were disease-free, four had a stable tumor residual, and only one patient died from the progression of the disease. **Conclusions**: Advanced preoperative tools allow one to define a safe surgical strategy. Due to the indolent behavior of thalamopeduncular tumors, surgery should be encouraged.

Keywords: thalamopeduncular tumor; pilocytic astrocytoma; transcranial magnetic stimulation; thalamopeduncular syndrome; DTI MRI; brain mapping

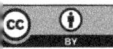

1. Introduction

Thalamopeduncular tumors are a new subgroup of lesions recently described by Puget et al. [1] that originate from the interface between the thalamus and the cerebral peduncles. They develop below a normal thalamus, pushing it upwards and displacing the corticospinal tract. Pediatric thalamopeduncular tumors represent less than 5% of all pediatric brain tumors. They can occur at all ages, rarely arise in adulthood, and mainly affect children in the first two decades of their life, with no gender preference. In the past, they were classified as tout court within a large group of tumors, defined as "thalamic", "brainstem" or "basal ganglia" tumors, without considering their different features in terms of clinical or radiological presentation and therapeutic strategies.

In most cases, the thalamopeduncular tumors are pilocytic astrocytoma. In the pediatric population, low-grade gliomas (LGG) have a very high chance of a long overall survival, reaching adulthood, and in the case of pilocytic astrocytoma and a histology without aggressive or infiltrative histopathological features, a complete recovery can be achieved with total resection, usually without the need for adjuvant oncological treatment.

If a more infiltrative tumor pattern is found, the recent molecular knowledge about genetic mutations such as KIAA1549-BRAF fusion and BRAF-V600E mutation could offer additional targets for therapies [2,3].

Frequently, thalamopeduncular tumors are responsible for a peculiar clinical syndrome named the "Thalamopeduncular syndrome of childhood", characterized by progressive spastic hemiparesis associated with pyramidal signs. Hydrocephalus may be present due to the proximity of the lesion to the ventricular system. Other signs such as visual impairment, cranial nerve palsy, and focal seizures are less common [4].

Before the nineties, these tumors were considered inoperable, due to the deep and complex areas involved. The lack of adequate neuroimaging and intraoperative tools made the cost–benefit ratio of thalamopeduncular surgery unfavorable. In most cases, patients were referred for radiotherapy with a poor prognosis due to early relapse, malignant transformation, or cognitive impairment.

Nowadays, new advanced neuroimaging techniques such as diffusion-tensor imaging tractography (DTI MRI) and neuronavigated transcranial magnetic stimulation (nTMS), together with neuronavigation system and intraoperative neurophysiological monitoring, allow one to plan an accurate surgical strategy to obtain good control of the disease with low morbidity and a favorable long-term outcome [5–7].

2. Materials and Methods

We retrospectively reviewed pediatric patients who underwent surgery for thalamopeduncular tumors at the Academic Pediatric Neurosurgery Department of Padova and at the Academic Neurosurgery Department of Verona from 2005 to 2022.

We collected eight cases, including four boys and four girls (M/F ratio 1:1) aged from 3 to 15 years with a mean age of 9 years. The clinical presentation at admission was progressive spastic hemiparesis in six patients, and in three of them, VII cranial nerve palsy was also observed. Other symptoms were ataxia in one case and headache in another one. In three patients, mild hydrocephalus was present (Table 1). For each patient, we assessed, sex, age at onset, the histopathological report (with Ki67 proliferation index), preoperative and postoperative brain MRI with gadolinium, DTI MRI to reconstruct the corticospinal spinal tracts, cortical motor mapping, white fiber reconstruction with nTMS (Nexstim®, Madison, WI, USA), the use of the neuronavigation system (Medtronic Stealth Station Navigation S7®, Lafayette, CO, USA), and the use of intraoperative neurophysiological monitoring (IONM).

The level of tumor resection was classified as a partial resection (<90% with the presence of residual tumor on postoperative MRI), a subtotal resection (>90% with small residual tumor on postoperative MRI), or a gross total resection (the absence of residual tumor on postoperative MRI).

Finally, we reported the surgical approaches performed, the additional surgery or eventual adjuvant therapies performed, the postoperative neurological status and the last clinical and neuroradiological follow-up available (Table 2).

Table 1. Data series.

Case	Sex; Age	Histology	Pre-Op EON	HY	Treatment	Post-Op EON	Relapse\Progression	2nd Treatment
A	F; 12	PA	HH	N	Surgery	HH Stable	N	-
B	F; 13	PA	Mild HP	Y	Surgery	HP improved	N	-
C	M; 7	PA	Moderate HP; VII CN palsy	N	Surgery	HP and VII CN palsy stable	N	-
D	F; 3	PA *	Ataxia	Y	Surgery	Worsened severe HP	Progression	Additional surgery + CH\RT
E	M; 15	PA	Mild HP	N	Surgery	HP stable	Progression	Additional surgery
F	F; 9	PA	Moderate HP	Y	Surgery	Transient HP Worsened **	N	-
G	M; 8	PA	Mild HP; VII CN palsy	N	Surgery	HP and VII CN palsy improved	N	-
H	M; 6	PA	HP	N	Surgery	HP stable	Progression	Additional surgery

EON, neurological exam; HP, hemiparesis; HH, headache; PA, pilocytic astrocytoma; PA *, more aggressive histopathological pattern (Ki67 > 5%); CN, cranial nerve; HY, hydrocephalus; Y, yes; N, no. Transient Worsened **, EON improved just during recovery and after a brief rehabilitation period.

Table 2. Surgical approaches performed, level of tumor resection and follow-up.

Case	Surgical Approach	EOR	FU (MO)	LTFU
A	Transsylvian	GTR	11	Disease free
B	Transtemporal T1–T2	STR	10	Stable residual
C	Transtemporal T1–T2	GTR	96	Disease free
D	Parietal transcortical	PR	36	Deceased
E	Transsylvian	STR	108	Stable residual
F	Transsylvian	STR	120	Stable residual
G	Transsylvian	STR	84	Stable residual
H	Transsylvian	STR	51	Stable residual

EOR, amount of tumor resection; GTR, gross total resection; STR, subtotal resection; PR, partial resection; FU, Follow-up; MO, months, LTFU, long-term follow-up.

3. Surgical Plan

Every patient underwent brain MRI with gadolinium (Gd) and DTI MRI tractography to reconstruct the cortical spinal bundles, and in recent cases, nTMS was used to reconstruct the cortical motor mapping.

Due to the deep sites and complex areas invaded by thalamopeduncular tumors, DTI MRI tractography (DTI) is an important tool used to identify the corticospinal tracts (CSTs) with the aim of planning a surgical approach and trying to obtain a gross total resection with respect to neurological function [8].

Neuronavigated transcranial magnetic stimulation (nTMS) was a recent neuroimaging tool introduced by the Academic Neurosurgery of Padova and Verona. nTMS is an innovative technique that allows one to obtain a preoperative functional mapping of the motor cortex, adding functional information on the CSTs with respect to the anatomic data obtained with DTI-MRI. nTMS requires collaboration from the patients, and for this reason, it is usually performed on adults [9].

DTI-MRI CST reconstruction combined with nTMS mapping allows for an accurate tridimensional visualization of the cortical spinal bundles and helps the surgeon to choose the safer surgical corridor (Figures 1 and 2).

In addition to the location and size of the lesions, the DTI MRI and the nTMS data are important tools used to decide the surgical approach.

We performed three main surgical approaches: transsylvian, transcortical transtemporal, and transcortical parietal.

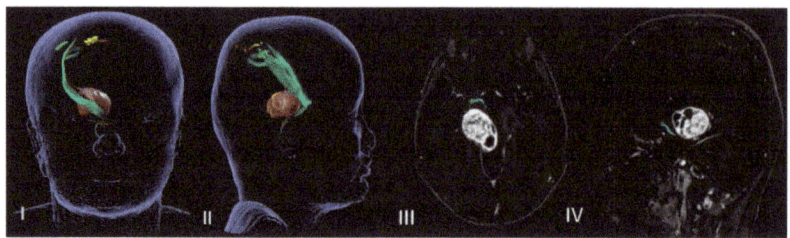

Figure 1. (**I–IV**) Neuronavigated transcranial magnetic stimulation pre-op study. (**I,II**) A 3D reconstruction of the nTMS data that shows cortical maps of the right spinal tract (CST) for the hand (green) and foot (yellow) and its relationship with the thalamopeduncular tumor of **Case B**. (**III,IV**): The brain MRI merged with the nTMS data shows that the cortical spinal tract (CST) runs antero-laterally with respect to a right thalamopeduncular tumor.

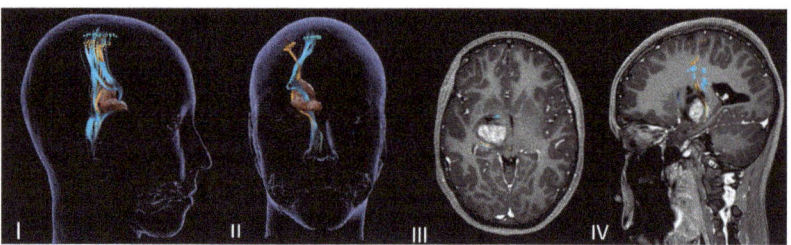

Figure 2. Neuronavigated transcranial magnetic stimulation pre-op study. (**I,II**) A 3D reconstruction of the nTMS data that shows cortical maps of the right spinal tract (CST) for the foot (blue) and hand (orange) and its relationship with the thalamopeduncular tumor of **Case A**. (**III,IV**) Brain MRI merged with nTMS data showing that the cortical spinal tract (CST) runs antero-medially respect to a right thalamopeduncular tumor.

Furthermore, intraoperative neurophysiological monitoring (corticospinal and corticobulbar SSEPs and MEPs) and cortical-subcortical mapping [10] guided all the intraoperative steps of the surgery.

Finally, in all cases, we performed a postoperative brain MRI with gadolinium within 24 h of the surgery (Figure 3).

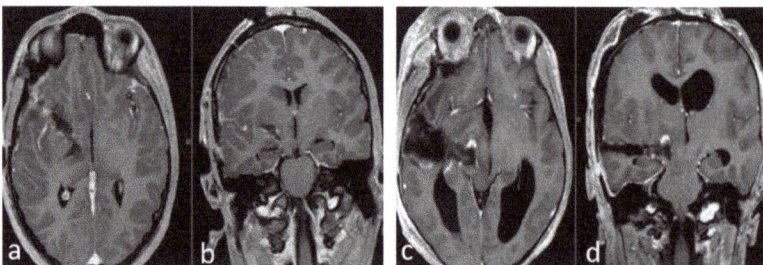

Figure 3. (**a–d**) Early postoperative brain MRI with gadolinium. (**a,b**) An early postoperative brain MRI, T1-weigthed with gadolinium in the axial (to the **left**) and coronal plane (to the **right**), for Case A in Figure 2. (**c,d**) An early post operative MRI, T1-weigthed with gadolinium, for Case B in Figure 1. **In detail**: In accordance with the nTMS data, we performed a transsylvian approach for Case A (**a,b**) obtaining a gross total resection (**GTR**). In Case B (**b–d**), we performed a trans-temporal approach, obtaining a subtotal resection (**STR**).

4. Results

In the last 17 years (from 2005 to 2022), a total of eight children with thalamopeduncular tumors underwent surgery in the Academic Pediatric Neurosurgery Department of Padova and in the Academic Neurosurgery Department of Verona.

In our series, the mean age was 9 years (range 3–15 years), with no gender prevalence, and the patients had not undergone any previous surgical intervention. Six patients developed "thalamo-peduncular syndrome" [11] with progressive spastic hemiparesis, and in three of them, facial cranial nerve palsy was observed. Other symptoms at onset were headache and an unstable gait. Indeed, three patients presented chronic hydrocephalus that did not require shunt surgery before the tumor resection.

In seven patients, the tumor was unilateral (in four on the left side and in three on the right side), and it was bilateral in one case. In all cases, the preoperative brain MRI with gadolinium showed mixed solid-cystic lesions with non-homogeneous contrast enhancement.

Preoperative DTI-MRI showed a posterior displacement of the cortical spinal tracts in three cases (posterolateral in) and anterior (four antero-lateral and one antero-medial) displacement in five cases.

In the most recent cases (**Case A–Case B**), the preoperative nTMS was performed to obtain a cortical motor mapping and the cortical spinal bundles reconstruction. The nTMS data confirmed the DTI MRI data for the motor bundles' displacement, adding functional information about cortical and subcortical motor areas of the mouth, arms and legs (Table 3).

Table 3. DTI and nTMS data for cortical spinal tracts' position with respect to the thalamopeduncular tumor.

Case	DTI CST	nTMS CST
A	AM	AM And P
B	AL	AL And P
C	AL	N\A
D	AL	N\A
E	PL	N\A
F	P	N\A
G	P	N\A
H	AL	N\A

DTI, diffusor tensor imaging; **nTMS**, neuronavigated transcranial magnetic stimulation; **CST**, cortical spinal tract; **AL**, antero-laterally; **AM**, antero-medially; **P**, posterior; **N\A**, data not available.

A total of 11 procedures were performed on eight patients. Two patients (**Case E–Case H**) required a second surgery for progression one and four years after surgery, respectively, and one required an early second-look surgery due to a partial resection (**Case D**).

The main surgical corridor used was the transsylvian approach (**Case A–E–F–G–H**). In two cases, we used the transcortical transtemporal route (**Case B–C**), and in one case, we used a posterior parietal approach (**Case D**) due to the greater posterior parietal development of the lesion. We achieved GTR in two cases (**Case A–Case C**), STR in five (**Case B–E–F–G–H**), and PR in one (**Case D**).

All the tumors were pilocytic astrocytoma, but in one, we found a more infiltrative and aggressive histopathological pattern with a higher proliferation index (Ki67) (**Case D**) (Table 4).

The location and the extension of the tumor together with the DTI-MRI and nTMS reconstruction CST data guided the preoperative surgical plan. In all cases, we used intraoperative neurophysiological monitoring of the SSEPs, MEPs, and cortical\subcortical mapping. The brainstem acoustic evoked responses (BAERs) were used in the presence of a great extension of the lesion to the midbrain and the pons and the visual evoked potentials (flash-VEPs) in cases of the involvement of the optic chiasm or optic tracts.

Table 4. Histopathological report and molecular features.

Case	Histology Features	ki67%	kiaa1549-braf	braf v600e
A	PA (Nos)	2%	positive	negative
B	PA (Nos)	1%	positive	negative
C	PA (Nos)	1%	(-)	(-)
D	PA (infiltrative)	5%	negative	negative
E	PA (Nos)	3%	(-)	(-)
F	PA (Nos)	1%	(-)	(-)
G	PA (Nos)	1%	negative	negative
H	PA (Nos)	3%	(-)	(-)

PA pilocytic astrocytoma; Nos not otherwise specified; (-) Data non avaible.

Two patients showed improved neurological status after the surgery (**Case B–G**) and four maintained stable (**Case A–C–E–H**). Two patients worsened immediately after the surgery (**Case D–F**), but one (**Case F**) improved during recovery, recovering to his pre-surgery neurological status after a period of rehabilitation.

Three patients had a progression of their disease (**Case E–D–H**). Two patients (**Case E–H**) experienced a regrowth of the lesion after 15 months and four years, respectively, and therefore underwent an additional surgery, obtaining a new subtotal resection with good clinical and radiological long-term outcomes.

In only one case (**Case D**), due to an important extension and aggressive histopathological pattern, a partial resection was achieved. For this reason, we performed an early second-look surgery to obtain a new partial resection. Therefore, this patient received additional adjuvant therapy (CHT\RT) after a multidisciplinary discussion with the oncologist group. Finally, this patient died due to a rapid progression of disease.

At the last neuroradiological and clinical follow-up, five patients had a stable residual tumor (**Case B–E–F–G–H**), two were disease-free (**Case A–C**), and one was deceased (**Case D**). The mean follow-up was 64.5 months (range 10–120 months).

5. Discussion

Thalamopeduncular tumors are lesions that arise at the junction between the thalamus and the cerebral peduncles [1] (Figure 4). Most of these tumors are slow-growing pilocytic astrocytoma and displaced the corticospinal bundle, leading to the typical contralateral progressive spastic hemiparesis described as "childhood thalamopeduncular syndrome" [11].

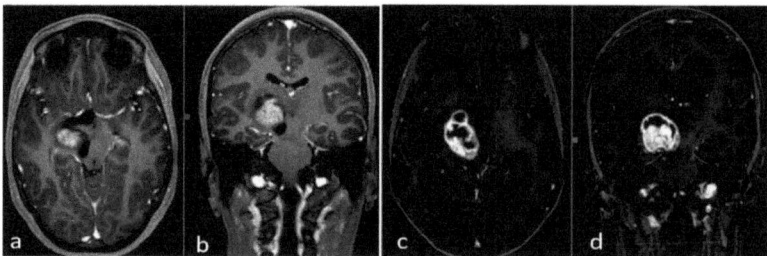

Figure 4. Preoperative brain MRI of the thalamopeduncular tumor of **Case A** (a,b) and of **Case B** (c,d). (a,b) Brain MRI, T1-weighted with gadolinium, showing solid-cystic right thalamopeduncular tumors in the axial plane (on the **left**) and coronal plane (on the **right**) in **Case A**. (c,d) Brain MRI, T1-weighted with gadolinium, showing a right thalamopeduncular lesion with disomogenous contrast enhancement in the axial (on the **left**) and coronal (on the **right**) plane in **Case B**.

The natural history of pediatric low-grade gliomas is favorable, and children have an excellent survival prognosis in comparison to adults. Overall survival rates at 10 and

20 years range from 80 to 90%. Therefore, in the pediatric population, these lesions rarely undergo malignant transformation during their lifetime and have a very low mortality rate [12,13]. For all these reasons, these patients can reach later adulthood.

Our series collected and retrospectively reviewed eight children with thalamopeduncular tumors who underwent surgery in the Academic Pediatric Neurosurgery Departments of Padova and Verona. In most cases, the clinical presentation observed was "childhood thalamopeduncular syndrome", as described in the literature [4–11]. Other symptoms such as headache and cranial nerve palsy were observed. Two cases (**Case B–F**), due to persistent hydrocephalus, required ventricular-peritoneal shunt surgery after tumor resection, unlike in the Baroncini and Cinalli series [14,15].

All patients in our series underwent elective surgery. We achieved gross total resection in two patients, subtotal resection in five, and a partial resection in one case (<90% removal). No mortality related to surgery occurred.

All tumors were pilocytic astrocytoma and were examined for their proliferation activity using a Ki67 marker with a mean of 2% (range 1–5%).

Three patients underwent an additional surgery for tumor progression, obtaining a new subtotal resection in two and a partial resection in one. This latter case presented a more infiltrative histopathological pattern, with a Ki67 of 5%, and a more rapid progression of the disease. For this reason, we performed an early second-look surgery and then an additional chemotherapy regime with carboplatin and vincristine followed by radiotherapy (SIOP-LGG 2004 protocol) [16].

Indeed, one patient died due to rapid progression of their disease, while the other seven patients in our series had a stable residual tumor or were disease-free at the last follow-up.

Our surgical series provides further evidence regarding the key role of surgical treatment with curative intent for challenging entities such as thalamopeduncular tumors with a low-grade histology.

According to the literature [17,18], due to the very low mortality rate of this condition and the rare possibility of undergoing malignant transformation, in low-grade thalamopeduncular tumors, we suggest maximizing tumor resection as the treatment of choice. The cornerstone of treatment of these lesions is surgery, even in cases of tumor regrowth.

Even a subtotal resection offers a good long-term outcome, as shown in our series. Five cases with subtotal resection were clinically and radiologically stable at long-term follow-up (Figure 5).

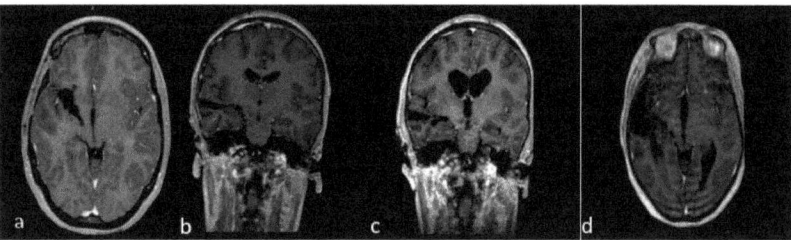

Figure 5. (**a–d**) Brain MRI, T1-weighted with gadolinium. Last follow-up of **Case A** (**a,b**) and **Case B** (**c,d**). (**a,b**) Brain MRI, T1-weighted with gadolinium, in the axial and coronal planes of **Case A**, showing good control of the disease (2021). (**b–d**): MRI, T1-weighted with gadolinium, in the coronal and axial planes of **Case B**, showing no evidence of relapse five years post-op.

Preoperative advanced techniques of neuroimaging, including the more recent nTMS, are important tools used to plan surgery and guide the intraoperative steps of tumor resection with a good risk–benefit ratio. Therefore, the surgical corridor is chosen according to the tumor location and size and according to the relationship between the tumor and the corticospinal tract, studied with DTI MRI and nTMS [19].

The introduction of nTMS for pediatric thalamopeduncular tumors has led to additional information about the topography of motor pathways from the brain cortex and provides functional information about the different components inside the cortical spinal bundles. Thus, the integration between anatomic and functional studies based on DTI MRI and nTMS allows for more precise and detailed knowledge of the motor bundles' position with respect to the tumor and consequently allows us to tailor a better surgical approach.

nTMS is also useful, as reported in the recent literature, for better understanding the benefits and risks of surgery in terms of neurological functional outcomes and to convey realistic expectations to families [7].

The use of an nTMS machine on children requires some precautions, such as the adaption of the nTMS seat workstation to the size of the children. The seat of the nTMS workstation is too large for a young patient, and so it must be adjusted to the height of the child in each individual case.

Therefore, nTMS is an exam that requires the patient's concentration and collaboration, which is difficult in the case of young patients, but we did not encounter any problems during mapping, and no side effects were registered for our patients, as the latest systematic review of the literature describes [5].

Even though further studies are needed to verify the utility of nTMS so as to improve surgical and functional outcomes in pediatric thalamopeduncular tumors, this paper and another one recently published by our work team describe the first surgical series where nTMS was applied in pediatric thalamopeduncular tumors for a preoperative study of the arrangement of the corticospinal bundles [20].

The technological tools described are valid instruments used to preserve and, in some cases, improve neurological function in patients with thalamopeduncular low-grade gliomas.

The limitations of this study must be kept in mind due to the small number of patients presented. Furthermore, our paper does not have statistical and comparative value with respect to overall survival with and without the use of these tools, but we wish to stress the utility of advanced presurgical tools for reconstructing cortical spinal bundles, as nTMS and DTI MR allow us to perform surgery on lesions located in deep and complex areas of the brain.

Indeed, we underline our surgical attitude to planning a maximal safe resection using DTI MRI, as described above, in children harboring thalamic and thalamopeduncular low-grade gliomas, as well as the use of innovative techniques as nTMS.

According to our experience, many residual tumors can be observed with serial MRI, and upon progression or clinical manifestation, further surgery and eventual oncological therapy can be considered depending on the histopathological and molecular tumor features, the location of the tumor and the patient's functional status.

The innovative technique described allows us to choose a safer surgical approach and helps the surgeon to obtain good control of the disease.

Another important aspect observed in children with thalamopeduncular tumors is that even though immediate worsening in the postoperative neurological exam is possible, in most patients, an improvement of their clinical status can occur during recovery or with a brief rehabilitation period.

As suggested in the literature [21], this clinical behavior in patients with thalamopeduncular tumors is probably due to a reduction in the compressive effects of the thalamopeduncular tumor on the thalamus and on the motor spinal tracts.

6. Conclusions

In the past, thalamopeduncular tumors were considered inoperable, and their surgery was characterized by elevated morbidity and mortality. Nowadays, safe surgical planning with advanced preoperative techniques, such as DTI MRI and nTMS, and intraoperative tools, such as intraoperative neurophysiological monitoring and neuronavigation systems, is the key to obtaining good control of the disease with acceptable surgery-related morbidity.

Therefore, due to the potential indolent behavior of thalamopeduncular low-grade gliomas, neurosurgical attitudes have changed, becoming more aggressive in recent years.

By using DTI MRI and nTMS for pediatric thalamopeduncular tumors, we showed a feasible and curative surgical approach which allowed us to navigate areas previously considered as a neurosurgical taboo, for it was impossible to conduct even a subtotal resection without severe complications, as supported by the recent literature.

Even if the use of nTMS is in its initial stages and further studies are needed to confirm its real potential for support in these kinds of tumors, our experience suggests the utility of nTMS as a preoperative instrument to provide functional information for cortical spinal bundles observed using DTI MRI, allowing us to improve the functional outcomes of patients with thalamopeduncular tumors.

Finally, we underline that a small residual tumor can be stable for many years, even after a subtotal resection; thus surgery for thalamopeduncular tumors should be encouraged.

Author Contributions: Manuscript conceptualization, data curation and original draft preparation, A.D.; investigation and figure preparation, G.M.F., V.B. and L.S.; methodology, manuscript review and editing, L.D. and A.L.; visualization and manuscript review, F.S. and D.d.; manuscript validation and project supervision, A.D. and L.D. All authors have read and agreed to the published version of the manuscript.

Funding: This research received no external funding.

Institutional Review Board Statement: Ethical approval was not required for this study.

Informed Consent Statement: All necessary consent forms were collected before the publication of this manuscript.

Data Availability Statement: Not applicable.

Conflicts of Interest: The authors declare no conflict of interest.

References

1. Puget, S.; Crimmins, D.W.; Garnett, M.R.; Grill, J.; Oliveira, R.; Boddaert, N.; Wray, A.; Lelouch-Tubiana, A.; Roujeau, T.; Di Rocco, F.; et al. Thalamic tumors in children: A reappraisal. *J. Neurosurg. Pediatr.* **2007**, *106* (Suppl. 5), 354–362. [CrossRef]
2. Lee, R.P.; Foster, K.A.; Lillard, J.C.; Klimo, P.; Ellison, D.W.; Orr, B.; Boop, F.A. Surgical and molecular considerations in the treatment of pediatric thalamopeduncular tumors. *J. Neurosurg. Pediatr.* **2017**, *20*, 247–255. [PubMed]
3. Wisoff, J.H.; Sanford, R.A.; Heier, L.A.; Sposto, R.; Burger, P.C.; Yates, A.J.; Holmes, E.J.; Kun, L.E. Primary neurosurgery for pediatric low-grade gliomas: A prospective multi-institutional study from the Children's Oncology Group. *Neurosurgery* **2011**, *68*, 1548–1554; discussion 1554–1545. [CrossRef]
4. Cuccia, V.; Monges, J. Thalamic tumors in children. *Child's Nerv. Syst.* **1997**, *13*, 514–521. [CrossRef] [PubMed]
5. Umana, G.E.; Scalia, G.; Graziano, F.; Maugeri, R.; Alberio, N.; Barone, F.; Crea, A.; Fagone, S.; Giammalva, G.R.; Brunasso, L.; et al. Navigated Transcranial Magnetic Stimulation Motor Mapping Usefulness in the Surgical Management of Patients Affected by Brain Tumors in Eloquent Areas: A Systematic Review and Meta-Analysis. *Front. Neurol.* **2021**, *12*, 644198.
6. Picht, T.; Mularski, S.; Kuehn, B.; Vajkoczy, P.; Kombos, T.; Suess, O. Navigated transcranial magnetic stimulation for preoperative functional diagnostics in brain tumor surgery. *Oper. Neurosurg.* **2009**, *65* (Suppl. 6), ons93–ons99. [CrossRef]
7. Rosenstock, T.; Picht, T.; Schneider, H.; Vajkoczy, P.; Thomale, U.W. Pediatric navigated transcranial magnetic stimulation motor and language mapping combined with diffusion tensor imaging tractography: Clinical experience. *J. Neurosurg. Pediatr.* **2020**, *26*, 583–593.
8. Celtikci, E.; Celtikci, P.; Fernandes-Cabral, D.T.; Ucar, M.; Fernandez-Miranda, J.C.; Borcek, A.O. High-Definition Fiber Tractography in Evaluation and Surgical Planning of Thalamopeduncular Pilocytic Astrocytomas in Pediatric Population: Case Series and Review of Literature. *World Neurosurg.* **2017**, *98*, 463–469.
9. Krieg, S.M.; Lioumis, P.; Mäkelä, J.P.; Wilenius, J.; Karhu, J.; Hannula, H.; Savolainen, P.; Lucas, C.W.; Seidel, K.; Laakso, A.; et al. Protocol for motor and language mapping by navigated TMS in patients and healthy volunteers; workshop report. *Acta Neurochir.* **2017**, *159*, 1187–1195.
10. Sala, F.; di Rocco, C. Intraoperative neurophysiological monitoring in neurosurgery: Moving the debate from evidence and cost-effectiveness to education and training. *World Neurosurg.* **2015**, *83*, 32–34. [CrossRef]
11. Broadway, S.J.; Ogg, R.J.; Scoggins, M.A.; Sanford, R.; Patay, Z.; Boop, F.A. Surgical management of tumors producing the thalamopeduncular syndrome of childhood. *J. Neurosurg. Pediatr.* **2011**, *7*, 589–595. [PubMed]

12. Bandopadhayay, P.; Bergthold, G.; London, W.B.; Goumnerova, L.C.; Morales La Madrid, A.; Marcus, K.J.; Guo, D.; Ullrich, N.J.; Robison, N.J.; Chi, S.N.; et al. Long-term outcome of 4,040 children diagnosed with pediatric low-grade gliomas: An analysis of the Surveillance Epidemiology and End Results (SEER) database. *Pediatr. Blood Cancer* **2014**, *61*, 1173–1179. [CrossRef] [PubMed]
13. Ryu, H.H.; Jung, T.Y.; Lee, G.J.; Lee, K.H.; Jung, S.H.; Jung, S.; Baek, H.J. Differences in the clinical courses of pediatric and adult pilocytic astrocytomas with progression: A single-institution study. *Child's Nerv. Syst.* **2015**, *31*, 2063–2069. [CrossRef]
14. Baroncini, M.; Vinchon, M.; Minéo, J.F.; Pichon, F.; Francke, J.P.; Dhellemmes, P. Surgical resection of thalamic tumors in children: Approaches and clinical results. *Child's Nerv. Syst.* **2007**, *23*, 753–760.
15. Cinalli, G.; Aguirre, D.T.; Mirone, G.; Ruggiero, C.; Cascone, D.; Quaglietta, L.; Aliberti, F.; Santi, S.D.; Buonocore, M.C.; Nastro, A.; et al. Surgical treatment of thalamic tumors in children. *J. Neurosurg. Pediatr.* **2018**, *21*, 247–257. [PubMed]
16. Thomale, U.W.; Gnekow, A.K.; Kandels, D.; Bison, B.; Hernáiz Driever, P.; Witt, O.; Pietsch, T.; Koch, A.; Capper, D.; Kortmann, R.D.; et al. Long-term follow-up of surgical intervention pattern in pediatric low-grade gliomas: Report from the German SIOP-LGG 2004 cohort. *J. Neurosurg. Pediatr.* **2022**, *30*, 316–329. [CrossRef]
17. Villarejo, F.; Amaya, C.; Pérez Díaz, C.; Pascual, A.; Alvarez Sastre, C.; Goyenechea, F. Radical surgery of thalamic tumors in children. *Child's Nerv. Syst.* **1994**, *10*, 111–114.
18. Beneš, V., 3rd; Zápotocký, M.; Libý, P.; Táborský, J.; Blažková, J., Jr.; Blažková, J., Sr.; Sumerauer, D.; Mišove, A.; Perníková, I.; Kynčl, M.; et al. Survival and functional outcomes in paediatric thalamic and thalamopeduncular low grade gliomas. *Acta Neurochir.* **2022**, *164*, 1459–1472. [CrossRef]
19. Moshel, Y.A.; Elliott, R.E.; Monoky, D.J.; Wisoff, J.H. Role of diffusion tensor imaging in resection of thalamic juvenile pilocytic astrocytoma. *J. Neurosurg. Pediatr.* **2009**, *4*, 495–505.
20. Baro, V.; Sartori, L.; Caliri, S.L.; Furlanis, G.M.; D'Amico, A.; Meneghini, G.; Facchini, S.; Ferreri, F.; Corbetta, M.; Denaro, L.; et al. Navigated Transcranial Magnetic Stimulation Motor Mapping and Diffusion Tensor Imaging Tractography for Diencephalic Tumor in Pediatric Patients. *Brain Sci.* **2023**, *13*, 234.
21. Memet Ozek, M.; Türe, U. Surgical approach to thalamic tumors. *Child's Nerv. Syst.* **2002**, *18*, 450–456.

Disclaimer/Publisher's Note: The statements, opinions and data contained in all publications are solely those of the individual author(s) and contributor(s) and not of MDPI and/or the editor(s). MDPI and/or the editor(s) disclaim responsibility for any injury to people or property resulting from any ideas, methods, instructions or products referred to in the content.

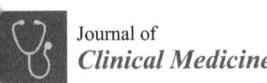

Article

Radiologically Defined Sarcopenia as a Biomarker for Frailty and Malnutrition in Head and Neck Skin Cancer Patients

Aniek T. Zwart [1,2,3,*,†], Laurence M. C. Kok [3], Julius de Vries [3], Marloes S. van Kester [4,5], Rudi A. J. O. Dierckx [2], Geertruida H. de Bock [1], Anouk van der Hoorn [2] and Gyorgy B. Halmos [3]

1. Department of Epidemiology, University Medical Center Groningen, University of Groningen, 9713 GZ Groningen, The Netherlands; g.h.de.bock@umcg.nl
2. Department of Radiology, University Medical Center Groningen, University of Groningen, 9713 GZ Groningen, The Netherlands
3. Department of Otolaryngology and Head and Neck Surgery, University Medical Center Groningen, University of Groningen, 9713 GZ Groningen, The Netherlands
4. Department of Dermatology, University Medical Center Groningen, University of Groningen, 9713 GZ Groningen, The Netherlands
5. Department of Dermatology, Haga Hospital Location Leyweg (Hagaziekenhuis), 2545 AA The Hague, The Netherlands
* Correspondence: a.t.zwart@umcg.nl; Tel.: +31-50-361-0738
† Current address: Department of Epidemiology, FA40, University Medical Center Groningen, University of Groningen, P.O. Box 30 001, 9700 RB Groningen, The Netherlands.

Abstract: The aim of this study was to evaluate whether radiologically defined sarcopenia, or a low skeletal muscle index (SMI), could be used as a practical biomarker for frailty and postoperative complications (POC) in patients with head and neck skin cancer (HNSC). This was a retrospective study on prospectively collected data. The L3 SMI (cm^2/m^2) was calculated with use of baseline CT or MRI neck scans and low SMIs were defined using sex-specific cut-off values. A geriatric assessment with a broad range of validated tools was performed at baseline. POC was graded with the Clavien–Dindo Classification (with a grade of > II as the cut-off). Univariate and multivariable regression analyses were performed with low SMIs and POC as the endpoints. The patients' (n = 57) mean age was 77.0 ± 9 years, 68.4% were male, and 50.9% had stage III–IV cancer. Frailty was determined according to Geriatric 8 (G8) score (OR 7.68, 95% CI 1.19–49.66, $p = 0.032$) and the risk of malnutrition was determined according to the Malnutrition Universal Screening Tool (OR 9.55, 95% CI 1.19–76.94, $p = 0.034$), and these were independently related to low SMIs. Frailty based on G8 score (OR 5.42, 95% CI 1.25–23.49, $p = 0.024$) was the only variable related to POC. However, POC was more prevalent in patients with low SMIs (Δ 19%, OR 1.8, 95% CI 0.5–6.0, $p = 0.356$). To conclude, a low SMI is a practical biomarker for frailty and malnutrition in HNSC. Future research should be focused on interventions based on low SMI scores and assess the effect of the intervention on SMI, frailty, malnutrition, and POC.

Keywords: head and neck neoplasms; skin neoplasms; postoperative complications; geriatric assessment; frail elderly; sarcopenia

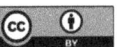

1. Introduction

Older patients have a higher chance of developing HNSC due to the cumulative damages from solar UV radiation, and this is a population that is expanding as our society ages [1–4]. Surgery is the primary treatment choice for HNSC; however, primary radiotherapy can be an alternative to surgery in selected cases. In general, surgical interventions for HNSC are relatively simple with local excision, but extensive surgery can be necessary for cases of advanced disease. Preoperative screening for this population is essential as older patients may have more comorbidities, functional impairments, psychological issues, and poorer social support, all of which can affect perioperative risk [5]. Hence, a multidisciplinary approach and personalized treatment are important for decision-making [6,7].

The Comprehensive Geriatric Assessment (CGA) is a multidimensional and interdisciplinary assessment and is the gold standard for identifying frail patients [6,8]. However, the CGA is time-intensive, partially subjective, requires the active participation of the patient, and can be strenuous for the patient or clinician. Therefore, shorter frailty screening questionnaires, such as the Geriatric 8 (G8) and the Groningen Frailty Indicator (GFI) are also available. Screening for frailty with the G8 is promising as it is related to postoperative complications (POC) [9], guideline deviations [10], and declined quality of life in HNSC patients [11]. Although shorter, these frailty screening tools still require the active participation of the patient, and the frailest patients tend to not return questionnaires [12]. A simple, objective method to assess frailty and the risk of POC could be helpful to overcome these problems.

SMI is considered a surrogate biomarker for total body skeletal muscle mass [13] and could be a fast, objective biomarker for frailty and POC in HNSC patients. Generally, neck imaging for HNSC is reserved for more complex or advanced cases. SMI can reliably be measured on CT and MRI neck scans that are conducted during oncological work-up [14,15], and it provides a convenient, objective, and less time-intensive tool relative to the CGA. A low SMI, also referred to as radiologically defined sarcopenia, has already emerged as a predictor for adverse clinical outcomes, including POC and frailty in patients with mucosal head and neck cancers (mHNC) [16–18]. The impact of a low SMI in HNSC could be considerable as a recent meta-analysis found that low SMIs were related to lower progression-free survival and lower overall survival in patients diagnosed with malignant cutaneous melanoma who had been treated with palliative immunotherapy [19].

However, the clinical value of SMI for predicting frailty and POC is unknown in HNSC, and insights could be beneficial for multidisciplinary teams when making treatment decisions or selecting patients for pre-habilitation, particularly in an older population. Therefore, in the present study, the aims were to: (1) determine SMI using baseline CT or MRI neck scans conducted during oncological work-up, (2) analyze the relationship between frailty and (low) SMI, and (3) investigate the impact of (low) SMI and frailty on the occurrence of POC in patients with HNSC.

2. Materials and Methods

Patients in this retrospective cohort study were prospectively enrolled in the Oncological Life Study (OncoLifeS) databiobank [20] after obtaining written informed consent. This large-scale, institutional oncological databiobank collects and stores the following details of adult patients diagnosed with cancer: clinical and treatment data, comorbidities, lifestyle, radiological and pathological findings, biomaterials, quality of life, and long-term outcomes. The OncoLifeS databiobank has been approved by the Medical Ethical Committee of the University Medical Center Groningen (UMCG) and is registered in the Dutch Trial Register under the registration number NL7839. The scientific board of OncoLifeS gave its permission for this study.

2.1. Patient Population and Data Collection

Between October 2014 and October 2018, 197 patients with HNSC were included in OncoLifeS. The patients were treated according to national guidelines within the multidisciplinary head and neck tumor board and, if applicable, the melanoma board. Eligibility criteria for the present study were patients who had been surgically treated for HNSC in the UMCG with follow-up data on POC, sufficient neck imaging at baseline, and a geriatric assessment at baseline (n = 65). Patients without imaging data at a level of C3 (n = 5), those with too small field of view (n = 2), or those with too much angulation in the cervical spine (n = 1) were excluded. In total, 57 patients (28.9% of the initial sample size) were included in this study.

The baseline patient, tumor, and treatment characteristics were extracted from the OncoLifeS databiobank, including age (years), sex, body mass index (BMI, kg/m^2), smoking status (never vs. former or current), alcohol usage (none or mild vs. heavy, as defined by the usage of two alcohol units or more per day), reason for referral (primary vs. residual or recurrent), primary tumor location, stage of disease (stage I–II vs. II–IV), tumor size (cm), tumor type, treatment intensity (minor vs. major, as defined by a surgery of > 120 min), type of anesthesia (local vs. general), and reconstructive surgery (yes vs. no). The seventh edition of the Union for International Cancer Control TNM Classification was used for defining tumor stage.

2.2. Frailty Screening and Geriatric Assessment

The included patients underwent a geriatric assessment on the first day of consultation using a range of validated tools (Table S1), and the outcomes were registered in OncoLifeS. The Geriatric 8 (G8) and Groningen Frailty Indicator (GFI) were used for frailty screening.

2.3. Quantification of Skeletal Muscle Mass

All scans were made for clinical purposes and performed using modern CT (n = 43) or MRI (1.5 Tesla, n = 9; 3 Tesla, n = 5) scanners. Most CT scans were performed with an intravenous iodine contrast (n = 42) and with the use of a soft tissue kernel of between 20 and 40 (n = 37). The CT slice thicknesses were 0.6–1.25 mm. Most MRI scans had a slice thickness of 3.0 mm without the use of an intravenous contrast (n = 13). Measurements on the MRI scans were completed on a T2, and if a T2 was not available, they were completed on a T1 (n = 4).

The SMIs were measured with CT and MRI neck scans using previously validated procedures [14,15]. In short, the third cervical vertebra (C3) was identified and the cross-sectional area (CSA, cm^2) of the neck musculature was measured [14]. The CSA at the C3 level was converted to the CSA at the third lumbar vertebra (L3) to calculate the SMI (cm^2/m^2) (see Equations 1 and 2) [13,14]. A low SMI was defined using sex-specific SMI cut-off values, with an SMI of < 42.4 cm^2/m^2 for males and an SMI of < 30.6 cm^2/m^2 for females [21]. One observer (LMC) took all of the measurements and was blinded for the baseline characteristics and clinical outcomes. Before making the CSA measurements in the dataset of the present study, the performance of this observer was tested in a separate training set (with the CT n = 25 and the MRI n = 25). In addition to the main observer, the observers for the inter-observer analyses included a PhD student (ATZ) with 5 years of experience doing these measurements, a board-certified radiologist, and three medical students. All CSA measurements taken by the main observer in the dataset of the present study were visually verified by ATZ. The equations used for the calculations were:

$$CSAatL3(\text{cm}^2) = 27.304 + 1.363 * CSAatC3(\text{cm}^2) + 0.640 * Weight(\text{kg}) \\ + 26.442 * Gender(Gender = 1\ for Female, 2\ for Female) - 0.671 * Age(\text{years}) \quad (1)$$

The lumbar SMI was then calculated using the formula published by Prado et al. see Formula (2) [5]

$$LumbarSMI\left(\text{cm}^2/\text{m}^2\right) = CMSAatL3/(height * height). \quad (2)$$

2.4. Postoperative Outcomes

POC was classified using the Clavien–Dindo Classification (CDC) with a grade of > II as a cut-off [22]. Unplanned readmission for any cause and duration of hospitalization (days) within thirty days post-surgery were recorded.

2.5. Statistical Analysis

Baseline characteristics, adverse postoperative outcomes, and frailty status were presented as means (standard deviations), medians (ranges), or values (%). Normality was analyzed in continuous data with a Kolmogorov–Smirnov analysis and Q–Q plots. Inter-rater observer reliability was analyzed with the Intraclass Correlation Coefficient (ICC). For the second research aim, the relationship between frailty and skeletal muscle mass was assessed by univariate and multivariable linear (with SMI being dependent) and logistic (with a low SMI being dependent) regression analyses. For the third research aim, the relationship between skeletal muscle mass, frailty, and POC was analyzed with univariate and multivariable logistic regression analyses (with a CDC grade of >II being dependent), and skeletal muscle mass, frailty, and the other baseline variables were the covariates. Statistically significant and clinically relevant variables ($\alpha < 0.05$, two-sided) from the univariate regression analyses with high impacts on the dependent variable, without multicollinearity (variance inflation factors of < 3), were selected for the multivariable regression analysis. To reduce overfitting, a multivariable model with only three covariates was built. Odds ratios (ORs) or beta (B) and 95% confidence intervals (CIs) were provided. SPSS version 28 (IBM, Armonk, NY, USA) was used for the analyses.

3. Results

3.1. General Patient Characteristics

In total, 57 patients with HNSC having neck imaging and a geriatric assessment at baseline were included in the present study. Table 1 shows the patients' baseline characteristics. The mean (SD) age of the study population was 77.1 ($\pm$ 9.0) years, and a majority of the patients were male (68.4%) and had stage III–IV disease classifications (50.9%). The tumors were mostly keratinocyte carcinoma (squamous and basal cell carcinoma) (73.7%) and located on the ears (36.8%). The prevalence levels of frailty were 20.0% and 41.9% for the GFI and the G8, respectively (Table 2).

3.2. Predictors for Skeletal Muscle Mass

The inter-rater reliability of the main observer was excellent for both the CT (ICC = 0.994, 95% CI 0.982–0.998, $p < 0.001$) and the MRI (ICC = 0.985, 95% CI 0.970–0.993, $p < 0.001$). The mean (SD) SMIs were 42.40 $\pm$ 6.75, 44.95 $\pm$ 6.01, and 26.87 $\pm$ 6.01 cm^2/m^2 for the total population, male patients, and female patients, respectively. Seventeen (29.8%) patients were diagnosed has having low SMIs. Figure 1 shows examples of patients with and without low SMIs. Frequencies, means, and medians for the clinical characteristics, frailty domains, and postoperative outcomes for the total population and for the patients with and without low SMIs are displayed in Tables 1–3, respectively.

The outcomes of the univariate regression analyses for low SMIs and SMIs are shown in Table 4 and Table S2. Adjusted for the type of anesthesia, the multivariable logistic regression identified frailty based on the G8 frailty screening tool scores (OR 7.68, 95% CI 1.19–49.66, $p = 0.032$), and medium-high malnutrition risk was determined according to the MUST (OR 9.55, 95% CI 1.19–76.94, $p = 0.034$) as significant variables associated with low SMIs (Table 5). After correction of alcohol usage, female sex (B −7.36, 95% CI −10.56−−4.16, $p < 0.001$) and (ex-) smokers (B 3.15, 95% CI 0.17–6.34, $p = 0.039$) remained significantly related to SMI according to the linear multivariable regression analysis (Table S3).

Table 1. Demographic and clinical characteristics of patients surgically treated for cutaneous malignancies of the head and neck area. The data are stratified for sarcopenia diagnosis. Disease stage was defined using the seventh edition of the Union for International Cancer Control TNM Classification. * indicates other malignancies, including angiosarcoma (n = 2), pleomorphic dermal sarcoma (n = 1), and dermatofibrosarcoma protuberans (n = 1). ** indicates instances defined as a surgery of > 120 min. *** indicates intraoperative reconstruction or subsequent reconstructive surgery. Due to missingness, not all numbers sum up to 57. BMI = body mass index and SD = standard deviation.

	Total n = 57	Normal SMI n = 40 (70.2%)	Low SMI n = 17 (29.8%)
Patient characteristics			
Age, mean ± SD, year	77.1 ± 9.0	75.5 ± 9.0	80.9 ± 7.9
Sex			
Male	39 (68.4%)	16 (40.0%)	2 (11.8%)
Female	18 (31.6%)	24 (60.0%)	15 (88.2%)
BMI, mean ± SD, kg/cm^2	26.9 ± 4.1	28.3 ± 3.9	23.6 ± 2.2
Smoking status			
Never	16 (34.0%)	11 (31.4%)	5 (41.7%)
Former or current	31 (66.0%)	24 (68.6%)	7 (58.3%)
Alcohol usage			
None or mild	37 (88.1%)	26 (86.7%)	11 (91.7%)
Heavy (>2 units/day)	5 (11.9%)	4 (13.3%)	1 (8.3%)
Tumor characteristics			
Reason for referral			
Primary	26 (45.6%)	20 (50%)	6 (35.3%)
Residual or recurrent	31 (54.4%)	20 (50%)	11 (64.7%)
Primary tumor location			
Ear	21 (36.8%)	15 (37.5%)	6 (35.3%)
Scalp	15 (26.3%)	9 (22.5%)	6 (35.3%)
Nose	5 (8.8%)	4 (10.0%)	1 (5.9%)
Temporal	3 (5.3%)	2 (5.0%)	1 (5.9%)
Cheek	3 (5.3%)	3 (7.5%)	-
Peri-orbital	3 (5.3%)	1 (2.5%)	2 (11.8%)
Neck	3 (5.3%)	2 (5.0%)	1 (5.9%)
Peri-oral	2 (3.5%)	2 (5.0%)	-
Frontal	2 (3.5%)	2 (5.0%)	-
Stage			
Stage I–II	28 (49.1%)	20 (50.0%)	8 (47.1%)
Stage III–IV	29 (50.9%)	20 (50.0%)	9 (52.9%)
Tumor size, median (range), cm	2.0 (0.2–12.0)	2.0 (0.2–12.0)	2.0 (1.0–6.5)
Tumor type			
Squamous cell carcinoma	36 (63.2%)	24 (60.0%)	12 (70.6%)
Basal cell carcinoma	6 (10.5%)	3 (7.5%)	3 (17.6%)
Malignant melanoma	7 (12.3%)	5 (15.5%)	2 (11.8%)
Merkel cell carcinoma	4 (7.0%)	4 (10.0%)	-
Other *	4 (7.0%)	4 (10.0%)	-
Treatment characteristics			
Treatment intensity **			
Minor	21 (38.9%0	13 (33.3%)	8 (53.3%)
Major	33 (61.1%)	26 (66.7%)	7 (46.7%)
Anesthesia			
Local	5 (8.8%)	1 (2.5%)	4 (23.5%)
General	52 (91.2%)	39 (97.5%)	13 (76.5%)
Reconstructive surgery ***			
No	25 (44.6%)	15 (38.5%)	10 (58.8%)
Yes	31 (55.4%)	24 (61.5%)	7 (41.2%)

Table 2. Outcomes of the geriatric assessments of patients surgically treated for cutaneous malignancies of the head and neck area. The data are stratified for low SMIs. Due to missingness, not all numbers sum up to 57. ACE-27 = Adult Comorbidity Evaluation 27, ADL = activities of daily living, G8 = Geriatric 8, GDS-15 = Geriatric Depression Scale 15, GFI = Groningen Frailty Indicator, IADL = instrumental activities of daily living, MMSE = Mini-Mental State Examination, MUST = Malnutrition Universal Screening Tool, ND = not determined, TUG = Timed Up and Go.

	Total $n = 57$	Normal SMI $n = 40$ (70.2%)	Low SMI $n = 17$ (29.8%)
Frailty indicators			
G8			
Non-frail (>14)	25 (58.1%)	21 (67.7%)	4 (33.3%)
Frail (≤14)	18 (41.9%)	10 (32.3%)	8 (66.7%)
GFI			
Non-frail (<4)	32 (80.0%)	23 (79.3%)	9 (81.8%)
Frail (≥4)	8 (20.0%)	6 (20.7%)	2 (18.2%)
Comorbidities			
ACE-27			
None or mild	14 (24.6%)	11 (27.5%)	3 (17.6%)
Moderate or severe	43 (75.4%)	29 (72.5%)	14 (82.4%)
Polypharmacy			
Medication count			
< 5 medications	29 (67.4%)	19 (61.3%)	10 (83.3%)
≥5 medications	14 (32.6%)	12 (38.7%)	2 (16.7%)
Nutritional status			
MUST			
Low risk	48 (84.2%)	37 (92.5%)	11 (64.7%)
Medium to high risk	9 (15.8%)	3 (7.5%)	6 (35.3%)
Functional status			
ADL			
Independent (<2)	53 (93.0%)	37 (92.5%)	16 (94.1%)
Moderate independent (2–4)	4 (7.0%)	3 (7.5%)	1 (5.9%)
IADL			
No restrictions (<1)	16 (37.2%)	10 (32.3%)	6 (50.0%)
Restrictions (≥1)	27 (62.8%)	21 (67.7%)	6 (50.0%)
TUG			
No restrictions (<20)	40 (95.2%)	30 (96.8%)	10 (90.9%)
Restrictions (≥20)	2 (4.8%)	1 (3.2%)	1 (9.1%)
History of falls			
No	46 (90.2%)	32 (88.9%)	14 (93.3%)
Yes	5 (9.8%)	4 (11.1%)	1 (6.7%)
Social support			
Education			
Low level	17 (37.0%)	13 (40.6%)	4 (28.6%)
Middle and high level	22 (56.4%)	15 (53.6%)	7 (63.6%)
Relationship			
No	15 (30.6%)	12 (34.3%)	3 (21.4%)
Yes	34 (69.4%)	23 (65.7%)	11 (78.6%)
Cognitive status			
MMSE			
Normal cognition (>24)	35 (81.4%)	26 (83.9%)	9 (75.0%)
Declined cognition (≤24)	8 (18.6%)	5 (16.1%)	3 (25.0%)
Risk of delirium			
No	47 (82.5%)	32 (80.0%)	15 (88.2%)
Yes	10 (17.5%)	8 (20.0%)	2 (11.8%)
Psychological status			
GDS-15			
No depression (<6)	40 (95.2%)	29 (96.7%)	11 (91.7%)
Depression (≥6)	2 (4.8%)	1 (3.3%)	1 (8.3%)

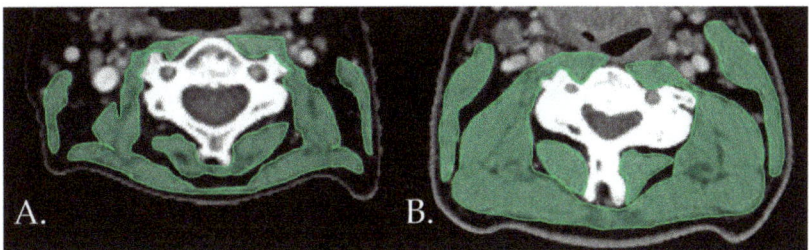

Figure 1. Examples of patients with (**A**) and without (**B**) low SMIs on the neck CT.s CT: computed tomography. SMI: skeletal muscle index.

3.3. Predictors for Postoperative Outcomes

Of all patients, 61.4% endured POCs (CDC > II) (Table 3). The univariate logistic regression with POC as the dependent variable (Table 4) showed that SMI as a continuous variable did not have a high or significant impact on POC (OR 1.02, 95% CI 0.94–1.10, $p = 0.703$). Although the occurrence of POC was more often seen in patients with low SMIs (70.6%) compared to patients with normal SMIs (51.5%), the association was not significant (OR 1.77 95% CI 0.53–5.99, $p = 0.356$). POCs did not occur in patients with local anesthesia. To generate an OR for anesthesia type, the occurrence of POC was randomly added to one patient with local anesthesia. Although not significant, general anesthesia may have had a high impact on POC (OR 8.24 95% CI 0.85–79.44, $p = 0.068$). The G8 frailty screening tool score (OR 5.42, 95% CI 1.25–23.49, $p = 0.024$) was the only variable significantly related to POC according to the univariate logistic regression analysis, and a multivariable regression analysis was therefore not conducted. Secondary outcomes showed that unplanned readmission and duration of hospitalization were equally distributed between patients with and without low SMIs.

Table 3. Postoperative outcomes for patients surgically treated for skin cancer of the head and neck region. The data are stratified for low SMIs. SMI = skeletal muscle index.

	Total $n = 57$	Normal SMI $n = 40$ (70.2%)	Low SMI $n = 17$ (29.8%)
Complications			
No complications	22 (38.6%)	17 (42.5%)	5 (29.4%)
Grade I	9 (15.8%)	6 (15.0%)	3 (17.6%)
Grade II	15 (26.3%)	10 (25.0%)	5 (29.4%)
Grade III	9 (15.8%)	6 (15.0%)	3 (17.6%)
Grade IV	2 (3.5%)	1 (2.5%)	1 (5.9%)
Grade >II (endpoint)	35 (61.4%)	23 (57.5%)	12 (70.6%)
Hospitalization			
Duration			
Median (range), days	4.0 (1.0–29.0)	4.0 (1.0–29.0)	3.0 (1.0–22.0)
Missing	1		
Unplanned readmission			
No	51 (89.5%)	36 (90.0%)	15 (88.2%)
Yes	6 (10.5%)	4 (10.0%)	2 (11.8%)

Table 4. Univariate linear regression analysis with SMI as the dependent variable and two univariate logistic regression analyses with low SMIs and POC as the dependent variables. Significant p-values (α < 0.05) are curved and bold. * indicates that one value was manually added into a blank cell to generate the odds ratios. 95% CI = 95% confidence interval, ACE-27 = Adult Comorbidity Evaluation 27, B = beta, ADL = activities of daily living, BMI = body mass index, G8 = Geriatric 8, GDS-15 = Geriatric Depression Scale 15, GFI = Groningen Frailty Indicator, MUST = Malnutrition Universal Screening Tool, OR = odds ratio, POC = postoperative complication, SD = standard deviation, SMI = skeletal muscle index, TUG = Timed Up and Go.

	SMI B (95% CI)	p-Value	Low SMI OR (95% CI)	p-Value	POC OR (95% CI)	p-Value
Age, year	−0.12 (−0.32–0.09)	0.255	1.09 (1.00–1.18)	*0.041*	0.99 (0.93–1.05)	0.750
Sex						
Male	Ref		Ref		Ref	
Female	−8.08 (−11.30–−4.86)	*>0.001*	0.20 (0.04–0.10)	*0.049*	0.50 (0.64–6.25)	0.233
BMI, kg/cm²	0.74 (0.33–1.14)	*0.001*	0.58 (0.42–0.80)	*0.001*	0.97 (0.85–1.11)	0.645
Smoking status						
Never	Ref		Ref		Ref	
Former or current	4.61 (1.20–8.02)	*0.009*	0.64 (0.17–2.48)	0.520	3.14 (0.90–11.03)	0.074
Alcohol usage						
None or mild	Ref		Ref		Ref	
Heavy (>2 units/day)	7.23 (1.14–13.31)	*0.021*	0.59 (0.06–5.91)	0.654	3.40 (0.35–33.40) *	0.294 *
Stage						
Stage I–II	Ref		Ref		Ref	
Stage III–IV	2.60 (−0.95–6.15)	0.148	1.13 (0.36–3.51)	0.839	1.93 (0.65–5.68)	0.235
Treatment intensity *						
Minor	Ref		Ref		Ref	
Major	2.76 (−0.83–6.34)	0.129	0.44 (0.13–1.47)	0.182	2.42 (0.77–7.65)	0.131
Anesthesia						
Local	Ref		Ref		Ref	
General	4.34 (−1.95–10.62)	0.172	0.08 (0.01–0.81)	*0.033*	8.24 (0.85–79.44) *	0.068 *
Reconstruction						
No	Ref		Ref		Ref	
Yes	−3.46 (−7.04–0.13)	0.058	0.44 (0.14–1.40)	0.163	1.94 (0.65–5.75)	0.233
G8						
Non-frail (>14)	Ref		Ref		Ref	
Frail (≤14)	−2.09 (−5.94–1.76)	0.281	4.20 (1.02–17.32)	*0.047*	5.42 (1.25–23.49)	*0.024*
GFI						
Non-frail (<4)	Ref		Ref		Ref	
Frail (≥4)	2.17 (−3.01–7.34)	0.405	0.85 (0.14–5.03)	0.860	6.18 (0.68–56.15)	0.106
ACE-27						
None or mild	Ref		Ref		Ref	
Moderate or severe	1.65 (−2.53–5.83)	0.433	1.77 (0.43–7.38)	0.433	1.27 (0.37–4.31)	0.706
MUST						
Low risk	Ref		Ref		Ref	
Medium to high risk	−3.40 (−8.27–1.48)	0.168	6.73 (1.44–31.40)	*0.015*	0.75 (0.18–3.16)	0.695
TUG						
No restrictions (<20 s)	Ref		Ref		Ref	
Restrictions (≥20 s)	−4.90 (−14.64–4.84)	0.318	3.00 (0.17–52.53)	0.452	0.60 (0.04–10.32)	0.725
SMI, cm²/m²	-	-	-	-	1.02 (0.94–1.10)	0.703
Low SMI						
No	-	-	-	-	Ref	
Yes	-	-	-	-	1.77 (0.53–5.99)	0.356

Table 5. A multivariable logistic regression analysis with a low SMI as the dependent variable. Significant p-values ($\alpha < 0.05$) are curved and bold. 95% CI = 95% confidence interval, G8 = Geriatric 8, MUST = Malnutrition Universal Screening Tool, OR = odds ratio.

	Low SMI OR (95% CI)	p-Value
Anesthesia		
General	Ref	
Local	0.06 (0.00–1.15)	0.062
G8		
Non-frail (>14)	Ref	
Frail (≤14)	7.68 (1.19–49.66)	***0.032***
MUST		
Low risk	Ref	
Medium to high risk	9.55 (1.19–76.94)	***0.034***

4. Discussion

To our knowledge, this is the first study that quantified skeletal muscle mass with SMI in HNSC patients using CT or MRI neck scans taken during oncological work-up and assessed its clinical value. The key findings were that malnutrition risk (MUST) and frailty (G8) were independently and significantly related to radiologically defined sarcopenia (low SMI), and further, frailty (G8) was the only variable significantly related to POC. Although the difference was not significant, patients with low SMIs more often had POCs compared to patients with normal SMIs. These key findings give new insights into the interrelation of low SMIs, frailty, and POCs in patients diagnosed with HNSC.

4.1. Frailty, Malnutrition, and Skeletal Muscle Mass

The results of the present study are in line with other studies on frailty and low SMIs in mHNC [18,23–25]. Frailty and sarcopenia are not the same, and frailty is considered a geriatric syndrome while sarcopenia a disease [26]. Both are, however, related to multiple adverse clinical outcomes [27,28], and they have been found to be related to each other [18]. In this present study, a low SMI was found to be related to G8 score and not GFI score. This discrepancy in outcomes can be explained by the content of the frailty indicators. Compared to the GFI, the G8 is more focused on weight loss, BMI, mobility, and food intake, and it leans more toward a physical definition of frailty, which has a tendency to overlap more with sarcopenia [26,29]. In mHNC, previous studies have also found a significant relationship between a low SMI (with or without low muscle strength) and G8 score [23] but not with GFI score [23]. Moreover, G8 score was found to be the most suitable frailty screening tool in older adults with skin cancer [30], highlighting the importance of the found relationship between a low SMI and G8 score in this study. Officially, sarcopenia is defined as low muscle performance/strength and low muscle mass [26]. Moreover, the specificity of the G8 has been debated, and Pottel et al. and Hamaker et al. concluded that the G8 frailty screening tool is very sensitive—but not very specific—in contrast to the CGA [6,7]. Meerkerk et al. further investigated the association between frailty as measured with a geriatric assessment and a low SMI with and without low muscle strength in mHNC [23]. They found that a low SMI (without consideration of low muscle strength) was related to frailty [23]. This implies that adding muscle strength into the sarcopenia diagnosis is not beneficial for identifying frail patients, but it should be investigated if this is also the case in HNSC. Patients with low SMIs had higher risks of malnutrition in this study, which was in line with other studies [18,31]. Moreover, low SMIs could be irreversible as studies have shown that nutritional and/or exercise interventions are feasible and able to improve skeletal muscle mass in patients with mHNC [32,33], which, in turn, may improve (nutritional) health outcomes and frailty status.

4.2. Frailty and Postoperative Complications

De Vries et al. also analyzed the value of geriatric assessment and frailty indicators for predicting postoperative outcomes in patients diagnosed with HNSC undergoing surgery, and they found the G8 frailty indicator to be related to POC [9], which was in line with the outcome of the present study. Despite an overlapping patient cohort between the present study and the study by de Vries et al., differences were apparent regarding the definitions for POC (CDC grade of > II vs. grade of > III) and stage of disease (50.9% vs. 25.9% stage III–IV cancers). Therefore, it could be concluded that the G8 is able to predict postoperative complications in different cohorts of heterogenic HNSC patients. Moreover, the G8 has been shown to be related to other adverse health outcomes in HNSC patients, including guideline deviation [10] and declined quality of life [11]. A recent study by Valdatta et al. also observed a significant association between frailty (measured with FRAIL scores) and surgical complications in elderly patients diagnosed with non-melanoma skin cancer [34]. Therefore, screening for frailty appears to have a predictive value for adverse postoperative outcomes in skin cancer patients and should be recommended before initiating major surgery.

4.3. Skeletal Muscle Mass and Postoperative Complications

In mHNC patients, pre-treatment diagnosed sarcopenia has already been associated with negative clinical outcomes [17,18,27,35,36]. In this cohort, the patients with low SMIs more often developed POCs, and therefore, it appears to be a promising predictor. However, the difference was not significant, which was very likely due to the small sample size and the fact that less general anesthesia was used in sarcopenic patients, which, in turn, possibly had a high impact on POC. Low SMIs appeared to have a greater impact than SMI as a continuous variable on POC in this cohort. Sabel et al. found in their cohort of stage III melanoma patients that skeletal muscle mass qualified with decreased psoas muscle density on CT, which was independently associated with decreased disease-free survival, distant disease-free survival, and higher rates of surgical complications [37]. Measuring muscle density or adding low muscle strength to a sarcopenia diagnosis may further improve the association between skeletal muscle and POC. However, muscle density analysis using CT images was not feasible as most CT scans in the present study were generated with an intravenous iodine contrast, which is known to affect the muscle density measurements [38], and thus, no data on muscle strength were available.

4.4. Limitations

First, our sample size was relatively small and heterogenic in terms of tumor characteristics with a high percentage of complex cases. Therefore, caution should be made when extrapolating our findings to patients diagnosed with less complex and low-risk HNSC. Heterogeneous image techniques could be regarded as another possible limitation; however, recent research has found that CT and MRI neck imaging could be used interchangeably for skeletal muscle analysis [15]. In the present study, low muscle strength was not a criterion for sarcopenia. This could be seen as a limitation; however, a low SMI without consideration of muscle strength has been found to be associated with inferior health outcomes [39]. Moreover, others have encouraged the use of SMI and not muscle strength at the core of nutritional management strategies as skeletal muscle mass is an important metabolically active and homeostatic indicator [40]. Nevertheless, low muscle strength as an additional criterion for sarcopenia may be beneficial in HNSC cases to predict clinical outcomes. Ideally, SMI cut-off values as generated in an HNSC population should be applied to define low SMIs.

4.5. Strengths

First, the association between frailty and sarcopenia was assessed and their impact on postoperative outcomes was analyzed, which is highly clinically relevant. Second, patients were included prospectively and were assessed with a broad range of validated geriatric assessments and screening tools at baseline. Third, high observer reliability scores were achieved, and the observer was furthermore blinded from the clinical outcome, preventing bias. Fourth, we evaluated skeletal muscle mass using both SMIs and low SMIs to examine if certain relationships existed with or without using an SMI cut-off value.

4.6. Future Research

Identifying patients with low SMIs and assessing their prognostic value is fairly new in dermato-oncology, which creates many opportunities. It would be interesting to see if the prognostic value of SMI on POC can be improved. For instance, a low SMI defined using HNSC-specific SMI cut-off values may better predict postoperative outcomes than a low SMI based on mHNC SMI cut-off values. Moreover, the effect of low muscle strength on POC should be assessed. Therefore, after optimizing SMI cut-off values in HNSC, the present study should be repeated at a large-scale multicenter study to analyze the relationship between frailty, a low SMI (with and without consideration of low muscle strength), and POC in HNSC. Ideally, a multivariable regression analysis on (major) POC should be performed, including relevant clinical variables related to POC. Additionally, randomized controlled trials with interventions on low SMIs (with or without consideration of low muscle strength) should be performed to assess the effect on frailty and POC.

5. Conclusions

Preoperative frailty screening of elderly patients at risk for POCs is highly recommended, but it is time-intensive and could be strenuous for the patients. The present study found that malnutrition risk and frailty were independently related to low SMIs (also radiologically defined sarcopenia). Frailty, not SMI, was related to POC. Although the difference was not significant, patients with low SMIs more often had had POCs compared to patients with normal SMIs. These outcomes implied that patients with low SMIs may benefit from interventions to improve their frailty and nutritional status, which, in turn, may result in fewer complications. Therefore, identifying patients with low SMIs at baseline may help multidisciplinary teams to make treatment decisions or select patients for pre-habilitation. Hence, a low SMI is a practical and objective radiological biomarker for screening for frailty and malnutrition. However, further research is needed to assess the capability of SMIs to predict postoperative outcomes. Preoperative screening for frailty should be advised for major surgeries as frailty was the only variable significantly related to POC in this cohort of HNSC patients.

Supplementary Materials: The following supporting information can be downloaded at: https://www.mdpi.com/article/10.3390/jcm12103445/s1, Table S1: The geriatric assessment at baseline showing a range of validated instruments on multiple domains with applied cut-off values. Table S2: Remaining variables of the univariate linear regression analysis with SMI as the dependent variable and two univariate logistic regression analyses with low SMIs and POC as the dependent variables. Table S3: Multivariable linear regression analysis with SMI as the dependent variable [41–51].

Author Contributions: Conceptualization, A.T.Z., M.S.v.K., R.A.J.O.D., G.H.d.B., A.v.d.H., and G.B.H.; data curation, A.T.Z., J.d.V., G.H.d.B., and G.B.H.; formal analysis, A.T.Z. and G.H.d.B.; funding acquisition, A.T.Z.; investigation, A.T.Z., L.M.C.K., M.S.v.K., R.A.J.O.D., G.H.d.B., A.v.d.H., and G.B.H.; methodology, A.T.Z., L.M.C.K., M.S.v.K., R.A.J.O.D., G.H.d.B., A.v.d.H., and G.B.H.; project administration, A.T.Z. and G.B.H.; resources, G.H.d.B. and G.B.H.; software, L.M.C.K., R.A.J.O.D., and G.H.d.B.; supervision, G.H.d.B., A.v.d.H., and G.B.H.; validation, A.T.Z. and L.M.C.K.; visualization, L.M.C.K. and R.A.J.O.D.; writing—original draft, A.T.Z. and G.B.H.; writing—review and editing, A.T.Z., L.M.C.K., J.d.V., M.S.v.K., R.A.J.O.D., G.H.d.B., A.v.d.H., and G.B.H. All authors have read and agreed to the published version of the manuscript.

Funding: The first author received a three-year PhD scholarship for excellent master students from the Graduate School of Medical Sciences of the University of Groningen.

Institutional Review Board Statement: Patients in this present retrospective cohort study were prospectively enrolled in the Oncological Life Study (OncoLifeS) databiobank [19] after obtaining written informed consent. This large-scale, institutional oncological databiobank collects and stores the following details of adult patients diagnosed with cancer: clinical and treatment data, comorbidities, lifestyle, radiological and pathological findings, biomaterials, quality of life, and long-term outcomes. The OncoLifeS databiobank has been approved by the Medical Ethical Committee of the University Medical Center Groningen and is registered in the Dutch Trial Register under the registration number NL7839. The scientific board of OncoLifeS gave its permission for the presented study.

Informed Consent Statement: Informed consent was obtained from all subjects involved in the study. Written informed consent has been obtained from the patients to publish this paper.

Data Availability Statement: The data that support the findings of this study are available from the corresponding author upon reasonable request.

Acknowledgments: The first author is grateful for receiving the three-years PhD scholarship for excellent master students from the Graduate School of Medical Sciences of the University of Groningen. All authors thank Hariet L. Lancaster for her English revision of the manuscript.

Conflicts of Interest: The authors declare no conflict of interest.

References

1. Leiter, U.; Eigentler, T.; Garbe, C. Epidemiology of skin cancer. *Adv. Exp. Med. Biol.* **2014**, *810*, 120–140. [PubMed]
2. Apalla, Z.; Lallas, A.; Sotiriou, E.; Lazaridou, E.; Ioannides, D. Epidemiological trends in skin cancer. *Dermatol. Pract. Concept.* **2017**, *7*, 1–6. [CrossRef] [PubMed]
3. Hughley, B.B.; Schmalbach, C.E. Cutaneous Head and Neck Malignancies in the Elderly. *Clin. Geriatr. Med.* **2018**, *34*, 245–258. [CrossRef] [PubMed]
4. Garcovich, S.; Colloca, G.; Sollena, P.; Andrea, B.; Balducci, L.; Cho, W.C.; Bernabei, R.; Peris, K. Skin Cancer Epidemics in the Elderly as an Emerging Issue in Geriatric Oncology. *Aging Dis.* **2017**, *8*, 643–661. [CrossRef] [PubMed]
5. Haisma, M.S.; Bras, L.; Aghdam, M.A.; Terra, J.B.; Plaat, B.E.C.; Rácz, E.; Halmos, G.B. Effect of Patient Characteristics on Treatment Decisions Regarding Keratinocyte Carcinoma in Elderly Patients: A Review of the Current Literature. *Acta Derm. Venereol.* **2020**, *100*, adv00189-3543. [CrossRef]
6. Pottel, L.; Lycke, M.; Boterberg, T.; Pottel, H.; Goethals, L.; Duprez, F.; Van Den Noortgate, N.; De Neve, W.; Rottey, S.; Geldhof, K.; et al. Serial comprehensive geriatric assessment in elderly head and neck cancer patients undergoing curative radiotherapy identifies evolution of multidimensional health problems and is indicative of quality of life. *Eur. J. Cancer Care* **2014**, *23*, 401–412. [CrossRef]
7. Hamaker, M.E.; Jonker, J.M.; de Rooij, S.E.; Vos, A.G.; Smorenburg, C.H.; van Munster, B.C. Frailty screening methods for predicting outcome of a comprehensive geriatric assessment in elderly patients with cancer: A systematic review. *Lancet Oncol.* **2012**, *13*, e437–e444. [CrossRef]
8. Rubenstein, L.Z.; Stuck, A.E.; Siu, A.L.; Wieland, D. Impacts of Geriatric Evaluation and Management Programs on Defined Outcomes: Overview of the Evidence. *J. Am. Geriatr. Soc.* **1991**, *39 Pt 2*, 8S–16S; discussion 17S. [CrossRef]
9. de Vries, J.; Heirman, A.N.; Bras, L.; Plaat, B.E.C.; Rácz, E.; van Kester, M.S.; Festen, S.; de Bock, G.H.; van der Laan, B.F.; Halmos, G.B. Geriatric assessment of patients for cutaneous head and neck malignancies in a tertiary referral center: Predictors of postoperative complications. *Eur. J. Surg. Oncol.* **2020**, *46*, 123–130. [CrossRef]
10. Leus, A.J.G.; Haisma, M.S.; Terra, J.B.; Sidorenkov, G.; Festen, S.; Plaat, B.E.C.; Halmos, G.B.; Racz, E. Influence of Frailty and Life Expectancy on Guideline Adherence and Outcomes in Cutaneous Squamous Cell Carcinoma of the Head and Neck: A Prospective Pilot Study. *Dermatology* **2023**, *239*, 148–157. [CrossRef]
11. de Vries, J.; Bras, L.; Sidorenkov, G.; Festen, S.; Steenbakkers, R.J.H.M.; Langendijk, J.A.; Witjes, M.J.; van der Laan, B.F.; de Bock, G.H.; Halmos, G.B. Frailty is associated with decline in health-related quality of life of patients treated for head and neck cancer. *Oral Oncol.* **2020**, *111*, 105020. [CrossRef] [PubMed]
12. Bras, L.; de Vries, J.; Festen, S.; Steenbakkers, R.J.H.M.; Langendijk, J.A.; Witjes, M.J.H.; van der Laan, B.F.; de Bock, G.H.; Halmos, G.B. Frailty and restrictions in geriatric domains are associated with surgical complications but not with radiation-induced acute toxicity in head and neck cancer patients: A prospective study. *Oral Oncol.* **2021**, *118*, 105329. [CrossRef] [PubMed]
13. Mourtzakis, M.; Prado, C.M.; Lieffers, J.R.; Reiman, T.; McCargar, L.J.; Baracos, V.E. A practical and precise approach to quantification of body composition in cancer patients using computed tomography images acquired during routine care. *Appl. Physiol. Nutr. Metab.* **2008**, *33*, 997–1006. [CrossRef] [PubMed]

14. Swartz, J.E.; Pothen, A.J.; Wegner, I.; Smid, E.J.; Swart, K.M.; de Bree, R.; Leenen, L.P.; Grolman, W. Feasibility of using head and neck CT imaging to assess skeletal muscle mass in head and neck cancer patients. *Oral Oncol.* **2016**, *62*, 28–33. [CrossRef] [PubMed]
15. Zwart, A.T.; Becker, J.-N.; Lamers, M.J.; Dierckx, R.A.J.O.; de Bock, G.H.; Halmos, G.B.; van der Hoorn, A. Skeletal muscle mass and sarcopenia can be determined with 1.5-T and 3-T neck MRI scans, in the event that no neck CT scan is performed. *Eur. Radiol.* **2020**, *31*, 4053–4062. [CrossRef] [PubMed]
16. Jones, A.J.; Campiti, V.J.; Alwani, M.; Novinger, L.J.; Bonetto, A.; Sim, M.W.; Yesensky, J.A.; Moore, M.G.; Mantravadi, A.V. Skeletal Muscle Index's Impact on Discharge Dis-position after Head and Neck Cancer Free Flap Reconstruction. *Otolaryngol. Head Neck Surg.* **2020**, *165*, 59–68. [CrossRef] [PubMed]
17. Bril, S.I.; Pezier, T.F.; Tijink, B.M.; Janssen, L.M.; Braunius, W.W.; De Bree, R. Preoperative low skeletal muscle mass as a risk factor for pharyngocutaneous fistula and decreased overall survival in patients undergoing total laryngectomy. *Head Neck* **2019**, *41*, 1745–1755. [CrossRef]
18. Zwart, A.T.; van der Hoorn, A.; van Ooijen, P.M.A.; Steenbakkers, R.J.H.M.; de Bock, G.H.; Halmos, G.B. CT-measured skeletal muscle mass used to assess frailty in patients with head and neck cancer. *J. Cachexia Sarcopenia Muscle* **2019**, *10*, 1060–1069. [CrossRef]
19. Surov, A.; Meyer, H.J.; Wienke, A. Role of Sarcopenia in Advanced Malignant Cutaneous Melanoma Treated with Immuno-therapy: A Meta-Analysis. *Oncology* **2022**, *100*, 498–504. [CrossRef]
20. Sidorenkov, G.; Nagel, J.; Meijer, C.; Duker, J.J.; Groen, H.J.M.; Halmos, G.B.; Oonk, M.H.; Oostergo, R.J.; van der Vegt, B.; Witjes, M.J.; et al. The OncoLifeS data-biobank for oncology: A com-prehensive repository of clinical data, biological samples, and the patient's perspective. *J. Transl. Med.* **2019**, *17*, 374. [CrossRef]
21. van Rijn-Dekker, M.I.; van den Bosch, L.; van den Hoek, J.G.M.; Bijl, H.P.; van Aken, E.S.M.; van der Hoorn, A.; Oosting, S.F.; Halmos, G.B.; Witjes, M.J.; van der Laan, H.P. Impact of sar-copenia on survival and late toxicity in head and neck cancer patients treated with radiotherapy. *Radiother. Oncol.* **2020**, *147*, 103–110. [CrossRef] [PubMed]
22. Dindo, D.; Demartines, N.; Clavien, P.A. Classification of surgical complications: A new proposal with evaluation in a cohort of 6336 patients and results of a survey. *Ann. Surg.* **2004**, *240*, 205–213. [CrossRef] [PubMed]
23. Meerkerk, C.D.A.; Chargi, N.; de Jong, P.A.; Bos, F.V.D.; de Bree, R. Sarcopenia measured with handgrip strength and skeletal muscle mass to assess frailty in older patients with head and neck cancer. *J. Geriatr. Oncol.* **2021**, *12*, 434–440. [CrossRef] [PubMed]
24. Meerkerk, C.D.A.; Chargi, N.; de Jong, P.A.; Bos, F.V.D.; de Bree, R. Low skeletal muscle mass predicts frailty in elderly head and neck cancer patients. *Eur. Arch. Otorhinolaryngol.* **2022**, *279*, 967–977. [CrossRef] [PubMed]
25. De Bree, R.; Meerkerk, C.D.A.; Halmos, G.B.; Mäkitie, A.A.; Homma, A.; Rodrigo, J.P.; López, F.; Takes, R.P.; Vermorken, J.B.; Ferlito, A. Measurement of Sarcopenia in Head and Neck Cancer Patients and Its Association with Frailty. *Front. Oncol.* **2022**, *12*, 884988. [CrossRef] [PubMed]
26. Cruz-Jentoft, A.J.; Bahat, G.; Bauer, J.; Boirie, Y.; Bruyère, O.; Cederholm, T.; Cooper, C.; Landi, F.; Rolland, Y.; Sayer, A.A.; et al. Sarcopenia: Revised European consensus on defi-nition and diagnosis. *Age Ageing* **2019**, *48*, 16–31. [CrossRef]
27. Hua, X.; Liu, S.; Liao, J.-F.; Wen, W.; Long, Z.-Q.; Lu, Z.-J.; Guo, L.; Lin, H.-X. When the Loss Costs Too Much: A Systematic Review and Meta-Analysis of Sarcopenia in Head and Neck Cancer. *Front. Oncol.* **2020**, *9*, 1561. [CrossRef]
28. Dwimartutie, N.; Yusnidar, P.; Chandra, S.; Harimurti, K. The Impact of Frailty on 30-day Post-Elective Surgery Complications in Elderly Patients: A Prospective Cohort Study. *Acta Med. Indones* **2020**, *52*, 344–351.
29. Fried, L.P.; Tangen, C.M.; Walston, J.; Newman, A.B.; Hirsch, C.; Gottdiener, J.; Seeman, T.; Tracy, R.; Kop, W.J.; Burke, G.; et al. Frailty in older adults: Evidence for a phenotype. *J. Gerontol. A Biol. Sci. Med. Sci.* **2001**, *56*, M146–M157. [CrossRef]
30. van Winden, M.E.C.; Garcovich, S.; Peris, K.; Colloca, G.; de Jong, E.M.G.J.; Hamaker, M.E.; van de Kerkhof, P.C.M.; Lubeek, S.F.K. Frailty screening in dermato-oncology practice: A modified Delphi study and a systematic review of the literature. *J. Eur. Acad. Dermatol. Venereol.* **2021**, *35*, 95–104. [CrossRef]
31. Ligthart-Melis, G.C.; Luiking, Y.C.; Kakourou, A.; Cederholm, T.; Maier, A.B.; de van der Schueren, M.A.E. Frailty, Sarcopenia, and Malnutrition Frequently (Co-)occur in Hospitalized Older Adults: A Systematic Review and Meta-analysis. *J. Am. Med. Dir. Assoc.* **2020**, *21*, 1216–1228. [CrossRef] [PubMed]
32. Cederholm, T.; Jensen, G.L.; Correia, M.I.T.D.; Gonzalez, M.C.; Fukushima, R.; Higashiguchi, T.; Baptista, G.; Barazzoni, R.; Blaauw, R.; Coats, A.J.S.; et al. GLIM criteria for the diagnosis of malnutrition—A consensus report from the global clinical nutrition community. *J. Cachexia Sarcopenia Muscle* **2019**, *10*, 207–217. [CrossRef] [PubMed]
33. Lønbro, S.; Dalgas, U.; Primdahl, H.; Johansen, J.; Nielsen, J.L.; Aagaard, P.; Hermann, A.P.; Overgaard, J.; Overgaard, K. Progressive resistance training rebuilds lean body mass in head and neck cancer patients after radiotherapy—Results from the randomized DAHANCA 25B trial. *Radiother. Oncol.* **2013**, *108*, 314–319. [CrossRef] [PubMed]
34. Sandmael, J.A.; Bye, A.; Solheim, T.S.; Stene, G.B.; Thorsen, L.; Kaasa, S.; Lund, J.; Oldervoll, L.M. Feasibility and preliminary effects of resistance training and nutritional supplements during versus after radiotherapy in patients with head and neck cancer: A pilot randomized trial. *Cancer* **2017**, *123*, 4440–4448. [CrossRef]
35. Valdatta, L.; Perletti, G.; Maggiulli, F.; Tamborini, F.; Pellegatta, I.; Cherubino, M. FRAIL scale as a predictor of complications and mortality in older patients undergoing reconstructive surgery for non-melanoma skin cancer. *Oncol. Lett.* **2019**, *17*, 263–269. [CrossRef] [PubMed]

36. Findlay, M.; White, K.; Lai, M.; Luo, D.; Bauer, J.D. The Association between Computed Tomography–Defined Sarcopenia and Outcomes in Adult Patients Undergoing Radiotherapy of Curative Intent for Head and Neck Cancer: A Systematic Review. *J. Acad. Nutr. Diet.* **2020**, *120*, 1330–1347.e8. [CrossRef]
37. Chargi, N.; Bril, S.I.; Emmelot-Vonk, M.H.; de Bree, R. Sarcopenia is a prognostic factor for overall survival in elderly patients with head-and-neck cancer. *Eur. Arch. Otorhinolaryngol.* **2019**, *276*, 1475–1486. [CrossRef] [PubMed]
38. Sabel, M.; Lee, J.; Cai, S.; Englesbe, M.; Holcombe, S.; Wang, S. Sarcopenia as a Prognostic Factor among Patients with Stage III Melanoma. *Ann. Surg. Oncol.* **2011**, *18*, 3579–3585. [CrossRef]
39. van Vugt, J.L.A.; Coebergh van den Braak, R.R.J.; Schippers, H.J.W.; Veen, K.M.; Levolger, S.; de Bruin, R.W.F.; Koek, M.; Niessen, W.J.; IJzermans, J.N.; Willemsen, F.E. Con-trast-enhancement influences skeletal muscle density, but not skeletal muscle mass, measurements on computed tomography. *Clin. Nutr.* **2018**, *37*, 1707–1714. [CrossRef]
40. Hilmi, M.; Jouinot, A.; Burns, R.; Pigneur, F.; Mounier, R.; Gondin, J.; Neuzillet, C.; Goldwasser, F. Body composition and sarcopenia: The next-generation of personalized oncology and pharmacology? *Pharmacol. Ther.* **2019**, *196*, 135–159. [CrossRef]
41. Bellera, C.A.; Rainfray, M.; Mathoulin-Pélissier, S.; Mertens, C.; Delva, F.; Fonck, M.; Soubeyran, P. Screening older cancer patients: First evaluation of the G-8 geriatric screening tool. *Ann. Oncol.* **2012**, *23*, 2166–2172. [CrossRef] [PubMed]
42. Schuurmans, H.; Steverink, N.; Lindenberg, S.; Frieswijk, N.; Slaets, J.P. Old or frail: What tells us more? *J. Gerontol. A Biol. Sci. Med. Sci.* **2004**, *59*, M962–M965. [CrossRef] [PubMed]
43. Piccirillo, J.F. Importance of Comorbidity in Head and Neck Cancer. *Laryngoscope* **2015**, *125*, 2242. [CrossRef] [PubMed]
44. Sharma, M.; Loh, K.P.; Nightingale, G.; Mohile, S.G.; Holmes, H.M. Polypharmacy and potentially inappropriate medication use in geriatric oncology. *J. Geriatr. Oncol.* **2016**, *7*, 346–353. [CrossRef] [PubMed]
45. Malnutrition Universal Screening Tool. 2011. Available online: https://www.bapen.org.uk/pdfs/must/ (accessed on 7 May 2018).
46. Katz, S.; Ford, A.B.; Moskowitz, R.W.; Jackson, B.A.; Jaffe, M.W. Studies of Illness in the Aged. the Index of Adl: A Stand-ardized Measure of Biological and Psychosocial Function. *JAMA* **1963**, *185*, 914–919. [CrossRef]
47. Lawton, M.P.; Brody, E.M. Assessment of older people: Self-maintaining and instrumental activities of daily living. *Gerontologist* **1969**, *9*, 179–186. [CrossRef] [PubMed]
48. Podsiadlo, D.; Richardson, S. The Timed "Up & Go": A Test of Basic Functional Mobility for Frail Elderly Persons. *J. Am. Geriatr. Soc.* **1991**, *39*, 142–148. [CrossRef]
49. Folstein, M.F.; Folstein, S.E.; McHugh, P.R. "Mini-Mental State". A Practical Method for Grading the Cognitive State of Patients for the Clinician. *J. Psychiatr. Res.* **1975**, *12*, 189–198. [CrossRef]
50. Oud, F.M.; de Rooij, S.E.; Schuurman, T.; Duijvelaar, K.M.; van Munster, B.C. Predictive value of the VMS theme 'Frail elderly': Delirium, falling and mortality in elderly hospital patients. *Ned. Tijdschr. Geneeskd.* **2015**, *159*, A8491.
51. Sheikh, J.I.; Yesavage, J.A. Geriatric Depression Scale (GDS): Recent evidence and development of a shorter version. *Clin. Gerontol. J. Aging Ment. Health* **1986**, *5*, 165–173.

Disclaimer/Publisher's Note: The statements, opinions and data contained in all publications are solely those of the individual author(s) and contributor(s) and not of MDPI and/or the editor(s). MDPI and/or the editor(s) disclaim responsibility for any injury to people or property resulting from any ideas, methods, instructions or products referred to in the content.

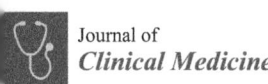

Article

EGFR-Driven Mutation in Non-Small-Cell Lung Cancer (NSCLC) Influences the Features and Outcome of Brain Metastases

Daniele Armocida [1,2,†], Alessandro Pesce [3,†], Mauro Palmieri [1], Fabio Cofano [4], Giuseppe Palmieri [4], Paola Cassoni [5], Carla Letizia Busceti [2], Francesca Biagioni [2], Diego Garbossa [4], Francesco Fornai [2,†], Antonio Santoro [1] and Alessandro Frati [2,*]

1. Human Neurosciences Department, Neurosurgery Division, "Sapienza" University, 00161 Rome, RM, Italy; danielearmocida@yahoo.it (D.A.); mauro.palmieri@uniroma1.it (M.P.); antonio.santoro@uniroma1.it (A.S.)
2. IRCCS "Neuromed", 86077 Pozzilli, IS, Italy; carla.busceti@neuromed.it (C.L.B.); francesca.biagioni@neuromed.it (F.B.); francesco.fornai@neuromed.it (F.F.)
3. Neurosurgery Unit, "Santa Maria Goretti" University Hospital, 04100 Latina, LT, Italy; ale_pesce83@yahoo.it
4. Neurosurgery Unit, Department of Neuroscience "Rita Levi Montalcini", University of Turin, 10126 Turin, TO, Italy; fabio.cofano@gmail.com (F.C.); giuseppe.palmieri@unito.it (G.P.); diego.garbossa@unito.it (D.G.)
5. Pathology Unit, Department of Medical Sciences, University of Turin, 10126 Turin, TO, Italy; paola.cassoni@unito.it
* Correspondence: alessandro.frati@uniroma1.it
† These authors contributed equally to this work.

Abstract: Background: Brain metastases (BMs) is one of the most frequent metastatic sites for non-small-cell lung cancer (NSCLC). It is a matter of debate whether EGFR mutation in the primary tumor may be a marker for the disease course, prognosis, and diagnostic imaging of BMs, comparable to that described for primary brain tumors, such as glioblastoma (GB). This issue was investigated in the present research manuscript. **Methods:** We performed a retrospective study to identify the relevance of EGFR mutations and prognostic factors for diagnostic imaging, survival, and disease course within a cohort of patients affected by NSCLC-BMs. Imaging was carried out using MRI at various time intervals. The disease course was assessed using a neurological exam carried out at three-month intervals. The survival was expressed from surgical intervention. **Results:** The patient cohort consisted of 81 patients. The overall survival of the cohort was 15 ± 1.7 months. EGFR mutation and ALK expression did not differ significantly for age, gender, and gross morphology of the BM. Contrariwise, the EGFR mutation was significantly associated with MRI concerning the occurrence of greater tumor (22.38 ± 21.35 cm^3 versus 7.68 ± 6.44 cm^3, p = 0.046) and edema volume (72.44 ± 60.71 cm^3 versus 31.92 cm^3, p = 0.028). In turn, the occurrence of MRI abnormalities was related to neurological symptoms assessed using the Karnofsky performance status and mostly depended on tumor-related edema (p = 0.048). However, the highest significant correlation was observed between EGFR mutation and the occurrence of seizures as the clinical onset of the neoplasm (p = 0.004). **Conclusions:** The presence of EGFR mutations significantly correlates with greater edema and mostly a higher seizure incidence of BMs from NSCLC. In contrast, EGFR mutations do not affect the patient's survival, the disease course, and focal neurological symptoms but seizures. This contrasts with the significance of EGFR in the course and prognosis of the primary tumor (NSCLC).

Keywords: brain metastases; lung cancer; NSCLC; EGFR; ALK; brain tumor

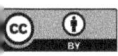

1. Introduction

Brain metastases (BM) are the most common intracranial tumors in adults and significantly affect lethality. Roughly, 40% of patients with malignancies develop intracranial metastases during the disease course. Lung cancer is the neoplasm, which leads to the highest percentage of brain metastases [1–3]. Among various lung cancers, non-small cell lung cancer (NSCLC) is the leading cause of BMs and represents the most frequent cancer-related death worldwide [1]. Approximately 5–30% of all BMs derive from NSCLC [4,5]. Over 40% of patients carrying an early diagnosis of lung cancer develop BMs during the disease course [1,2,6,7], which significantly worsens the life expectancy and the quality of life (QoL) [8].

The increase in BMs, which was registered in the last decades, is likely due to prolonged life duration, which is achieved in the general population affected by neoplasm [9,10], and mainly due to advances in the treatment of primary cancer, and an earlier diagnosis of BM due to an improvement in neuroimaging techniques [11]. However, despite current standard treatments represented by microsurgical resection, focal fractionated radiotherapy, stereotactic radiosurgery, and BM from NSCLC continues to be associated with a poor prognosis [12–16]. Therefore, at present, intense research activity is dedicated to unravelling the key molecular targets of NSCLC to develop novel therapeutic strategies to treat NSCLC-derived BMs. A key molecule characterizing NSCLC is epidermal growth factor receptor (EGFR), along with anaplastic lymphokinase (ALK), and PD-L1 [17]. In fact, it has been observed that the incidence of BM is higher in patients with ALK fusions [18–20] and EGFR mutations [18–22]. In detail, EGFR positivity or ALK-1 rearrangements (which are mutually exclusive in their occurrence) are associated with the worsening of tumor progression. The ability to identify these targets prompted specific therapies that modified the prognosis of the primary tumor. Therefore, at present, EGFR positivity represents a therapeutic advantage to delay tumor progression by using specific tyrosine-kinase inhibitors, which improves survival and reduces the relapse of lung cancer, thus leading to a better prognosis [23,24], even considering that EGFR positivity is often associated with PD-L1 negativity [25]. When considering the therapeutic development achieved via treating EGFR-positive primary NSCLC, one may argue that the same outcome may apply to NSCLC-derived BMs. Unfortunately, NSCLC-derived EGFR-positive metastasis does not respond positively to the specific treatment [26,27]. To understand the significance of EGFR positivity for the natural course of NSLC-derived BMs, we carried out the present study.

With this aim, we retrospectively analyzed a consecutive series of patients who had resection surgery of NSCLC-derived BMs from January 2015 to January 2019 at the Department of Neurosurgery of Policlinico Umberto I of Rome (Italy) and Hospital Molinette of Turin (Italy). In this study, we retrospectively identify the significance of the occurrence of EGFR mutations by assessing life expectancy, neurological symptoms in the disease course, and neuroimaging (to assess neoplasm and edema volume measured on FLAIR sequences) in a cohort of 81 surgically treated patients.

2. Materials and Methods

2.1. Participants and Eligibility

All the patients included in the final cohort meet the following inclusion criteria:

1. A preoperative KPS scale score >50%.
2. An estimated overall survival of >3 months (according to the radiation therapy oncology group and the grade prognostic assessment rankings) [28,29]
3. The estimated target of the surgical procedure was the gross-total, near-total, or sub-total resection of the lesions: no biopsies were included. We included those patients where complete surgical resection could be guaranteed by pre-operative planning, thus excluding cases with multiple deep-site metastases that could not be surgically treated by definition. Patients with sub-centimetric heteroplastic lesions were included after dedicated conformational radiotherapy regimens.
4. The molecular analysis of EGFR mutations was carried out in the brain metastases in addition to the primary NSCLC.
5. Only patients who may undergo post-surgical adjuvant chemo-radiotherapy and a follow-up program were included.

6. Patients were included if they received standard conformational planning with a linear accelerator (LINAC).
7. Once the progression of the disease was noticed, the patient and the relevant imaging were referred again to our attention to evaluate the feasibility of a second surgery or to address the patient to the second line of adjuvant treatment.

All patients underwent a general medical, neurological, and oncological evaluation at admission. For all patients, we recorded gender; age; peri- and post-operative KPS; clinical presentation; survival; antiepileptic prophylaxis and treatment; the incidence of postoperative seizures; and tumor- and surgery-related variables: number, location and side of the lesions, tumor and edema volume, morphology, the onset of the primary tumor, and molecular profile (EGFR, ALK, and PD-L1).

In particular, the specimens used in this study were examined for EGFR. DNA mutations in EGFR were detected using polymerase chain reaction (PCR) to identify mutations within exons 19 and 21. Immunohistochemistry for CDX-2, CK7, CK20, TTF-1, and Napsin-A was routinely carried out. Overall survival (OS) was recorded in months; it was measured from the date of diagnosis to the fatality considering the last contact when alive. Clinical information was obtained using the digital institutional database. A particular focus was centered on the performance status expressed as KPS results, which were used as dichotomy data (either more or less than score 70, KPS). This score was chosen since it is critical for a patient's survival when BM are present [13,30–32]. KPS was recorded before surgery at the time of diagnosis and it was repeated 30 days after surgery (early post-operative evaluation and it was further recorded at the end of the adjuvant treatment, the last outpatient evaluation).

2.2. Preoperative and Operative Protocol

All patients received a pre-operative brain MRI scan, including a 3 Tesla volumetric study with the following sequences: T2w, fluid-attenuated inversion recovery (FLAIR), and isotropic volumetric T1-weighted magnetization-prepared rapid acquisition gradient echo (MPRAGE) before and after intravenous administration of paramagnetic contrast agent; diffusion tensor sequences (DTI) with 3D tractography and functional MRI (fMRI) completed our protocol for what concerns lesions affecting eloquent locations. The volume of the contrast-enhancing lesion was calculated by drawing a region of interest (ROI) in a volumetric enhancing post-contrast study weighted in T1 (a multi-voxel study), conforming to the margins of the contrast-enhancing lesion. In contrast, the volume of edema was measured by drawing an ROI in a FLAIR-weighted research, from which the previously calculated lesion was subtracted. The study was carried out using the Horos Dicom Viewer (v 3.36, opensource software, Pixmeo SARL, Bernex, Switzerland; https://horosproject.org/) [33]. Moreover, we routinely performed total-body sodium-enhanced CT and bone scintigraphy to complete the oncology staging protocol.

In a standard neurosurgical theatre, all the procedures were performed with an infrared-based Neuro-navigator (Brainlab, Kick® Purely Navigation), with a standard operative microscope. During the first post-operative day, as routine, the patients underwent a CT scan to exclude major complications and a volumetric brain MRI scan to evaluate the EOR. For both groups, in the case of lesions placed within non-eloquent areas, a standard total intravenous anesthesia protocol with Propofol (1 mg/kg) and Remifentanil (0.5 mg/kg/min) was applied. For lesions involving the sensory-motor and language-related cortex, a standard full awake surgery protocol was routinely performed with the aid of intraoperative neuro-monitoring realized using bi- and monopolar stimulating probes, respectively, for the cortical and sub-cortical mapping. No muscle relaxants were administered when intra-operative neuromonitoring or no awake surgery was performed [34]. During surgery, tumor excision was arrested when:

1. Despite a directly visualized or navigation-proven remnant, neuromonitoring or intraoperative neuropsychological testing outlined a risk for postoperative sensory-motor damage,

2. The white matter appeared free of disease in each aspect of the surgical cavity.

2.3. Data Sources and Quantitative Variables

The extent of resection (EOR) was determined by comparing the MR images obtained before surgery and the first early MRI after surgery, following the RANO criteria [35]. EOR was coded in a 3-step ordinal variable as reported elsewhere [11]: gross-total resection (GTR) <2 mm^3 residual lesions; near-total resection (NTR) ($\geqq$2 to <5 mm^3), and sub-total resection (STR) ($\geqq$5 mm^3).

In the case of GTR, "tumor progression" was defined as the first MRI scan demonstrating the presence of pathologically enhancing tissue characterized using an MRI pattern (mainly relying on perfusion-weighted imaging) inconsistent with a cerebral radiation injury (which is, in fact, a "pseudo-progression"). In incomplete resections (NTR/STR), a volumetric increase in the residual disease detected at the first postoperative MRI scan was considered as disease progression. A close-range dedicated neuro-imaging follow-up program was routinely performed at our institution. This program included:

A standard early (maximum 24 h after surgery) postoperative volumetric brain MRI; at approximately one month from surgery (25–35 days), a volumetric brain MRI scan was repeated for a first step follow-up control and information for the radiation treatment planning; a volumetric brain MRI scan was performed every three months at the end of irradiation; and we performed a complete medical and neurological outpatient re-evaluation at every radiological reevaluation.

2.4. Size, Statistics, and Potential Source of Bias

The study size was determined based on the selection of the inclusion criteria. The sample was analyzed with SPSS v18 (SPSS Inc., released 2009, PASW Statistics for Windows, Version 18.0, Chicago, IL, USA) to outline potential correlations between variables under investigation. Comparisons between nominal variables were carried out using the Chi^2 test. EOR, OS, PFS mean, edema, lesion volume, and their correlations with EGFR mutations were compared with one-way and multivariate ANOVA analysis and contrast analysis and post-hoc tests. Kaplan–Meier survival analysis was carried out. Continuous variable correlations were investigated using Pearson's bivariate correlation. The threshold of statistical significance was considered $p < 0.05$.

2.5. Ethical Issue

The Institutional Review Board approved the informed consent at our Institution (IRB 6168 Prot. 0935/2020). Before the surgical procedure, all the patients gave informed written explicit consent after appropriate information. The data reported in the study have been completely anonymized. No treatment randomization was carried out. This study is perfectly consistent with the Helsinki Declaration of Human Rights in Medical Research.

3. Results

In a period ranging from January 2015 to January 2019, a total of 81 patients suffering from NSCLC brain metastases have been operated on in our Neurosurgical Departments. A total of 27 patients were female (33.3%), and 54 were male (66.7%) with a 1:2 ratio. The average age of the cohort was 62.1 years ± 10.9. In this cohort, brain metastasis favored frontal (32 patients, 39.5%) and cerebellar (18 patients, 22.2%) localization; in general, the lesions were more commonly found in the supratentorial compartment (77.8%) with no infratentorial involvement but the cerebellum. The frontal placement is statistically significant ($p < 0.001$). Thirty-six patients had a right lesion, 43 left, while just 2 involved the midline. No statistically significant side-specificity was evident. The tumor morphology was mostly solid and compact (61.7%), whereas BMs presented as cystic lesions in 19.7% of cases. The average volume of the lesions and perilesional edema were, respectively, 14.62 ± 18.5 cm^3 and 54.21 ± 45.76 cm^3. The diagnosis and clinical presentation were more commonly synchronous (60.5%) rather than metachronous and with sensory-motor dysfunction (41.9%) or with seizures (27.2%). In 59 cases (72.8%), a GTR was achieved. A total of 67 patients presented a preoperative KPS over 70 before surgery, whereas 73 had the same performance status at the 30th post-operative day re-evaluation ($p = 0.001$). The overall survival of the cohort was 15 ± 17 months (data reassumed in Table 1).

Table 1. Patient's demographics.

		N = 81 Patients
Sex		Male N = 54–66.7%
		Female N = 27–33.3%
Age		62.1 years ± 10.9
KPS at admission		>70 = 67–82.7%
		<70 = 14–17.3%
GPA for 80 pts (1 missing datum)		3 = 4 pts
		2.5 = 14 pts
		2 = 16 pts
		1.5 = 22 pts
		1 = 22 pts
		0.5 = 2 pts
KPS after surgery (30 d)		>70 = 73–90.1%
		<70 = 9–11.1%
KPS at last Evaluation		>70 = 49–60.5%
		<70 = 32–39.5%
Dead 68/81 pts at 09/20		48 dead
		20 alive
Overall Survival		15 ± 1.7 months
Volume (cm^3)		14.62 ± 18.5
Edema Volume (cm^3)		54.21 ± 45.76
Periventricular		11 pts–15.1%
Location		Supratentorial = 63–77.8%
		Subtentorial = 18–22.2%
Major Lobe involved		Frontal 32 (39.5%)
		Temporal 5 (6.1%)
		Occipital 10 (12.34%)
		Parietal 16 (19.75%)
		Cerebellar 18 (22.22%)
Side		Left 43 (53.1%)
		Right 36 (44.4%)
		Midline 2 (2.47%)

Table 1. Cont.

	N = 81 Patients
Symptoms at onset	Seizures 22 (27.16%)
	Sensory-Motor Dysfunction 34 (41.9%)
	Asymptomatic (follow-up) 25 (30.8%)
Antiepileptic Profilaxis and Treatment	43 pts (53.1%)
Post-operative Seizure	25 pts (30.86%)
Surgical Resection	GTR = 59 (72.84%)
	STR = 22 (27.16%)
Morphology of Tumors	Solid = 50 (61.73%)
	Cystic = 16 (19.75%)
	Hemorragic = 8 (9.87%)
	Mixed = 7 (8.6%)
Onset	Synchronous = 49 pts (60.5%)
	Metachronous = 32 pts (39.5%)
Extracranial metastases	5 pts (6.2%)
Immunohystochemical/molecular features	
EGFR mutation	Expressed = 56.25%
	Not expressed = 43.75%
ALK mutation	Expressed = 17%
	Not expressed = 83%
PD-L1 expression with tumor proportion score (TPS) ≥1%	(TPS) ≥1% = 54% of pts
	Not Expressed = 46% of pts

Abbreviations: Karnofsky performance status (KPS), Graded Prognostic Assessment (GPA), Gross-total resection (GTR), Sub-total resection (STR), tumor proportion score (TPS).

3.1. Volume and Edema

Tumor volume and edema demonstrated a significant reciprocal association (r = 0.369, p = 0.010) (Figure 1), and the more significant edema was associated with supratentorial placement (p = 0.034, Figure 2a). The tumor-related edema demonstrates an association with neurological symptoms at the beginning of the disease (p = 0.048) rather than with the volume of the lesion per se (p = 0.891), outlining that the tumor-associated edema is more commonly responsible for the neurological symptoms rather than a greater tumor volume itself. Moreover, a greater tumor volume was associated with a higher incidence of complications (p = 0.031, Figure 2b), which, in turn, was also associated with significantly shorter survival (p = 0.018 Figure 2c). This finding is exciting when observing, on a multivariate ANOVA analysis, that complications, per se, negatively affect survival, independently of tumor volume (p = 0.002, Figure 2d). Furthermore, on a repeated measures ANOVA analysis, edema was demonstrated to play a statistically significant role (p = 0.049, Figure 3a) affecting the early post-operative period: patients with edema volume greater than 30 cm^3 had a poorer outcome on post-operative day 30th at KPS when compared with pre-operative and late follow up time intervals.

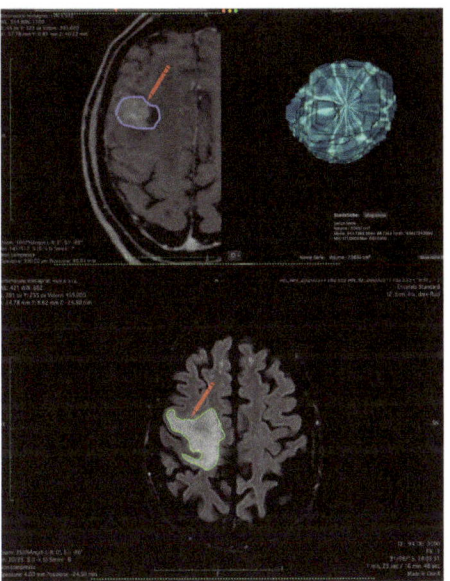

Figure 1. Figure shows tumor reconstruction using Horos software with volumetric calculation of contrast capturing lesion and peritumoral edema.

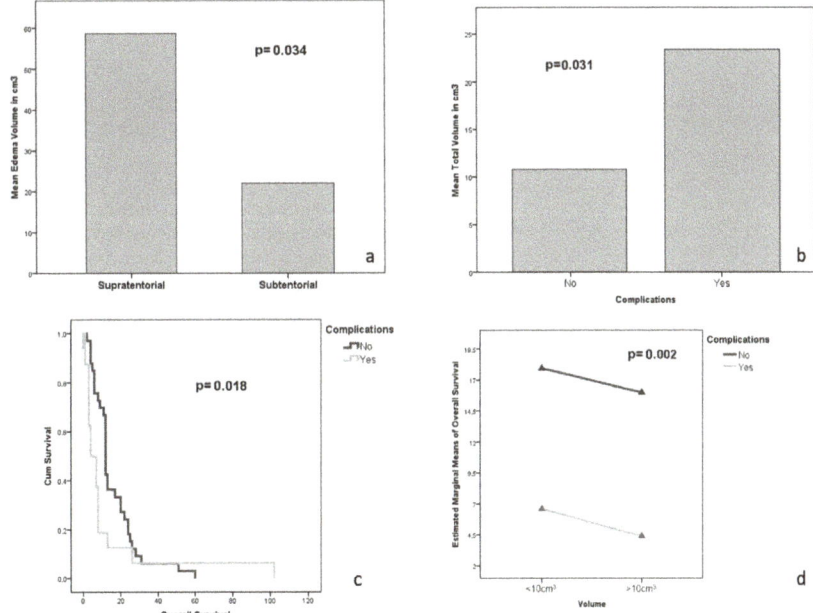

Figure 2. (a) One-way ANOVA analysis demonstrating the association between edema volume and the intracranial compartment. (b) One-way ANOVA analysis demonstrating the association between total volume and the incidence of complications. (c) Kaplan–Meier survival curve demonstrating the impact of complications on survival. (d) Multivariate ANOVA analysis demonstrating the association between complications and survival independently from the volume of the lesion.

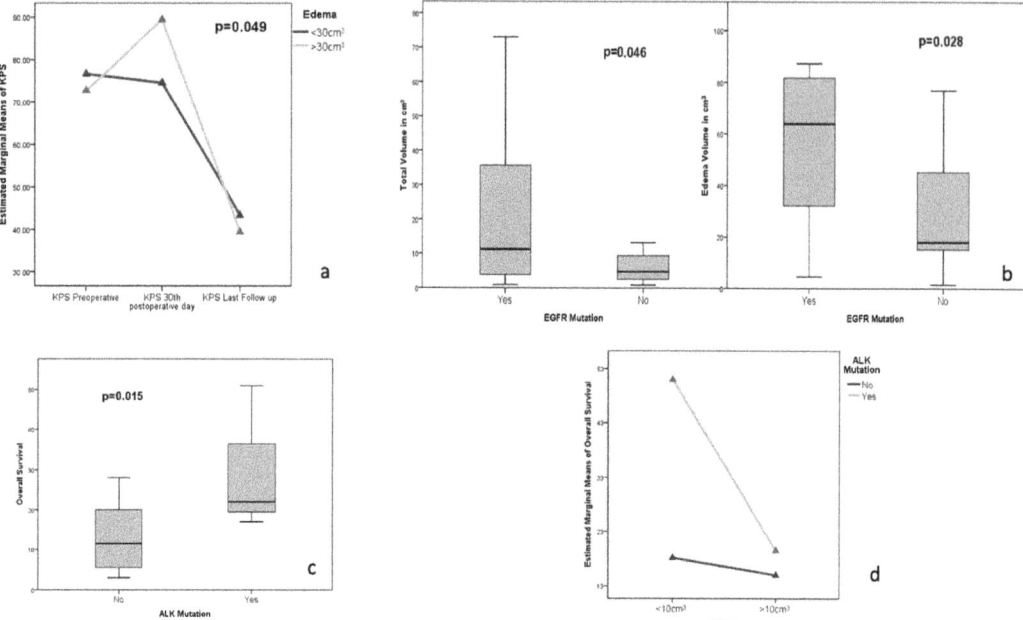

Figure 3. (**a**) Repeated measures ANOVA analysis demonstrating the impact of edema on the functional status (**b**) One-way ANOVA analysis demonstrating the association between EGFR mutation status and the lesion and edema volumes. (**c**) One-way ANOVA analysis demonstrating the association between ALK mutation status and Overall Survival. (**d**) Multivariate ANOVA analysis demonstrating the association between ALK mutation status and survival with respect to the volume of the lesion: the survival advantage disappears for the greater lesions.

3.2. EGFR-Related Parameters

In all cases, the presence of EGFR was confirmed both within the primary tumor and its BM. This is important since some cases may possess EGFR mutations in the primary tumor but not within its BM, while in the presence of an EGFR-positive BM, the primary tumor necessarily expresses EGFR as well. EGFR mutations were neither significantly associated with gender, age, nor with the shape and number of the BM (Table 2); in contrast, the size and peri-lesion edema were significantly associated with the EGFR mutations (for BM's volume 22.38 ± 21.35 cm^3 in EGFR expressing BMs versus 7.68 ± 8.44 cm^3 in non-EGFR expressing BMs while for peri-lesion edema was 72.44 ± 60.71 cm^3 versus 31.92 cm^3; $p = 0.046$ and $p = 0.028$, respectively. Figure 3b). Remarkably, in our series, EGFR was not associated with any specific neurological symptoms apart from the incidence of pre-operative seizures ($p = 0.004$). EGFR was not associated with survival, while the expression of ALK, as previously reported [36], was strongly associated with survival. In fact, the cumulative survival of patients presenting ALK mutation was 30.0 ± 18.36 months compared with 12.88 ± 8.31 months in the wild-type ALK phenotype ($p = 0.015$, Figure 3c). ALK mutation was associated with better survival in patients harboring smaller lesions, possibly with smaller edema volumes. In great lesions (>10 cm^3) with bigger edema (>30 cm^3), the survival advantage of ALK mutation disappears (Figure 3d).

Table 2. EGFR mutation groups analysis.

Total 81	EGFR +	EGFR −	p-Value
N° of cases	45	36	
Age	61.34 ± 11.11	63.1 ± 9	1
Volume (cm^3)	22.38 ± 21.35	7.68 ± 6.44	0.046
Edema volume (cm^3)	72.44 ± 60.71	31.92	0.028
Clinical debut			
Seizure	20	2	0.004
Sensory-Motor Dysfunction	16	18	1
Asymptomatic (follow-up)	9	16	0.41
Morphology			1
Hemorragic	25	21	
Cistic	7	9	
Solid	6	2	
Mixed	3	4	
Overall Survival	12 ± 4.3	16 ± 6.5	0.77

4. Discussion

So far, the current treatment of BMs is represented by RT (or radiosurgery) or microsurgery followed by RT [37,38]. Concerning NSCLC, treatment protocols have been radically changed by discovering molecular targets, such as EGFR and ALK, and the subsequent development of specific drugs aimed to block these receptors. However, their efficacy in patients affected by BMs is not fully understood because this group of patients is usually excluded from clinical studies, especially when neurologically symptomatic [8,39]. Therefore, a standard treatment schedule for these patients needs to be identified [40].

Recent findings suggest that driver mutations in NSCLC would be at least partly associated with the development of BMs in NSCLC. More specifically, EGFR mutations have been detected in 64% and 31% of patients with and without BMs, respectively, suggesting that brain metastases would be more frequent in tumors bearing EGFR mutations [41]. Recent evidence regarding anaplastic lymphoma kinase (ALK) translocations also indicates that they may predispose to brain metastasis formation [42].

Although ALK translocations might correlate with the development of BMs, they may represent a beneficial event for prognosis. Nevertheless, the association between ALK positivity and prognosis is widely debated [43]. Further studies are needed to establish a correlation between ALK mutation and better survival in patients with small brain lesions. Despite the occurrence of EGFR mutations that improve the prognosis of primary lung neoplasm [44], such an association could not be confirmed in these studies concerning EGFR-positive BMs. Further evidence is needed to confirm this finding and specific correlative studies should consider lesion volumes and amount of brain edema. In fact, as described in this study, the presence of larger volumes of edema is associated with a higher incidence of neurological symptoms. Treatment of both the primary neoplasms and the BMs is not contraindicated solely by a single BM, and complete resection of all diseases should be attempted whenever safe and feasible. Operative mortality and morbidity for this combined approach are low [45]. In fact, given the encouraging results in terms of survival, primary tumor resection and treatment (neurosurgical intervention or irradiation) for synchronous lung and brain lesions appear to be justified [15,32–34,46]. In our cohort, we defined two groups of patients harboring BMs: those with a single lesion synchronous with the primary tumor and those with a solitary lesion that develops months or years after successfully managing the primary tumor. Some authors observed that the synchronous presentation of lung cancer and BMs is a negative prognosis factor [14,17,47].

In the present study, several factors (functional status, general health conditions, morphological and histological features of the lesions, and prognostic indices) have been investigated to analyze their association with the risk of death at 12 weeks and at one year. Among these, only the KPS score (>70%) and RT application appear to be significant protective factors [47–51]. Moreover, morbidity and mortality rates have decreased significantly with improved neurosurgical techniques and perioperative care. Most single BMs are manageable by total resection, performed on 72.84% of the patients with low mortality and morbidity rates, in line with data reported in the literature [44]. Nevertheless, the surgical indication in debilitated patients with advanced systemic disease should be carefully considered because the morbidity and deaths in our study were primarily due to systemic and infectious complications.

In BMs without surgical indication, treatment options, such as SRS or SRS and whole-brain radiotherapy (WBRT), should be performed whenever feasible by tailoring the treatment protocol to both the patient's and the diseases' specificity. Prophylactic cranial irradiation (PCI) has been abandoned due to complications, such as cognitive disorders and neurological deficits [52]. This strengthens the need to develop accurate approaches to identify those patients affected by lung cancer-bearing an increased risk of developing BMs. In this scenario, the role of ALK and EGFR could be relevant in the immediate future [26,27,35].

The main limitation of the present paper is its retrospective nature. Moreover, the current investigation was conducted on a subset of BMs patients, which met the criteria for surgical indication, and who had relatively good functional status. Therefore, this may affect the general outcome of all the patients suffering from BMs from NSCLC of the present findings. Another potential bias is the limited availability of the ALK and EGFR status in the entire cohort (41 ALK and 37 EGFR-investigated patients). Nevertheless, the conclusions reported here are statistically significant, thus, providing exciting clues concerning the use of ALK and EGFR in patients' stratification.

The occurrence of high correlation between EGFR mutations and seizure incidence may extend the significance of this study making EGFR more than a mere disease marker to disclose novel avenues in the pathophysiology of BMs and epilepsy. In fact, in a very recent paper, where patients affected by mesial temporal lobe sclerosis and limbic seizures were analyzed, abnormal EGFR signaling was measured [26], which poses a causal relationship between EGFR mutations in BMs, primary tumors, and seizure onset.

5. Conclusions

According to the results of the present study, the presence of EGFR mutations correlates with edema, volumes of the lesion, and a higher incidence of seizures, while no effects were noticed on prognosis. Contrariwise, the presence of ALK translocations in BMs deriving from NSCLC could be associated with a better prognosis. Given the dense scientific debate on the role of EGFR and ALK mutations in NSCLC, aimed studies on BMs derived from this specific family of lung cancer should be carried out to explore their impact on diagnosis and treatment prognosis.

Author Contributions: Conceptualization, F.F. and D.A.; methodology, F.B., F.C. and C.L.B.; validation, F.F. investigation, C.L.B., P.C., G.P.; resources, A.F.; data curation, F.F., M.P.; writing—original draft preparation, D.A. and A.P.; writing—review and editing, A.F.; visualization and supervision, A.F. and D.G.; project administration, F.F., A.F., A.S. All authors have read and agreed to the published version of the manuscript.

Funding: This work was supported by the Italian Ministry of Health (Current Research 2023).

Institutional Review Board Statement: The data reported in the study have been completely anonymized. Because of its retrospective nature, no treatment randomization was performed. No deviation, even minimal in respect to the world-recognized gold standard treatments, has been performed in the preoperative or postoperative therapies or diagnostic tools. The Institutional Review Board of our Institution approved the informed consent with appropriate ethics committee approbation (IRB 6168 Prot. 0935/2020). This study is consistent with the Helsinki Declaration of Ethical principles for human medical research.

Informed Consent Statement: Informed consent was obtained from all subjects involved in the study. Written informed consent has been obtained from the patient(s) to publish this paper.

Data Availability Statement: Data are available on request to the corresponding author.

Conflicts of Interest: The authors declare no conflict of interest.

References

1. Picarelli, H.; Oliveira, M.L.; Marta, G.N.; Solla, D.J.F.; Teixeira, M.J.; Figueiredo, E.G. Mortality, Morbidity, and Prognostic Factors in the Surgical Resection of Brain Metastases: A Contemporary Cohort Study. *J. Neurol. Surg. A Cent. Eur. Neurosurg.* **2020**, *81*, 279–289. [CrossRef]
2. Al-Shamy, G.; Sawaya, R. Management of brain metastases: The indispensable role of surgery. *J. Neurooncol.* **2009**, *92*, 275–282. [CrossRef]
3. Wang, G.; Xu, J.; Qi, Y.; Xiu, J.; Li, R.; Han, M. Distribution of Brain Metastasis from Lung Cancer. *Cancer Manag. Res.* **2019**, *11*, 9331–9338. [CrossRef]
4. Lee, H.; Jeong, S.H.; Jeong, B.H.; Park, H.Y.; Lee, K.-J.; Um, S.-W.; Kwon, O.J.; Kim, H. Incidence of brain metastasis at the initial diagnosis of lung squamous cell car- cinoma on the basis of stage, excluding brain metastasis. *J. Thorac. Oncol.* **2016**, *11*, 426–431. [CrossRef]
5. Putora, P.M.; Fischer, G.F.; Früh, M.; Califano, R.; Fin-Faivre, C.; Van Houtte, P.; McDonalnd, F.; Nestele, U.; Dziadziuszko, R.; Le Pechoux, C.; et al. Treatment of brain metastases in small cell lung cancer: Decision-making amongst a multidisciplinary panel of European experts. *Radiother. Oncol.* **2020**, *149*, 84–88. [CrossRef] [PubMed]
6. Yang, H.; He, D.; Wang, F.; Deng, Q.; Xie, Z. A study on different therapies and prognosis-related factors for brain metastases in lung adenocarcinoma patients with driver mutation. *Clin. Exp. Metastasis* **2020**, *37*, 391–399. [CrossRef] [PubMed]
7. Saad, A.G.; Yeap, B.Y.; Thunnissen, F.B.; Pinkus, G.S.; Pinkus, J.L.; Loda, M.; Sugarbaker, D.J.; Johnson, B.E.; Chirieac, L.R. Imuno-histochemical markers associated with brain metastases in patients with non- small cell lung carcinoma. *Cancer* **2008**, *113*, 2129–2138. [CrossRef] [PubMed]
8. Yoshida, H.; Kim, Y.H.; Iwatsubo, S.; Sakaguchi, C.; Sakamori, Y.; Nagai, H.; Ozasa, H.; Mio, T.; Hirai, T. Management and Outcomes of Newly Diagnosed Non-Small Cell Lung Cancer Patients with Brain Metastases: A Real-World Study in Japan. *Oncology* **2020**, *98*, 460–467. [CrossRef] [PubMed]
9. Bonnette, P.; Puyo, P.; Gabriel, C.; Giudicelli, R.; Regnard, J.F.; Riquet, M.; Brichon, P.Y.; Groupe Thorax. Surgical management of non-small cell lung cancer with synchronous brain metastases. *Chest* **2001**, *119*, 1469–1475. [CrossRef]
10. Iwasaki, A.; Shirakusa, T.; Yoshinaga, Y.; Enatsu, S.; Yamamoto, M. Evaluation of the treatment of non-small cell lung cancer with brain metastasis and the role of risk score as a survival predictor. *Eur. J. Cardiothorac. Surg.* **2004**, *26*, 488–493. [CrossRef]
11. Frati, A.; Pesce, A.; Palmieri, M.; Celniku, M.; Raco, A.; Salvati, M. Surgical Treatment of the Septuagenarian Patients Suffering from Brain Metastases: A Large Retrospective Observational Analytic Cohort-Comparison Study. *World Neurosurg.* **2018**, *114*, e565–e572. [CrossRef] [PubMed]
12. Penel, N.; Brichet, A.; Prevost, B.; Duhamel, A.; Assaker, R.; Dubois, F.; Lafitte, J.J. Pronostic factors of synchro- nous brain metastases from lung cancer. *Lung Cancer* **2001**, *33*, 143–154. [CrossRef] [PubMed]
13. Antuña, A.R.; Vega, M.A.; Sanchez, C.R.; Fernandez, V.M. Brain Metastases of Non-Small Cell Lung Cancer: Prognostic Factors in Patients with Surgical Resection. *J. Neurol. Surg. A Cent. Eur. Neurosurg.* **2018**, *79*, 101–107. [CrossRef]
14. Granone, P.; Margaritora, S.; D'Andrilli, A.; Cesario, A.; Kawamukai, K.; Meacci, E. Non-small cell lung cancer with single brain metastasis: The role of surgical treatment. *Eur. J. Cardiothorac. Surg.* **2001**, *20*, 361–366. [CrossRef]
15. Lo, C.K.; Yu, C.H.; Ma, C.C.; Ko, K.M.; Leung, S.C. Surgical management of primary non-small-cell carcinoma of lung with synchronous solitary brain metastasis: Local experience. *Hong Kong Med. J.* **2010**, *16*, 186–191. [PubMed]
16. Travis, W.D.; Brambilla, E.; Nicholson, A.G.; Yatabe, Y.; Austin, J.; Beasley, M.B.; Chirieac, L.; Dacic, S.; Duhig, E.; Flieder, D.; et al. The 2015 World Health Organization Classification of Lung Tumors: Impact of Genetic, Clinical and Radiologic Advances Since the 2004 Classification. *J. Thorac. Oncol.* **2015**, *10*, 1243–1260. [CrossRef]
17. Fleckenstein, J.; Petroff, A.; Schäfers, H.-J.; Wehler, T.; Schöpe, J.; Rübe, C. Long-term outcomes in radically treated synchronous vs. metachronous oligometastatic non-small-cell lung cancer. *BMC Cancer* **2016**, *16*, 348. [CrossRef] [PubMed]
18. Toyokawa, G.; Seto, T.; Takenoyama, M.; Ichinose, Y. Insights into brain metastasis in patients with ALK+ lung cancer: Is the brain truly a sanctuary? *Cancer Metastasis. Rev.* **2015**, *34*, 797–805. [CrossRef]
19. Patil, T.; Smith, D.E.; Bunn, P.A.; Aisner, D.L.; Le, A.; Hancock, M.; Purcell, W.; Bowles, D.; Camidge, R.; Doebele, R. The Incidence of Brain Metastases in Stage IV ROS1-Rearranged Non-Small Cell Lung Cancer and Rate of Central Nervous System Progression on Crizotinib. *J. Thorac. Oncol.* **2018**, *13*, 1717–1726. [CrossRef]

20. Grinberg-Rashi, H.; Ofek, E.; Perelman, M.; Skarda, J.; Yaron, P.; Hajdúch, M.; Jacob-Hirsch, J.; Amariglio, N.; Krupsky, M.; Simansky, D.; et al. The expression of three genes in primary non-small cell lung cancer is associated with metastatic spread to the brain. *Clin. Cancer Res.* **2009**, *15*, 1755–1761. [CrossRef]
21. Iuchi, T.; Shingyoji, M.; Itakura, M.; Yokoi, S.; Moriya, Y.; Tamura, H.; Yoshida, Y.; Ashinuma, H.; Kawasaki, K.; Hasegawa, Y.; et al. Frequency of brain metastases in non-small-cell lung cancer, and their association with epidermal growth factor receptor mutations. *Int. J. Clin. Oncol.* **2015**, *20*, 674–679. [CrossRef] [PubMed]
22. Rangachari, D.; Yamaguchi, N.; VanderLaan, P.A.; Folch, E.; Mahadevan, A.; Floyd, S.; Uhlmann, E.; Wong, E.; Dahlberg, S.; Huberman, M.; et al. Brain metastases in patients with EGFR-mutated or ALK-rearranged non-small-cell lung cancers. *Lung Cancer* **2015**, *88*, 108–111. [CrossRef]
23. Fridman, W.H.; Zitvogel, L.; Sautès-Fridman, C.; Kroemer, G. The immune contexture in cancer prognosis and treatment. *Nat. Rev. Clin. Oncol.* **2017**, *14*, 717–734. [CrossRef] [PubMed]
24. Haratani, K.; Hayashi, H.; Tanaka, T.; Kaneda, H.; Togashi, Y.; Sakai, K.; Hayashi, K.; Tomida, S.; Chiba, Y.; Yonesaka, K.; et al. Tumor immune microenvironment and nivolumab efficacy in EGFR mutation-positive non-small-cell lung cancer based on T790M status after disease progression during EGFR-TKI treatment. *Ann. Oncol.* **2017**, *28*, 1532–1539. [CrossRef]
25. Liu, S.Y.; Dong, Z.Y.; Wu, S.P.; Xie, Z.; Yan, L.-X.; Li, Y.-F.; Yan, H.-H.; Su, J.; Yang, J.-J.; Zhou, Q.; et al. Clinical relevance of PD-L1 expression and CD8+ T cells infiltration in patients with EGFR-mutated and ALK-rearranged lung cancer. *Lung Cancer* **2018**, *125*, 86–92. [CrossRef] [PubMed]
26. Maurer-Morelli, C.V.; de Vasconcellos, J.F.; Bruxel, E.M.; Rocha, C.S.; do Canto, A.M.; Tedeschi, H.; Yasuda, C.L.; Cendes, F.; Lopes-Cendes, I. Gene expression profile suggests different mechanisms underlying sporadic and familial mesial temporal lobe epilepsy. *Exp. Biol. Med.* **2022**, *247*, 2233–2250. [CrossRef] [PubMed]
27. Nardone, V.; Romeo, C.; D'Ippolito, E.; Pastina, P.; D'Apolito, M.; Pirtoli, L.; Caraglia, M.; Mutti, L.; Bianco, G.; Falzea, A.C.; et al. The role of brain radiotherapy for EGFR- and ALK-positive non-small-cell lung cancer with brain metastases: A review. *Radiol. Med.* **2023**, *128*, 316–329. [CrossRef]
28. Bethune, G.; Bethune, D.; Ridgway, N. Epidermal growth factor receptor (EGFR) in lung cancer: An overview and update. *J. Thorac. Dis.* **2010**, *2*, 48–51.
29. Sperduto, P.W.; Kased, N.; Roberge, D.; Xu, Z.; Shanley, R.; Luo, X.; Sneed, P.; Chao, S.; Weil, R.; Suh, J.; et al. Summary report on the graded prognostic assessment: An accurate and facile diagnosis-specific tool to estimate survival for patients with brain metastases. *J. Clin. Oncol.* **2012**, *30*, 419–425. [CrossRef]
30. Gaspar, L.E.; Scott, C.; Murray, K.; Curran, W. Validation of the RTOG recursive partitioning analysis (RPA) classification for brain metastases. *Int. J. Radiat. Oncol. Biol. Phys.* **2000**, *47*, 1001–1006. [CrossRef]
31. Xu, Q.; Wang, Y.; Liu, H.; Meng, S.; Zhou, S.; Xu, J.; Schmid-Bindert, G.; Zhou, C. Treatment outcome for patients with primary NSCLC and synchronous solitary metastasis. *Clin. Transl. Oncol.* **2013**, *15*, 802–809. [CrossRef] [PubMed]
32. Gray, P.J.; Mak, R.H.; Yeap, B.Y.; Cryer, S.; Pinnell, N.; Christianson, L.; Sher, D.; Arvold, N.; Baldini, E.; Chen, A.; et al. Aggressive therapy for patients with non-small cell lung carcinoma and synchronous brain-only oligometastatic disease is associated with long-term survival. *Lung Cancer* **2014**, *85*, 239–244. [CrossRef] [PubMed]
33. Tensaouti, F.; Khalifa, J.; Lusque, A.; Plas, B.; Lotterie, J.A.; Berry, I.; Laprie, A.; Cohen-Jonathan Moyal, E.; Lubrano, V. Response Assessment in Neuro-Oncology criteria, contrast enhancement and perfusion MRI for assessing progression in glioblastoma. *Neuroradiology* **2017**, *59*, 1013–1020. [CrossRef]
34. Paglia, F.; Caporlingua, A.; Armocida, D.; Rizzo, F.; Santoro, A.; D'angelo, L. Preoperative 3D volume reconstruction of the posterior wall of the sphenoid sinus with Horos: A free, simple and reliable tool in endoscopic endonasal trans-sphenoidal surgery. *Neurocirugia* **2022**, *33*, 219–226. [CrossRef]
35. Bernhardt, D.; Adeberg, S.; Bozorgmehr, F.; Opfermann, N.; Hörner-Rieber, J.; König, L.; Kappes, J.; Thomas, M.; Unterberg, A.; Herth, F.; et al. Outcome and prognostic factors in single brain metastases from small-cell lung cancer. Outcome und Prognose faktoren bei singulären Hirnmetastasen des kleinzelligen Bronchialkarzinoms. *Strahlenther Onkol.* **2018**, *194*, 98–106. [CrossRef] [PubMed]
36. Frati, A.; Pesce, A.; Palmieri, M.; Iasanzaniro, M.; Familiari, P.; Angelini, A.; Salvati, M.; Rocco, M.; Raco, A. Hypnosis-Aided Awake Surgery for the Management of Intrinsic Brain Tumors versus Standard Awake-Asleep-Awake Protocol: A Preliminary, Promising Experience. *World Neurosurg.* **2019**, *121*, e882–e891. [CrossRef]
37. Armocida, D.; Pesce, A.; Di Giammarco, F.; Frati, A.; Santoro, A.; Salvati, M. Long Term Survival in Patients Suffering from Glio-blastoma Multiforme: A Single-Center Observational Cohort Study. *Diagnostics* **2019**, *9*, 209. [CrossRef]
38. Costa, D.B.; Shaw, A.T.; Ou, S.H.; Solomon, B.; Riely, G.; Ahn, M.-J.; Zhou, C.; Shreeve, M.; Selaru, P.; Polli, A.; et al. Clinical experience with crizotinib in patients with advanced ALK-re- arranged non-small-cell lung cancer and brain metastases. *J. Clin. Oncol.* **2015**, *33*, 1881–1888. [CrossRef]
39. D'Andrea, G.; Palombi, L.; Minniti, G.; Pesce, A.; Marchetti, P. Brain Metastases: Surgical Treatment and Overall Survival. *World Neurosurg.* **2017**, *97*, 169–177. [CrossRef]
40. Carden, C.P.; Agarwal, R.; Saran, F.; Judson, I.R. Eligibility of patients with brain metastases for phase I trials: Time for a rethink? *Lancet Oncol.* **2008**, *9*, 1012–1017. [CrossRef]
41. Qin, H.; Wang, C.; Jiang, Y.; Zhang, X.; Zhang, Y.; Ruan, Z. Patients with single brain metastasis from non-small cell lung cancer equally benefit from stereotactic radiosurgery and surgery: A systematic review. *Med. Sci. Monit.* **2015**, *21*, 144–152.

2. Pao, W.; Girard, N. New driver mutations in non-small-cell lung cancer. *Lancet Oncol.* **2011**, *12*, 175–180. [CrossRef]
3. Preusser, M.; Berghoff, A.S.; Ilhan-Mutlu, A.; Magerle, M.; Dinhof, C.; Widhalm, G.; Dieckmann, K.; Marosi, C.; Wöhrer, A.; Hackl, M.; et al. ALK gene translocations and amplifications in brain metastases of non-small cell lung cancer. *Lung Cancer* **2013**, *80*, 278–283. [CrossRef] [PubMed]
4. Liu, Y.; Ye, X.; Yu, Y.; Lu, S. Prognostic significance of anaplastic lymphoma kinase rearrangement in patients with completely resected lung adenocarcinoma. *J. Thorac. Dis.* **2019**, *11*, 4258–4270. [CrossRef]
5. Li, W.Y.; Zhao, T.T.; Xu, H.M.; Wang, Z.-N.; Xu, Y.-Y.; Han, Y.; Song, Y.-X.; Wu, J.-H.; Xu, H.; Yin, S.-C.; et al. The role of EGFR mutation as a prognostic factor in survival after diagnosis of brain metastasis in non-small cell lung cancer: A systematic review and meta-analysis. *BMC Cancer* **2019**, *19*, 145. [CrossRef] [PubMed]
6. Endo, C.; Hasumi, T.; Matsumura, Y.; Sato, N.; Deguchi, H.; Oizumi, H.; Sagawa, M.; Tsushima, T.; Takahashi, S.; Shibuya, J.; et al. A prospective study of surgical procedures for patients with oligometastatic non-small cell lung cancer. *Ann. Thorac. Surg.* **2014**, *98*, 258–264. [CrossRef] [PubMed]
7. Billing, P.S.; Miller, D.L.; Allen, M.S.; Deschamps, C.; Trastek, V.F.; Pairolero, P.C. Surgical treatment of primary lung cancer with synchronous brain metastases. *J. Thorac. Cardiovasc. Surg.* **2001**, *122*, 548–553. [CrossRef]
8. Fuentes, R.; Bonfill, X.; Exposito, J. Surgery versus radiosurgery for patients with a solitary brain metastasis from non-small cell lung cancer. *Cochrane Database Syst. Rev.* **2006**, *2006*, CD004840. [CrossRef] [PubMed]
9. Salvati, M.; Armocida, D.; Pesce, A.; Palmieri, M.; Venditti, E.; D'Andrea, G.; Frati, A.; Santoro, A. No prognostic differences between GBM-patients presenting with postoperative SMA-syndrome and GBM-patients involving cortico-spinal tract and primary motor cortex. *J. Neurol. Sci.* **2020**, *419*, 117188. [CrossRef]
10. Armocida, D.; Frati, A.; Salvati, M.; Santoro, A.; Pesce, A. Is Ki-67 index overexpression in IDH wild type glioblastoma a predictor of shorter Progression Free survival? A clinical and Molecular analytic investigation. *Clin. Neurol. Neurosurg.* **2020**, *198*, 106126. [CrossRef]
11. Armocida, D.; Pesce, A.; Di Giammarco, F.; Frati, A.; Salvati, M.; Santoro, A. Histological, molecular, clinical and outcomes characteristics of Multiple Lesion Glioblastoma. A retrospective monocentric study and review of literature. *Neurocirugia* **2021**, *32*, 114–123. [CrossRef] [PubMed]
12. Armocida, D.; Pesce, A.; Frati, A.; Santoro, A.; Salvati, M. EGFR amplification is a real independent prognostic impact factor between young adults and adults over 45yo with wild-type glioblastoma? *J. Neurooncol.* **2020**, *146*, 275–284. [CrossRef] [PubMed]

Disclaimer/Publisher's Note: The statements, opinions and data contained in all publications are solely those of the individual author(s) and contributor(s) and not of MDPI and/or the editor(s). MDPI and/or the editor(s) disclaim responsibility for any injury to people or property resulting from any ideas, methods, instructions or products referred to in the content.

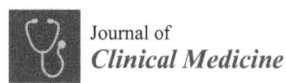

Article

Impact of Alcohol and Smoking on Outcomes of HPV-Related Oropharyngeal Cancer

Yu-Hsuan Lai [1,2,3], Chien-Chou Su [2], Shang-Yin Wu [1,3], Wei-Ting Hsueh [1], Yuan-Hua Wu [1], Helen H. W. Chen [1], Jenn-Ren Hsiao [4], Ching-Hsun Liu [5] and Yi-Shan Tsai [2,6,*]

1. Department of Oncology, National Cheng Kung University Hospital, College of Medicine, National Cheng Kung University, Tainan 704302, Taiwan
2. Clinical Innovation and Research Center, National Cheng Kung University Hospital, College of Medicine, National Cheng Kung University, Tainan 704302, Taiwan
3. Institute of Clinical Medicine, College of Medicine, National Cheng Kung University, Tainan 701401, Taiwan
4. Department of Otolaryngology, National Cheng Kung University Hospital, College of Medicine, National Cheng Kung University, Tainan 704302, Taiwan
5. Department of Pathology, National Cheng Kung University Hospital, College of Medicine, National Cheng Kung University, Tainan 704302, Taiwan
6. Department of Medical Imaging, National Cheng Kung University Hospital, College of Medicine, National Cheng Kung University, Tainan 704302, Taiwan
* Correspondence: n506356@mail.hosp.ncku.edu.tw; Tel.: +886-6-2353535 (ext. 2401)

Abstract: Background: The aim of this study was to evaluate the impact of adverse lifestyle factors on outcomes in patients with human papillomavirus (HPV)-related oropharyngeal squamous cell carcinoma (OPSCC). Methods: From 2010 to 2019, 150 consecutive non-metastatic OPSCC patients receiving curative treatment in our institution were retrospectively enrolled. HPV positivity was defined as p16 expression ≥75%. The effects of adverse lifestyle factors on overall survival (OS) and disease-free survival (DFS) on OPSCC patients were determined. Results: The median follow-up duration was 3.6 years. Of the 150 OPSCCs, 51 (34%) patients were HPV-positive and 99 (66%) were HPV-negative. The adverse lifestyle exposure rates were 74.7% (n = 112) alcohol use, 57.3% (n = 86) betel grid chewing, and 78% (n = 117) cigarette smoking. Alcohol use strongly interacted with HPV positivity (HR, 6.00; 95% CI, 1.03–35.01), leading to an average 26.1% increased risk of disease relapse in patients with HPV-positive OPSCC. Heavy smoking age ≥30 pack-years was associated with increased risk of death (HR, 2.05; 95% CI, 1.05–4.00) and disease relapse (HR, 1.99; 95% CI, 1.06–3.75) in OPSCC patients. In stratified analyses, the 3-year absolute risk of disease relapse in HPV-positive OPSCC patients reached up to 50% when alcohol use and heavy smoking for ≥30 pack-years were combined. Conclusions: Alcohol acted as a significant treatment-effect modifier for DFS in HPV-positive OPSCC patients, diluting the favorable prognostic effect of HPV positivity. Heavy smoking age ≥30 pack-years was an independent adverse prognostic factor of OS and DFS in OPSCC patients. De-intensification treatment for HPV-related OPSCC may be avoided when these adverse lifestyle factors are present.

Keywords: alcohol; smoking; betel nut; human papillomavirus (HPV); oropharyngeal cancer; treatment-effect modifier; prognostic factor

Citation: Lai, Y.-H.; Su, C.-C.; Wu, S.-Y.; Hsueh, W.-T.; Wu, Y.-H.; Chen, H.H.W.; Hsiao, J.-R.; Liu, C.-H.; Tsai, Y.-S. Impact of Alcohol and Smoking on Outcomes of HPV-Related Oropharyngeal Cancer. *J. Clin. Med.* **2022**, *11*, 6510. https://doi.org/10.3390/jcm11216510

Academic Editors: Marco Zeppieri, Tamara Ius, Filippo Flavio Angileri, Antonio Pontoriero and Alessandro Tel

Received: 17 October 2022
Accepted: 1 November 2022
Published: 2 November 2022

Publisher's Note: MDPI stays neutral with regard to jurisdictional claims in published maps and institutional affiliations.

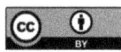

Copyright: © 2022 by the authors. Licensee MDPI, Basel, Switzerland. This article is an open access article distributed under the terms and conditions of the Creative Commons Attribution (CC BY) license (https://creativecommons.org/licenses/by/4.0/).

1. Introduction

Over the past few decades, the prevalence of human papillomavirus (HPV)-related oropharyngeal squamous cell carcinoma (OPSCC) has increased rapidly—particularly in high-income countries [1,2]. Unlike other head and neck squamous cell carcinomas (HNSCCs), HPV-related OPSCCs have distinct clinical presentations: the patients tend to be younger and the cancers are less associated with smoking and more associated with primary tonsillar tumors and cystic cervical lymph node metastasis [3]. HPV-16 accounts for at least 85% of all HPV-related OPSCCs [4]. Two HPV oncogenes, E6 and E7, are key drivers of HPV-mediated carcinogenesis. E6 and E7 involve increased degradation of the tumor suppressor proteins p53 and Rb, respectively, resulting in the loss of cell-cycle checkpoint activation in response to DNA damage and uncontrolled licensing of DNA replication—which together result in genomic instability and resistance to apoptosis [5,6]. p16 is upregulated during the process of E7-directed epigenetic reprogramming [7]. Thus, p16 overexpression is a surrogate marker for HPV-related OPSCC [8]. The cutoff of p16 positivity by immunohistochemistry (IHC) staining is nuclear expression $\geq$+2/+3 intensity and $\geq$75% distribution [9].

The prognostic significance of HPV status in OPSCC has been established; patients with HPV-related OPSCC have a more favorable treatment response and longer survival time than HPV-unrelated OPSCC [10–12]. The American Joint Committee on Cancer (AJCC) has defined HPV-positive and HPV-negative OPSCCs as separate entities because of their distinct tumor characteristics, biological behaviors, and treatment outcomes [9,13].

Asian OPSCC patients have poorer treatment outcomes than other ethnicities [14,15]. One suspected reason for this is the lower rate of HPV positivity in OPSCC, which is about 30% to 50% in Asians but 70% to 85% in Western populations [2]. Higher rates of alcohol use, betel grid chewing, and cigarette smoking (ABC lifestyle factors) in Asia also might contribute to poorer prognosis [14]. The ABC lifestyle factors are especially common in Southeast Asia—especially in low socioeconomic and less-educated populations [16]. ABC lifestyle factors usually coexist, which may contribute to a dramatically increased risk of developing HNSCC in multi-user persons compared with that in persons who have never been exposed to ABC factors [17]. Although the role of ABC lifestyle factors has been well established in the development of HNSCC [18,19], less is known about their prognostic significance in patients with HPV-positive OPSCC. Epidemiologic studies of HPV-positive OPSCC have been conducted mostly in Western countries and are therefore not generalizable to non-Western countries [20], where factors such as cultural and behavioral differences might result in different etiologies in HPV-positive OPSCC. Wider geographically based investigations are necessary to guide region-specific clinical treatments and public health policies.

As de-intensification treatment protocols in patients with HPV-positive OPSCC are currently applied [21–23], it is important to identify patients where such attempts may not be safe. We hypothesized that ABC lifestyle factors moderate the effects of p16 status on survival in OPSCC patients. This study aimed to evaluate the impact of ABC lifestyle factors on treatment outcomes in patients with HPV-positive OPSCC and to optimize the selection of a subgroup of HPV-positive OPSCC patients for de-intensification treatment.

2. Materials and Methods

2.1. Patients

One hundred and fifty OPSCC patients who had completed a course of curative treatment, consisting of surgery and radiotherapy (RT)-based therapy from January 2010 to October 2019, were consecutively collected and analyzed. All patients had received a complete staging work-up before treatment and were followed to determine their treatment response and survival. The exclusion criteria were: (1) other underlying malignancy or distant metastasis at the time that OPSCC was diagnosed; (2) lack of available pretreatment primary tumor specimens to re-evaluate p16 expression by IHC staining; (3) lack of pretreatment contrast-enhanced computed tomography (CT) images of the head and neck to re-evaluate clinical staging. The Institutional Review Board approved this retrospective study.

2.2. Demographic and Clinical Data

Patient data—including age, gender, tumor subsites, history of ABC lifestyle (alcohol consumption, betel grid chewing, cigarette smoking), smoking age (number of cumulative pack-years of smoking), treatment-related profiles (surgery, radiotherapy, chemotherapy), and outcome data—were gathered by retrospective chart review. The clinical and pathological staging that had been determined previously were re-evaluated and revised based on the seventh and eighth editions of the AJCC staging system [9,13].

HPV status was determined by re-examination of p16 nuclear expression in the pretreatment primary tumor by IHC staining. After tissue specimens from our human biobank were collected, all the slides were re-evaluated by a head and neck pathologist with 30-years' experience to determine the HPV status. HPV positivity was defined as the presence of p16 expression in $\geq 75\%$ of carcinoma cells, with nuclear reactivity on IHC staining [9].

2.3. Treatments

The standard primary treatments for OPSCC were surgery and RT-based therapy. Definitive concurrent chemoradiotherapy (CCRT) with a platinum-based chemotherapeutic regimen was most often used in locally advanced OPSCC. The curative-intent radiation dose to the primary tumor and grossly involved lymph nodes was 60–74 Gy in 1.8–2.2 Gy per fraction, delivered daily with intensity-modulated radiotherapy or volumetric-modulated arc therapy techniques. Induction chemotherapy was allowed before primary treatments. Adjuvant treatments after primary surgery were indicated when patients with adverse pathological features—including positive/close surgical margin, extranodal extension, pT3–pT4 disease, positive lymph node metastasis, perineural invasion, lymphovascular space invasion, or any other concern—when determined to be appropriate by multidisciplinary discussion.

2.4. Statistical Analysis

Baseline characteristics were presented as mean (standard deviation) for continuous variables and number (frequency) for categorical variables. The Kaplan–Meier survival method was used to depict the curves for the distribution of time to death or relapse and log-rank tests were carried out to evaluate differences between HPV-positive and HPV-negative OPSCC patients. Overall survival (OS) was defined as the date of initial treatment to the date of death or last follow-up. Disease-free survival (DFS) was defined as the date of initial treatment to the date of disease relapse (locoregional recurrence and/or distant metastasis) or death. The p-value of continuous variables was calculated by the two-sample t-test whereas the p-value of categorical variables was calculated by the chi-square test and Fisher's exact test.

Among patients with OPSCC, univariable Cox proportional hazard models were applied to identify significant patient characteristics associated with OS and DFS—including p16 status, gender, age, clinical stage, tumor subsites, initial treatment, and ABC lifestyle factors. We hypothesized that ABC lifestyle factors could modify the effects of p16 status for OS and DFS. We used multivariable Cox proportional hazard models with patient characteristics and p16 status and lifestyle factors as interaction terms by using the stepwise variable selection method to select relevant variables for OS and DFS. The criteria for the model fitting were based on the Akaike information criterion. Furthermore, multivariate models were constructed with interaction terms that were selected by the stepwise method and significant and clinically relevant variables from univariate analyses. The multicollinearity and proportional hazard assumption of the models were checked; none of the models showed high multicollinearity and the proportional hazard assumption was met.

The stratified analyses were made according to alcohol use and smoking age to estimate 3-year and 5-year cumulative risks of disease relapse in HPV-positive patients using multivariate models. The interaction plot was depicted by HPV status and alcohol use to show changes in the cumulative risk of disease relapse, which was estimated using multivariate models, in different situations. A two-tailed p value < 0.05 was considered statistically significant. All statistical results were carried out with R (version 4.1.0) software and Quanta for Medical Care AI: AI Medical Platform (QOCA AIM) 2.0 version (Quanta Computer Inc., Taoyuan, Taiwan).

3. Results

3.1. Patient Characteristics

One hundred and fifty patients were analyzed in this study; 99 (66%) had HPV-negative OPSCC and 51 (34%) were HPV-positive OPSCC patients. The mean age at diagnosis of OPSCC was 54.4 years; most were locally advanced OPSCCs. The ABC lifestyle exposure rates were: 112/150 (74.7%) patients showed alcohol consumption, 86/150 (57.3%) betel grid chewing, and 117/150 (78%) cigarette smoking. More than half of all patients (79/150; 52.7%) had concomitant ABC lifestyle exposure. Among the 150 patients, 39 (26%) were treated with primary surgery and 111 (74%) were treated with primary RT-based therapy (106 CCRT and 5 RT only). In the primary surgery group, 10 patients underwent induction chemotherapy before surgery and 35 underwent adjuvant RT/CCRT after surgery. In the primary RT-based therapy group, 22 patients underwent induction chemotherapy before definitive RT/CCRT. The baseline characteristics of the study population are summarized in Table 1.

Table 1. Baseline characteristics of the study population.

Variable	p16 (−), n = 99		p16 (+), n = 51		p-Value
	n	%	n	%	
Male, n, %	93	93.94	37	72.55	<0.001
Female, n, %	6	6.06	14	27.45	<0.001
Age, mean, SD	53.3	9.22	56.7	9.71	0.036
Age, n, %					0.085
<50	36	36.36	10	19.61	
50–59	35	35.35	20	39.22	
≥60	28	28.28	21	41.18	
Cigarette smoking, n, %	91	91.92	26	50.98	<0.001
Smoking age (pack-years), mean, SD	31.8	26.8	14.4	17.9	<0.001
Smoking age (pack-years), n, %					<0.001
0	8	8.08	25	49.02	
1–9	7	7.07	3	5.88	
10–19	14	14.14	0	0.00	
20–29	18	18.18	10	19.61	
≥30	52	52.53	13	25.49	
Alcohol use, n, %	86	86.87	26	50.98	<0.001
Betel quid chewing, n, %	76	76.77	10	19.61	<0.001
ABC concomitant use, n, %					<0.001
3	70	70.7	9	17.65	
2 of 3	20	20.2	12	23.53	
Tumor subsite, n, %					0.002
Tonsil	47	47.47	40	78.43	
Soft palate	22	22.22	6	11.76	
Tongue base	23	23.23	5	9.80	
Posterior pharyngeal wall	7	7.07	0	0.00	
Clinical stage (AJCC 7th ed.), n, %					0.041
Stage I	2	2.02	1	1.96	
Stage II	7	7.07	0	0.00	
Stage III	6	6.06	9	17.65	
Stage IVA	68	68.69	37	72.55	
Stage IVB	16	16.16	4	7.84	

Table 1. Cont.

Variable	p16 (−), n = 99		p16 (+), n = 51		p-Value
	n	%	n	%	
Clinical stage (AJCC 8th ed.), n, %					<0.001
Stage I	2	2.02	26	50.98	
Stage II	7	7.07	15	29.41	
Stage III	5	5.05	10	19.61	
Stage IVA	55	55.56	0 *	0.00 *	
Stage IVB	30	30.3	0 *	0.00 *	
Initial treatment, n, %					0.024
Surgery	32	32.32	7	13.73	
RT-based therapy	67	67.68	44	86.27	
CCRT	66	66.67	40	78.43	
RT only	1	1.01	4	7.84	
Disease relapse, n, %	58	58.59	13	25.49	<0.001
LRR	25	25.25	6	11.76	
DM	18	18.18	5	9.80	
LRR + DM	15	15.15	2	3.92	
Mortality, n, %	61	61.62	9	17.65	<0.001
DOD	47	47.47	5	9.80	
Dead, other reason	14	14.14	4	7.84	

* The clinical stage of nonmetastatic HPV-positive OPSCC was downstaged to stage III or less in the eighth edition of the American Joint Committee on Cancer (AJCC) staging system. Abbreviations: n, number of patients; SD, standard deviation; ABC, alcohol/betel nut/cigarette; AJCC, American Joint Committee on Cancer; ed., edition; RT, radiotherapy; CCRT, concurrent chemoradiotherapy; LRR, locoregional recurrence; DM, distant metastasis; DOD, died of disease.

Between the two groups of HPV-positive and HPV-negative OPSCC patients, there was no significant difference in the age distribution and clinical stage. In patients with HPV-positive OPSCC, the dominant tumor subsite was the tonsil and the majority received primary RT-based therapy. Patients with HPV-negative OPSCC had a significantly higher proportion of male gender, a higher exposure rate to ABC lifestyle factors, and a higher smoking age (Table 1).

3.2. Treatment Outcomes

The median follow-up time was 3.6 years. The recurrence rate was 47.3%, with 71 of the 150 patients developing disease relapse (locoregional recurrence and/or distant metastasis). The mortality rate was 46.7%, which meant that 70 of the 150 patients had expired by the time of analysis. Patients with HPV-positive OPSCC had significantly lower disease relapse and mortality rates than those with HPV-negative OPSCC ($p < 0.001$; Table 1). The 3-year overall survival (OS) and disease-free survival (DFS) rates for HPV-positive versus HPV-negative OPSCC patients were 90% versus 52% and 74.5% versus 42.9%, respectively (both p values < 0.0001; Figure 1).

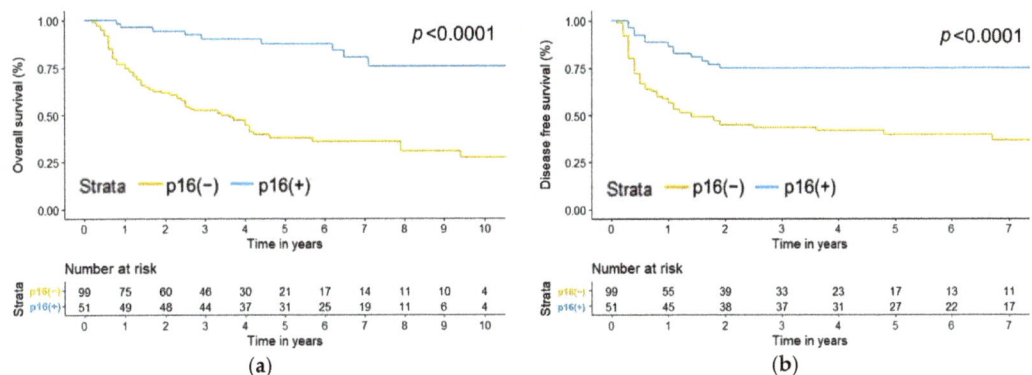

Figure 1. Kaplan–Meier estimate of (**a**) overall survival ($p < 0.0001$) and (**b**) disease-free survival ($p < 0.0001$) by p16 status.

3.3. Factors Affecting Overall Survival (OS)

In the multivariate analysis, the HPV status (positive: hazard ratio, 0.09; 95% CI, 0.02–0.44), clinical stage (stage IVA: hazard ratio, 2.72; 95% CI, 1.05–7.00; stage IVB: hazard ratio, 15.62; 95% CI, 5.29–46.13), and smoking age ($\geq$30 pack-years: hazard ratio, 2.05; 95% CI, 1.05–4.00) were significant prognostic factors for OS in OPSCC patients (Table 2). There was no significant interaction between HPV positivity and ABC lifestyle factors; that is, ABC lifestyle factors were not significant treatment-effect modifiers for OS in HPV-positive OPSCC (Table 2).

Table 2. Univariate and multivariate analyses for overall survival.

Variable	Univariate		Multivariate			
			Stepwise Selection *		Selected Predictors #	
	HR	95% CI	HR	95% CI	HR	95% CI
	Covariate					
p16 (ref. = negative)	0.18	(0.09, 0.37)	0.08	(0.02, 0.35)	0.09	(0.02, 0.44)
Gender (ref. = male)	0.15	(0.04, 0.60)			0.52	(0.12, 2.33)
Age (5-year increments)	0.89	(0.78, 1.02)				
Clinical stage (ref. = stage I–III) &						
Stage IVA	2.69	(1.07, 6.76)	2.55	(1.00, 6.49)	**2.72**	**(1.05, 7.00)**
Stage IVB	12.11	(4.41, 33.26)	16.26	(5.76, 45.86)	**15.62**	**(5.29, 46.13)**
Tumor subsite (ref. = other sites than tonsil)	0.46	(0.28, 0.73)			0.77	(0.45, 1.33)
Initial treatment (ref. = surgery)	0.88	(0.52, 1.48)			1.02	(0.58, 1.81)
Smoking age (ref. = <20 pack-years)						
20–29	1.78	(0.85, 3.70)	0.96	(0.41, 2.23)	1.15	(0.46, 2.90)
$\geq$30	2.98	(1.67, 5.32)	1.90	(1.02, 3.54)	**2.05**	**(1.05, 4.00)**
Alcohol use (ref. = none)	3.19	(1.58, 6.44)			0.90	(0.39, 2.08)
Betel quid chewing (ref. = none)	2.35	(1.40, 3.96)			0.85	(0.45, 1.61)
	Interaction term					
p16: Smoking age (20–29 pack-years)			8.00	(1.16, 55.01)	5.74	(0.79, 41.53)
p16: Smoking age ($\geq$30 pack-years)			2.94	(0.43, 19.93)	2.53	(0.36, 17.85)
p16: Alcohol use						
p16: Betel quid chewing						

* Variable selection employed the stepwise method by the Akaike information criterion. # The Cox proportional hazard model was constructed with interaction terms that were selected by the stepwise method and significant and clinically relevant variables from univariate analyses. & The clinical stage was defined by the 7th edition of the American Joint Committee on Cancer (AJCC) staging system. Significant values of HR and 95% CI are in bold. Abbreviations: HR, hazard ratio; CI, confidence interval; ref., reference.

3.4. Factors Affecting Disease-Free Survival (DFS)

In the multivariate analysis, the HPV status (positive: hazard ratio, 0.10; 95% CI, 0.02–0.49), clinical stage (stage IVA: hazard ratio, 2.87; 95% CI, 1.11–7.41; stage IVB: hazard ratio, 8.43; 95% CI, 2.83–25.08), tumor subsite (tonsil: hazard ratio, 0.46; 95% CI, 0.27–0.80), and smoking age ($\geq$30 pack-years: hazard ratio, 1.99; 95% CI, 1.06–3.75) were significant prognostic factors for DFS in OPSCC patients (Table 3). Moreover, there was a strong interaction between HPV positivity and alcohol use (alcohol use: hazard ratio, 6.00; 95% CI, 1.03–35.01), which meant that alcohol was a significant treatment-effect modifier for DFS in HPV-positive OPSCC patients (Table 3). The presence of alcohol exposure diluted the favorable prognostic effect of HPV positivity in OPSCC patients. In a median follow-up duration of 3.6 years, alcohol use contributed to an average 26.1% increased risk of disease relapse in patients with HPV-positive OPSCC, whereas there was no risk increment in those with HPV-negative OPSCC (Figure 2). By stratification of smoking age among HPV-positive OPSCC patients with alcohol use, the 3-year absolute risk of disease relapse was 33% in those with smoking age <20 pack-years and up to 50% in those $\geq$30 pack-years (Table 4).

Table 3. Univariate and multivariate analyses for disease-free survival.

Variable	Univariate		Multivariate			
			Stepwise Selection *		Selected Predictors #	
	HR	95% CI	HR	95% CI	HR	95% CI
Covariate						
p16 (ref. = negative)	0.31	(0.17, 0.56)	0.12	(0.03–0.58)	**0.10**	**(0.02, 0.49)**
Gender (ref. = male)	0.32	(0.12, 0.88)			1.12	(0.36, 3.42)
Age (5-year increments)	0.98	(0.87, 1.11)	1.12	(0.97–1.28)		
Clinical stage (ref. = stage I–III) &						
Stage IVA	2.75	(1.09, 6.90)	3.6	(1.37–9.45)	**2.87**	**(1.11, 7.41)**
Stage IVB	10.68	(3.88, 29.41)	12.35	(4.09–37.26)	**8.43**	**(2.83, 25.08)**
Tumor subsite (ref. = other sites than tonsil)	0.34	(0.21, 0.55)	0.49	(0.26–0.83)	**0.46**	**(0.27, 0.80)**
Initial treatment (ref. = surgery)	1.05	(0.62, 1.78)			1.21	(0.68, 2.16)
Smoking age (ref. = <20 pack-years)						
20–29	1.43	(0.71, 2.88)	1.69	(0.77–3.70)	1.64	(0.74, 3.63)
$\geq$30	2.07	(1.20, 3.55)	1.88	(1.01–3.49)	**1.99**	**(1.06, 3.75)**
Alcohol use (ref. = none)	2.68	(1.37, 5.23)	0.66	(0.27–1.62)	0.57	(0.23, 1.39)
Betel quid chewing (ref. = none)	1.77	(1.08, 2.92)			0.91	(0.48, 1.72)
Interaction term						
p16: Smoking age (20–29 pack-years)						
p16: Smoking age ($\geq$30 pack-years)						
p16: Alcohol use			4.4	(0.78–24.7)	**6.00**	**(1.03, 35.01)**
p16: Betel quid chewing						

* Variable selection employed the stepwise method by the Akaike information criterion. # The Cox proportional hazard model was constructed with interaction terms that were selected by the stepwise method and significant and clinically relevant variables from univariate analyses. & The clinical stage was defined by the 7th edition of the American Joint Committee on Cancer (AJCC) staging system. Significant values of HR and 95% CI are in bold. Abbreviations: HR, hazard ratio; CI, confidence interval; ref., reference.

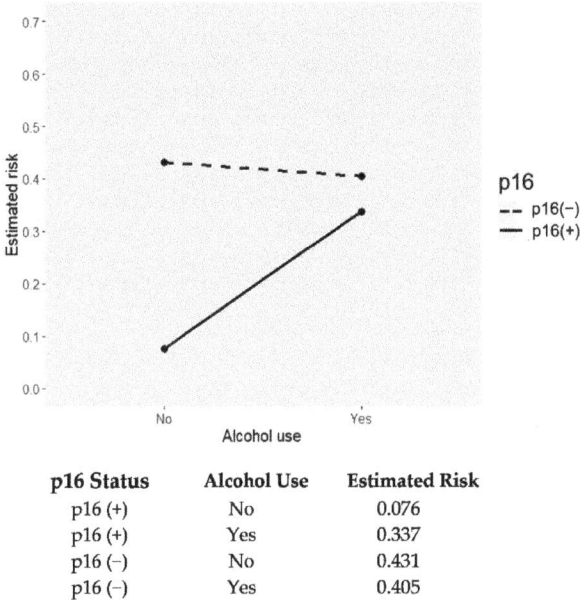

Figure 2. Interaction plot for estimated risk of disease relapse according to p16 status and alcohol use.

Table 4. The cumulative risks of disease relapse in HPV-related oropharyngeal cancer by alcohol and smoking age.

		p16 (+)	
Smoking Age	Follow-Up	Absolute Risk (95% CI)	Absolute Risk (95% CI)
		Alcohol (−)	Alcohol (+)
<20 pack-years	3 years	0.12 (0.11, 0.14)	0.33 (0.24, 0.39)
	5 years	0.14 (0.12, 0.15)	0.35 (0.26, 0.42)
20–29 pack-years	3 years	0.19 (0.18, 0.20)	0.45 (0.35, 0.51)
	5 years	0.21 (0.20, 0.21)	0.47 (0.37, 0.54)
≥30 pack-years	3 years	0.22 (0.21, 0.24)	0.50 (0.38, 0.57)
	5 years	0.24 (0.22, 0.25)	0.52 (0.41, 0.59)

Abbreviations: HPV, human papilloma virus; CI, confidence interval.

4. Discussion

In this study, we demonstrated that alcohol was a significant treatment-effect modifier for DFS in HPV-positive OPSCC patients. The presence of alcohol use diluted the favorable prognostic effect of HPV positivity in OPSCC patients, leading to an average 26.1% increased risk of disease relapse. A heavy smoking age of ≥30 pack-years was a poor prognostic factor of all-cause and disease-specific mortality among OPSCC patients, regardless of HPV status. On the other hand, betel grid chewing made no contribution to effect modification or the prediction of treatment outcomes in patients with OPSCC.

Confusion between treatment-effect modifiers and prognostic factors is common. Effect modifiers, also called effect moderators, are factors that influence how well an intervention affects the outcome. Prognostic factors are factors that predict the outcome of a disease [24]. Scientifically, effect modifiers must be differentiated from prognostic factors, but it is more challenging to claim that a factor is an effect modifier rather than a prognostic factor. Prognostic factors are familiar to oncologists and are used to provide patients with a more accurate prognosis, but they do not help identify which patients will respond best to a specific intervention. Effect modification has recently become of particular interest in oncology in the era of targeted therapy and immunotherapy, where the effectiveness of a treatment might largely depend on host or tumor factors [25,26]—as does HPV-related OPSCC. Due to the heterogeneous tumor behavior present in HPV-positive and HPV-negative OPSCCs, the variety of variables affecting treatment outcomes may play different roles as effect modifiers or prognostic factors. Determining the treatment-effect modifiers in HPV-positive OPSCC helps to identify subgroups of patients who respond better or worse to de-escalation treatments.

Our data indicate that alcohol is a significant treatment-effect modifier for DFS in HPV-positive OPSCC patients. Exposure to alcohol is well-known as a dominant etiologic factor of HNSCC. A large case-control study conducted by Lee et al. involved 740 HNSCC patients in Taiwan [25]; although the patients enrolled in this study were heterogeneous, the results showed a significant positive dose–response relationship between pre-diagnosis alcohol use and worse OS in HNSCC. This association was more significant for non-oral cavity HNSCC than for oral HNSCC. A possible mechanism for this is the polymorphism of the ethanol-metabolizing genes ADH1B and ALDH2, which modify the relationship between pre-diagnosis alcohol use and the OS of HNSCC patients—providing a possible biological explanation [27]. However, unlike our study, this analysis did not adjust for HPV status (due to a lack of access to the tumor tissues to test for HPV)—thus prohibiting its generalization to HPV-positive OPSCC. A recent study in Belgium demonstrated that alcohol use was a poor prognostic factor for OS in OPSCC patients and established a simplified scoring system composed of p16 status, smoking, and alcohol [28]. Another study showed that alcohol consumption was an independent factor for survival among patients with HPV-negative OPSCC rather than for those with HPV-positive OPSCC [29]. So far, relevant studies on the impact of alcohol use on HPV-positive OPSCC are scanty and contradictory. To the best of our knowledge, our study was the first to highlight the role of alcohol use as a treatment-effect modifier for HPV-positive OPSCC, which had not been previously evaluated and reported. The findings of our provided supporting evidence that p16 expression is not the only key factor for survival in OPSCC patients and demonstrated that the favorable prognostic effect of HPV positivity in OPSCC patients can be diluted by alcohol use.

Our study also demonstrated that smoking was not a treatment-effect modifier for HPV-positive OPSCC, but heavy smoking age ≥ 30 pack-years was a significant prognostic indicator of worse OS and DFS in OPSCC patients. A considerable amount of literature has explored the association between smoking and HPV-positive OPSCC. First, the association between smoking and the pathogenesis of HPV-positive OPSCC was suggested. The potential pathways of smoking-related carcinogenesis were likely attributed to cellular alterations and DNA damage, promoting infection by and the persistence of HPV [30]. By pooling two large head and neck cancer studies with HPV serology data, Anantharaman et al. demonstrated that smoking was consistently associated with increased risks of both HPV-positive and HPV-negative OPSCC [31]. Second, the association between smoking and treatment-related outcomes in HPV-positive OPSCC has been widely explored. The results remained somewhat controversial, with some studies reporting smoking as a poor prognostic factor independent of HPV status, which is consistent with our findings [32,33], and others reporting smoking exposure as a poor prognostic factor within the context of HPV-positive OPSCC [34,35]. Though there are some conflicting results, most studies agree that smoking is associated with worse OS and a trend towards worse DFS in HPV-positive OPSCC [36]. Third, the association between the amount of smoking and worse survival outcomes in HPV-positive OPSCC has been investigated. There is no consensus on the cutoff for high-risk smokers. Several previous studies have reported smoking age >10 pack-years as a cutoff delineating higher risk HPV-positive OPSCC patients [10,37]. Other smoking metrics reported in the literature have included smoking age >20 pack-years, >20 cigarettes daily, total pack-years, current smoking, and ever smoking—with variable prognostic effects on survival outcomes [38–40]. The divergence in outcomes determined by these smoking metrics might be due to heterogeneous patient populations, various sample sizes, and different lifestyle factors, with exposure influenced by different cultures. However, most studies have agreed that the heavier the smoking, the worse the survival outcomes [36]. Our study recommended a cutoff of ≥30 pack-years smoking age for risk stratification in Asian OPSCC populations. As more than three-quarters of our study population had a smoking history—with the majority being heavy smokers—and more than half also had ABC lifestyle exposure, our study populations were more reflective of current conditions among OPSCC patients in Southeast Asia [14,16,41].

Compared to previous studies, the strength of our study was the clear definition of HPV positivity as the presence of p16 expression in ≥75% of carcinoma cells, showing nuclear reactivity on IHC staining [9]. We repeated p16 immunostaining tests in all the pretreatment primary tumor tissues, which were reviewed by a 30-year-experienced head and neck pathologist to accurately discriminate between HPV positivity and negativity. Furthermore, all the pretreatment CT images of the head and neck region were reviewed by a 15-year-experienced radiologist to revise clinical staging based on the seventh and eighth editions of the AJCC staging system to accurately display disease status. Detailed ABC lifestyle exposure histories and an adequate follow-up duration (median 3.6 years) made our results more convincing. Despite the retrospective study design, the consecutive enrollment of qualified OPSCC participants made the internal validity of patient selection solid and reliable. Finally, and most importantly, this was the first study providing the new concept, with convincing evidence, that alcohol is a treatment-effect modifier for HPV positivity.

The limitation of this study was the lack of quantification of alcohol consumption. Detailed quantification of alcohol consumption can include information on drinking status, frequency, the level of drinking, and drink-years [27]. Due to the retrospective nature of this study, our information on alcohol use relied on medical record reviews. There might be some inaccurate reporting due to recall bias when taking histories, or potential falsification of alcohol history due to guilt or shame. Further studies would benefit from including more objective measures of alcohol quantification such as questionnaires or prospective study designs.

5. Conclusions

Alcohol acted as a significant treatment-effect modifier for DFS in HPV-positive OPSCC patients, diluting the favorable prognostic effect of HPV positivity. A heavy smoking age of ≥30 pack-years was an independent adverse prognostic factor for OS and DFS in OPSCC patients. The 3-year absolute risk of disease relapse reached up to 50% in HPV-positive OPSCC patients when alcohol use and a heavy smoking age of ≥30 pack-years were combined. The presence of alcohol use and a history of heavy smoking should be considered critical factors when making treatment decisions between standard and de-intensification protocols among HPV-positive OPSCC patients. Further large-scale studies are warranted to confirm these findings.

Author Contributions: Conceptualization, Y.-H.L. and Y.-S.T.; methodology, Y.-H.L. and C.-C.S.; software, C.-C.S.; formal analysis, C.-C.S.; writing—original draft preparation, Y.-H.L., C.-C.S., S.-Y.W., W.-T.H., Y.-H.W. and Y.-S.T.; writing—review and editing, Y.-S.T.; supervision, H.H.W.C., J.-R.H. and C.-H.L.; funding acquisition, Y.-H.L. All authors have read and agreed to the published version of the manuscript.

Funding: This research was funded by National Cheng Kung University Hospital, College of Medicine, National Cheng Kung University, Tainan, Taiwan (grant number NCKUH-11005005).

Institutional Review Board Statement: The study was approved by the Institutional Review Board of National Cheng Kung University Hospital (A-ER-108-477) for studies involving humans.

Informed Consent Statement: Patient consent was waived due to the retrospective nature of the study.

Data Availability Statement: The data presented in this study are available on reasonable request from the corresponding author. The data are not publicly available due to privacy.

Acknowledgments: We are grateful for the technical services provided by the Bioinformatics Group of the Smart Healthcare Solution in National Cheng Kung University Hospital. We also give thanks for the support from the Human Biobank, Research Center of Clinical Medicine, National Cheng Kung University Hospital.

Conflicts of Interest: The authors declare no conflict of interest.

References

1. Lechner, M.; Liu, J.; Masterson, L.; Fenton, T.R. HPV-associated oropharyngeal cancer: Epidemiology, molecular biology and clinical management. *Nat. Rev. Clin. Oncol.* **2022**, *19*, 306–327. [CrossRef]
2. Carlander, A.F.; Jakobsen, K.K.; Bendtsen, S.K.; Garset-Zamani, M.; Lynggaard, C.D.; Jensen, J.S.; Grønhøj, C.; Buchwald, C.V. A Contemporary Systematic Review on Repartition of HPV-Positivity in Oropharyngeal Cancer Worldwide. *Viruses* **2021**, *13*, 1326. [CrossRef]
3. Goldenberg, D.; Begum, S.; Westra, W.H.; Khan, Z.; Sciubba, J.; Pai, S.I.; Califano, J.A.; Tufano, R.P.; Koch, W.M. Cystic lymph node metastasis in patients with head and neck cancer: An HPV-associated phenomenon. *Head Neck* **2008**, *30*, 898–903. [CrossRef]
4. Kreimer, A.R.; Clifford, G.M.; Boyle, P.; Franceschi, S. Human papillomavirus types in head and neck squamous cell carcinomas worldwide: A systematic review. *Cancer Epidemiol. Biomark. Prev.* **2005**, *14*, 467–475. [CrossRef]
5. Scheffner, M.; Werness, B.A.; Huibregtse, J.M.; Levine, A.J.; Howley, P.M. The E6 oncoprotein encoded by human papillomavirus types 16 and 18 promotes the degradation of p53. *Cell* **1990**, *63*, 1129–1136. [CrossRef]
6. Huh, K.; Zhou, X.; Hayakawa, H.; Cho, J.Y.; Libermann, T.A.; Jin, J.; Harper, J.W.; Munger, K. Human papillomavirus type 16 E7 oncoprotein associates with the cullin 2 ubiquitin ligase complex, which contributes to degradation of the retinoblastoma tumor suppressor. *J. Virol.* **2007**, *81*, 9737–9747. [CrossRef]
7. McLaughlin-Drubin, M.E.; Crum, C.P.; Münger, K. Human papillomavirus E7 oncoprotein induces KDM6A and KDM6B histone demethylase expression and causes epigenetic reprogramming. *Proc. Natl. Acad. Sci. USA* **2011**, *108*, 2130–2135. [CrossRef]
8. Larsen, C.G.; Gyldenløve, M.; Jensen, D.H.; Therkildsen, M.H.; Kiss, K.; Norrild, B.; Konge, L.; von Buchwald, C. Correlation between human papillomavirus and p16 overexpression in oropharyngeal tumours: A systematic review. *Br. J. Cancer* **2014**, *110*, 1587–1594. [CrossRef]
9. Lydiatt, W.M.; Patel, S.G.; O'Sullivan, B.; Brandwein, M.S.; Ridge, J.A.; Migliacci, J.C.; Loomis, A.M.; Shah, J.P. Head and Neck cancers-major changes in the American Joint Committee on cancer eighth edition cancer staging manual. *CA Cancer J. Clin.* **2017**, *67*, 122–137. [CrossRef]
10. Ang, K.K.; Harris, J.; Wheeler, R.; Weber, R.; Rosenthal, D.I.; Nguyen-Tân, P.F.; Westra, W.H.; Chung, C.H.; Jordan, R.C.; Lu, C.; et al. Human papillomavirus and survival of patients with oropharyngeal cancer. *N. Engl. J. Med.* **2010**, *363*, 24–35. [CrossRef]
11. Fakhry, C.; Westra, W.H.; Li, S.; Cmelak, A.; Ridge, J.A.; Pinto, H.; Forastiere, A.; Gillison, M.L. Improved survival of patients with human papillomavirus-positive head and neck squamous cell carcinoma in a prospective clinical trial. *J. Natl. Cancer Inst.* **2008**, *100*, 261–269. [CrossRef]
12. Nguyen-Tan, P.F.; Zhang, Q.; Ang, K.K.; Weber, R.S.; Rosenthal, D.I.; Soulieres, D.; Kim, H.; Silverman, C.; Raben, A.; Galloway, T.J.; et al. Randomized phase III trial to test accelerated versus standard fractionation in combination with concurrent cisplatin for head and neck carcinomas in the Radiation Therapy Oncology Group 0129 trial: Long-term report of efficacy and toxicity. *J. Clin. Oncol.* **2014**, *32*, 3858–3866. [CrossRef]
13. O'Sullivan, B.; Huang, S.H.; Su, J.; Garden, A.S.; Sturgis, E.M.; Dahlstrom, K.; Lee, N.; Riaz, N.; Pei, X.; Koyfman, S.A.; et al. Development and validation of a staging system for HPV-related oropharyngeal cancer by the International Collaboration on Oropharyngeal cancer Network for Staging (ICON-S): A multicentre cohort study. *Lancet Oncol.* **2016**, *17*, 440–451. [CrossRef]
14. Chen, T.C.; Wu, C.T.; Ko, J.Y.; Yang, T.L.; Lou, P.J.; Wang, C.P.; Chang, Y.L. Clinical characteristics and treatment outcome of oropharyngeal squamous cell carcinoma in an endemic betel quid region. *Sci. Rep.* **2020**, *10*, 526. [CrossRef]
15. Tsai, M.H.; Cheng, Y.J.; Pao, T.H.; Hsueh, W.T.; Chen, H.H.W.; Wu, Y.H. Association of Primary Treatment Modality for Advanced-Stage Oropharyngeal Squamous Cell Carcinoma With Survival Outcomes. *JAMA Netw. Open* **2021**, *4*, e2112067. [CrossRef]
16. Ko, Y.C.; Chiang, T.A.; Chang, S.J.; Hsieh, S.F. Prevalence of betel quid chewing habit in Taiwan and related sociodemographic factors. *J. Oral Pathol. Med.* **1992**, *21*, 261–264. [CrossRef]
17. Hsu, W.L.; Chien, Y.C.; Chiang, C.J.; Yang, H.I.; Lou, P.J.; Wang, C.P.; Yu, K.J.; You, S.L.; Wang, L.Y.; Chen, S.Y.; et al. Lifetime risk of distinct upper aerodigestive tract cancers and consumption of alcohol, betel and cigarette. *Int. J. Cancer* **2014**, *135*, 1480–1486. [CrossRef]
18. Auguste, A.; Deloumeaux, J.; Joachim, C.; Gaete, S.; Michineau, L.; Herrmann-Storck, C.; Duflo, S.; Luce, D. Joint effect of tobacco, alcohol, and oral HPV infection on head and neck cancer risk in the French West Indies. *Cancer Med.* **2020**, *9*, 6854–6863. [CrossRef]

9. Kumar, R.; Rai, A.K.; Das, D.; Das, R.; Kumar, R.S.; Sarma, A.; Sharma, S.; Kataki, A.C.; Ramteke, A. Alcohol and Tobacco Increases Risk of High Risk HPV Infection in Head and Neck Cancer Patients: Study from North-East Region of India. *PLoS ONE* **2015**, *10*, e0140700. [CrossRef]
10. Fakhry, C.; Westra, W.H.; Wang, S.J.; van Zante, A.; Zhang, Y.; Rettig, E.; Yin, L.X.; Ryan, W.R.; Ha, P.K.; Wentz, A.; et al. The prognostic role of sex, race, and human papillomavirus in oropharyngeal and nonoropharyngeal head and neck squamous cell cancer. *Cancer* **2017**, *123*, 1566–1575. [CrossRef]
11. Marur, S.; Li, S.; Cmelak, A.J.; Gillison, M.L.; Zhao, W.J.; Ferris, R.L.; Westra, W.H.; Gilbert, J.; Bauman, J.E.; Wagner, L.I.; et al. E1308: Phase II Trial of Induction Chemotherapy Followed by Reduced-Dose Radiation and Weekly Cetuximab in Patients With HPV-Associated Resectable Squamous Cell Carcinoma of the Oropharynx- ECOG-ACRIN Cancer Research Group. *J. Clin. Oncol.* **2017**, *35*, 490–497. [CrossRef] [PubMed]
12. Hegde, J.V.; Shaverdian, N.; Felix, C.; Wang, P.C.; Veruttipong, D.; Hsu, S.; Riess, J.W.; Rao, S.D.; Daly, M.E.; Chen, A.M. Functional Outcomes After De-escalated Chemoradiation Therapy for Human Papillomavirus-Positive Oropharyngeal Cancer: Secondary Analysis of a Phase 2 Trial. *Int. J. Radiat. Oncol. Biol. Phys.* **2018**, *100*, 647–651. [CrossRef] [PubMed]
13. Chen, A.M.; Felix, C.; Wang, P.C.; Hsu, S.; Basehart, V.; Garst, J.; Beron, P.; Wong, D.; Rosove, M.H.; Rao, S.; et al. Reduced-dose radiotherapy for human papillomavirus-associated squamous-cell carcinoma of the oropharynx: A single-arm, phase 2 study. *Lancet Oncol.* **2017**, *18*, 803–811. [CrossRef]
14. Vickers, A.J.; Steineck, G. Prognosis, Effect Modification, and Mediation. *Eur. Urol.* **2018**, *74*, 243–245. [CrossRef] [PubMed]
15. Principe, D.R.; Kamath, S.D.; Korc, M.; Munshi, H.G. The immune modifying effects of chemotherapy and advances in chemo-immunotherapy. *Pharmacol. Ther.* **2022**, *236*, 108111. [CrossRef]
16. Clark, G.M. Prognostic factors versus predictive factors: Examples from a clinical trial of erlotinib. *Mol. Oncol.* **2008**, *1*, 406–412. [CrossRef]
17. Lee, W.T.; Hsiao, J.R.; Ou, C.Y.; Huang, C.C.; Chang, C.C.; Tsai, S.T.; Chen, K.C.; Huang, J.S.; Wong, T.Y.; Lai, Y.H.; et al. The Influence of Prediagnosis Alcohol Consumption and the Polymorphisms of Ethanol-Metabolizing Genes on the Survival of Head and Neck Cancer Patients. *Cancer Epidemiol. Biomark. Prev.* **2019**, *28*, 248–257. [CrossRef]
18. Bouland, C.; Dequanter, D.; Lechien, J.R.; Hanssens, C.; De Saint Aubain, N.; Digonnet, A.; Javadian, R.; Yanni, A.; Rodriguez, A.; Loeb, I.; et al. Prognostic Significance of a Scoring System Combining p16, Smoking, and Drinking Status in a Series of 131 Patients with Oropharyngeal Cancers. *Int. J. Otolaryngol.* **2021**, *2021*, 8020826. [CrossRef]
19. Saito, Y.; Yoshida, M.; Ushiku, T.; Omura, G.; Ebihara, Y.; Shimono, T.; Fukayama, M.; Yamasoba, T.; Asakage, T. Prognostic value of p16 expression and alcohol consumption in Japanese patients with oropharyngeal squamous cell carcinoma. *Cancer* **2013**, *119*, 2005–2011. [CrossRef]
20. Sinha, P.; Logan, H.L.; Mendenhall, W.M. Human papillomavirus, smoking, and head and neck cancer. *Am. J. Otolaryngol.* **2012**, *33*, 130–136. [CrossRef]
21. Anantharaman, D.; Muller, D.C.; Lagiou, P.; Ahrens, W.; Holcátová, I.; Merletti, F.; Kjærheim, K.; Polesel, J.; Simonato, L.; Canova, C.; et al. Combined effects of smoking and HPV16 in oropharyngeal cancer. *Int. J. Epidemiol.* **2016**, *45*, 752–761. [CrossRef] [PubMed]
22. Gillison, M.L.; Zhang, Q.; Jordan, R.; Xiao, W.; Westra, W.H.; Trotti, A.; Spencer, S.; Harris, J.; Chung, C.H.; Ang, K.K. Tobacco smoking and increased risk of death and progression for patients with p16-positive and p16-negative oropharyngeal cancer. *J. Clin. Oncol.* **2012**, *30*, 2102–2111. [CrossRef] [PubMed]
23. Hong, A.M.; Martin, A.; Chatfield, M.; Jones, D.; Zhang, M.; Armstrong, B.; Lee, C.S.; Harnett, G.; Milross, C.; Clark, J.; et al. Human papillomavirus, smoking status and outcomes in tonsillar squamous cell carcinoma. *Int. J. Cancer* **2013**, *132*, 2748–2754. [CrossRef] [PubMed]
24. Hafkamp, H.C.; Manni, J.J.; Haesevoets, A.; Voogd, A.C.; Schepers, M.; Bot, F.J.; Hopman, A.H.; Ramaekers, F.C.; Speel, E.J. Marked differences in survival rate between smokers and nonsmokers with HPV 16-associated tonsillar carcinomas. *Int. J. Cancer* **2008**, *122*, 2656–2664. [CrossRef]
25. Lassen, P.; Lacas, B.; Pignon, J.P.; Trotti, A.; Zackrisson, B.; Zhang, Q.; Overgaard, J.; Blanchard, P. Prognostic impact of HPV-associated p16-expression and smoking status on outcomes following radiotherapy for oropharyngeal cancer: The MARCH-HPV project. *Radiother. Oncol.* **2018**, *126*, 107–115. [CrossRef]
26. Chen, S.Y.; Massa, S.; Mazul, A.L.; Kallogjeri, D.; Yaeger, L.; Jackson, R.S.; Zevallos, J.; Pipkorn, P. The association of smoking and outcomes in HPV-positive oropharyngeal cancer: A systematic review. *Am. J. Otolaryngol.* **2020**, *41*, 102592. [CrossRef]
27. Chidambaram, S.; Nakken, E.R.; Kennedy, W.; Thorstad, W.L.; Chen, S.Y.; Pipkorn, P.; Zevallos, J.P.; Mazul, A.L. Prognostic Significance of Smoking in Human Papillomavirus-Positive Oropharyngeal Cancer Under American Joint Committee on Cancer Eighth Edition Stage. *Laryngoscope* **2020**, *130*, 1961–1966. [CrossRef]
28. Chen, S.Y.; Last, A.; Ettyreddy, A.; Kallogjeri, D.; Wahle, B.; Chidambaram, S.; Mazul, A.; Thorstad, W.; Jackson, R.S.; Zevallos, J.P.; et al. 20 pack-year smoking history as strongest smoking metric predictive of HPV-positive oropharyngeal cancer outcomes. *Am. J. Otolaryngol.* **2021**, *42*, 102915. [CrossRef]
29. Huang, S.H.; Xu, W.; Waldron, J.; Siu, L.; Shen, X.; Tong, L.; Ringash, J.; Bayley, A.; Kim, J.; Hope, A.; et al. Refining American Joint Committee on Cancer/Union for International Cancer Control TNM stage and prognostic groups for human papillomavirus-related oropharyngeal carcinomas. *J. Clin. Oncol.* **2015**, *33*, 836–845. [CrossRef]

40. Vawda, N.; Banerjee, R.N.; Debenham, B.J. Impact of Smoking on Outcomes of HPV-related Oropharyngeal Cancer Treated with Primary Radiation or Surgery. *Int. J. Radiat. Oncol. Biol. Phys.* **2019**, *103*, 1125–1131. [CrossRef]
41. Hsiao, J.R.; Huang, C.C.; Ou, C.Y.; Chang, C.C.; Lee, W.T.; Tsai, S.T.; Huang, J.S.; Chen, K.C.; Lai, Y.H.; Wu, Y.H.; et al. Investigating the health disparities in the association between lifestyle behaviors and the risk of head and neck cancer. *Cancer Sci.* **2020**, *111*, 2974–2986. [CrossRef] [PubMed]

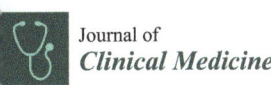

Review

Understanding and Managing Pineal Parenchymal Tumors of Intermediate Differentiation: An In-Depth Exploration from Pathology to Adjuvant Therapies

Andrea Bianconi [1,*], Flavio Panico [1], Bruna Lo Zito [2], Andrea Do Trinh [3], Paola Cassoni [3], Umberto Ricardi [2], Diego Garbossa [1], Fabio Cofano [1], Cristina Mantovani [2] and Luca Bertero [3]

1. Neurosurgery Unit, Department of Neuroscience, University of Turin, 10126 Turin, Italy
2. Radiation Oncology Unit, Department of Oncology, University of Turin, 10126 Turin, Italy
3. Pathology Unit, Department of Medical Sciences, University of Turin, 10126 Turin, Italy
* Correspondence: andrea.bianconi@edu.unito.it

Abstract: Background: Pineal parenchymal cell tumors constitute a rare group of primary central nervous system neoplasms (less than 1%). Their classification, especially the intermediate subtype (PPTIDs), remains challenging. Methods: A literature review was conducted, navigating through anatomo-pathological, radiotherapy, and neurosurgical dimensions, aiming for a holistic understanding of these tumors. Results: PPTIDs, occupying an intermediate spectrum of malignancy, reveal diverse histological patterns, mitotic activity, and distinct methylation profiles. Surgical treatment is the gold standard, but when limited to partial removal, radiotherapy becomes crucial. While surgical approaches are standardized, due to the low prevalence of the pathology and absence of randomized prospective studies, there are no shared guidelines about radiation treatment modalities. Conclusion: Surgical removal remains pivotal, demanding a personalized approach based on the tumor extension. This review underscores the considerable variability in treatment approaches and reported survival rates within the existing literature, emphasizing the need for ongoing research to better define optimal therapeutic strategies and prognostic factors for PPTIDs, aiming for further and more detailed stratification among them.

Keywords: pineal region; pineal parenchymal tumor; pineal gland; biopsy; intensity modulation radiation therapy; stereotactic radiosurgery; craniospinal irradiation

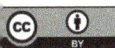

1. Introduction

Pineal parenchymal cell tumors (PPT) are a rare group of tumors representing less than 1% of all primary central nervous system neoplasms. Originating from pineocytes or their precursor cells, these tumors pose unique challenges both during the diagnostic assessment and clinical management. The World Health Organization (WHO) classification stratifies PPTs into distinct entities, ranging from the well-differentiated pineocytomas to the highly malignant pineoblastomas [1]. Among them, the intermediate category of pineal parenchymal cell tumors of intermediate differentiation (PPTID) remains a critically debated subset, presenting a spectrum of histologic features that defy easy categorization [2].

Tackling the management of these tumors remains a complex endeavor, primarily due to their rarity and the resulting limited pool of comprehensive studies. The inherent clinical heterogeneity exhibited by PPTs adds an additional layer of complexity. In this review, we delve into the intricacies of PPTs, emphasizing the histologic and immunohistochemical nuances that underpin their classification, and consequently their treatment. From the initial characterization by Schild et al. in 1993 to their formal inclusion in the WHO classification in 2000, PPTIDs have emerged as a distinct subgroup, encompassing both low and high-grade variants [3,4].

This review places a particular emphasis on the importance of a multidisciplinary approach, exploring anatomo-pathological, radiotherapeutic, and neurosurgical aspects. Through this lens, we aim to provide a comprehensive understanding of the clinical landscape, shedding light on the challenges in diagnosis and management while paving the way for future research endeavors.

2. Pathological Features of Pineal Parenchymal Tumors

According to the latest 2021 WHO classification of central nervous systems, two entities are defined at the opposite ends of the spectrum of pineal parenchyma tumors: pineocytoma (PC), a well-differentiated neoplasm, and pineoblastoma (PB), a poorly differentiated, aggressive neoplasm [1]. The pineal tumor of intermediate differentiation (PPTID) is located in the middle, representing a less defined group of neoplasms [5,6].

2.1. Pineocytomas

Pineocytoma was defined by the WHO in 2021 as a Grade 1 entity—a well-differentiated pineal parenchymal neoplasm exhibiting expansile growth that can result in compression of adjacent structures, leading to variable signs and symptoms [7]. The cut surface shows a well-circumscribed homogeneous or granular mass with a greyish-tan appearance. Histologically, it presents as a moderately cellular neoplasm composed of small, round, blue, and mature cells organized in sheets or showing large pineocytomatous rosettes, a hallmark feature, not present in the normal pineal gland. Gangliocytic differentiation can be variably present and a pleomorphic variant has also been described [8].

Mitotic figures are rarely present in pineocytomas [9–11]. The mean Ki67, in most cases, is <1% [11–13]. Pineocytomas exhibit strong positivity for synaptophysin, neuron-specific enolase, and NFP [2,9,13–16]. Other markers have shown variable positivity, including class III beta-tubulin, microtubule-associated protein tau, and chromogranin-A [2,9,14,15]. On average, the interval between the onset of symptoms and surgery was four years for pineocytomas [5]. To date, there have been no reported cases of metastasis in patients affected by pineocytoma [8,17]. The five-year survival in this group ranges from 86% to 91% [8,17]. A review highlighted that the extent of surgical resection is the main independent prognostic factor [18]. Immunoexpression of CRX, a transcription factor, and ASMT, a fundamental enzyme in the synthesis of melatonin, serves as a sign of a biological link to pinealocytes [19–21]. There are no recurrent genetic mutations in pineocytomas [22,23], but they exhibit a distinct methylation profile [24].

2.2. Pineal Parenchymal Tumors of Intermediate Differentiation

Pineal tumors of intermediate differentiation are characterized by intermediate malignancy between pineocytoma and pineoblastoma [4,7]. Histologically, they are composed of diffuse sheets or large lobules of monomorphic round cells that appear more differentiated than those observed in pineoblastomas. They can show two main microscopic patterns: they can be densely lobulated with an endocrine-arranged vascularity or diffuse, mimicking oligodendroglioma or neurocytoma. The nuclei are round with moderate atypia and "salt and pepper" chromatin [3,8]. According to the WHO in 2021, Grade 2 or 3 can be assigned based on histopathological features, highlighting the intrinsic heterogeneity of this neoplasm [1].

PPTIDs are positive for synaptophysin [9,13,25], while showing variable positivity for NFP and chromogranin-A [2,9,16,26]. As in pineocytoma, CRX is expressed as well as ASMT/HIOMT, which acts as both a diagnostic and prognostic marker [19–21]. Mitotic activity ranges from low to moderate [7]. The mean proliferation index Ki67 is significantly different from pineocytomas and pineoblastomas, with values ranging from 3.5% to 16.1% [22,25,27,28]. PPTIDs are less aggressive neoplasms compared to pineoblastoma, with a higher probability of localized disease at diagnosis. A more favorable prognostic difference between these entities can be observed by comparing the median overall survival of PPTID against PB (165 months vs. 77 months) and progression-free survival (93 months vs. 46 months) [29]. Jouvet et al. and Fauchon et al. have proposed a prognosis-oriented classification of PPTIDs with mitotic count and neuronal differentiation assessed by anti-NFP immunohistochemistry [9,17]. Low-grade PPTID, corresponding to WHO grade 2, was defined as having <6 mitosis per 10 HPF and expression of NFP in many cells [9]. Five-year survival in this group was 74%, and relapse occurred in 26%, mostly in the first site of the neoplasm after some delay [17]. High-grade PPTID, corresponding to WHO grade 3, was defined as having <6 mitosis without NFP expression by immunohistochemistry or >6 mitosis with NFP expression. Five-year survival in this group was 39%, and relapse occurred in 53%, mostly outside the pineal region [9,17]. Low-grade and high-grade prognostic groups showed a difference in the Ki67 proliferation index (5.2% vs. 11.2%) [10]. Nevertheless, the latest WHO classification of CNS tumors acknowledges that definite histological grading criteria are still missing.

It has been demonstrated that PPTIDs can harbor KBTBD4 small in-frame insertions [30]. The copy-number profile of PPTIDs is relatively flat, with some cases of broad gains or losses, particularly chromosome imbalances resembling those observed in pineoblastomas, though minor [22,24]. PPTIDs have a distinct methylation profile that can be further distinguished into two subtypes whose prognosis is still to be established: PPTID-A and PPTID-B [24].

2.3. Pinealoblastomas

Pineoblastoma is a malignant Grade 4 neoplasm—a poorly differentiated, highly cellular, malignant embryonal neoplasm arising in the pineal gland. Upon gross examination, they appear as partially defined invasive masses—soft and friable, pinkish-grey. Pineoblastomas appear as small round blue tumors composed of highly cellular sheets of small cells without a defined pattern. They show irregular, hyperchromatic nuclei with an occasional small nucleolus, high nuclear-to-cytoplasmic ratio, scant cytoplasm, and faint cell borders [3,7].

Pinealoblastomas exhibit positivity for synaptophysin and NSE [9]. Staining positivity for NFP and chromogranin A is significantly less frequent compared to pineocytomas [9,16,31]. There is no loss of SMARCB1/INI1 staining in pineoblastomas, a useful feature to distinguish them from atypical teratoid rhabdoid tumors [32]. Pineoblastoma is a neoplasm characterized by a high mean proliferation index, ranging from 16.9% to 50.1% [10,13,21,22]. It stands out as the most aggressive neoplasm of the pineal region, with frequent craniospinal dissemination and extracranial metastasis [3,17,33,34]. In older series, overall survival in pineoblastoma was reported to be as low as 1.3 years; however, recent studies indicate a better median overall survival time, reaching 4.1–8.7 years [35,36]. Negative prognostic predictors for pineoblastoma include disseminated disease at diagnosis, young age, and partial surgical resection [37]. The prognosis of pineoblastoma is extremely unfavorable, with patients often succumbing within two years from diagnosis [5].

From a cytogenetic perspective, structural alterations of chromosome 1 have been observed, and there may be losses of chromosomes [2,6,7,14,17] with some rare focal gains [22,38,39]. Reports also mention copy number variations and/or mutually exclusive mutations of DICER1, DROSHA, and DGCR8 [24,40–43]. DNA methylation profiling has identified four subgroups of pineoblastomas: miRNA processing altered type 1, miRNA processing altered type 2, RB1 altered, and MYC/FOXR activated [24,41,43]. These subgroups carry prognostic implications, with the miRNA processing altered type 2 subtype showing an overall good prognosis, while the outcomes of RB1-altered and the MYC/FOXR2-activated subgroups are notably poor.

3. Clinical Insights and Radiological Aspects

PPTID clinical presentation is not different from other PPTs and the main symptoms are linked to the increase in the intracranial pressure caused by obstructive hydrocephalus [44]. Developing hydrocephalus is a direct consequence of the extension of the tumor in the posterior part of the third ventricle and the obstruction of the cerebrospinal fluid flow through the acqueduct of Sylvius. Less common are symptoms from compression of the superior colliculus, with eye movement disorders such as Parinaud syndrome [3].

Also regarding radiological aspects, PPTIDs serve as a bridge entity between pineocytomas and pineoblastomas, exhibiting intermediate characteristics between the two. Pineocytomas commonly appear as well-defined, homogeneous masses measuring less than 3 cm on CT, exhibiting hypo- to isointense signal intensity on T1-weighted MRI sequences, and matching the intensity of brain parenchyma on T2-weighted sequences, occasionally with cystic or calcified areas [45,46]. In contrast, pineoblastomas are often larger and irregular, invading adjacent brain tissue, leading to hydrocephalus. On CT, they appear slightly hyperdense with post-contrast enhancement and possible calcifications. MRI findings for pineoblastomas include isointensity to hypointensity on T1-weighted images, isointensity on T2-weighted images with areas of cyst formation or necrosis, vivid heterogeneous enhancement on post-contrast T1 images, and restricted diffusion on DWI (diffusion weighted imaging)/ADC (Apparent Diffusion Coefficient) with ADC values around 400–800 mm^2/s [47]. In MR spectroscopy, an increase in choline and a decrease in N-acetylaspartate can be observed, with the possibility of detecting myoinositol. However, limited data exist regarding cerebral blood flow and cerebral blood volume, which may be increased in pineoblastomas [48].

The PPTIDs, being able to exhibit characteristic features of both the aforementioned tumors, typically present as well-defined, isodense to hyperdense masses on CT scans, often with observable calcifications, which, like all pineal parenchymal tumors, tend to be present and dispersed peripherally. On T1-weighted MRI, they appear isointense to slightly hyperintense, while T2-weighted images may show hyperintensity. Contrast-enhanced MRI may reveal heterogeneous enhancement [7]. PPTIDs may demonstrate local invasion and can obstruct cerebrospinal fluid flow, leading to obstructive hydrocephalus [49,50]. Heterogeneous signal intensity, reflecting variations in cellularity and tissue composition, and different patterns, such as lobulated or diffuse, may be observed [51].

4. Role of Neurosurgery

4.1. Management of Hydrocephalus

In the case of these tumors, obstructive hydrocephalus, a common issue with pineal region tumors, remains a primary concern at diagnosis. Addressing hydrocephalus promptly is essential. Treatment options include the use of a ventricular internal shunt or, preferably, an endoscopic third ventriculostomy (ETV) [52,53]. ETV is preferred because, in addition to relieving hydrocephalus, it offers the opportunity to perform a biopsy if the tumor protrudes into the posterior part of the third ventricle [54]. ETV is a safe procedure with a very low risk of complications, mostly related to the challenging control of potential bleeding in highly vascularized lesions [55].

4.2. Biopsy

Before engaging in multidisciplinary therapeutic discussions, obtaining tissue samples is of paramount importance. In many patients with hydrocephalus, a biopsy can be performed during the third ventriculostomy itself, particularly in cases of large tumors extending forward within the third ventricle cavity [53,56,57]. For other patients, a stereotactic biopsy is typically conducted under neuronavigation guidance [58]. However, performing biopsies in PRTs carries the risk of obtaining non-representative samples, especially in cases of mixed tumors containing different tumoral components [55,59]. Despite the complex venous anatomy in the vicinity (including the Galen vein and tributaries), the morbidity and mortality associated with PRT biopsies are comparable to those of other brain locations [60].

4.3. Surgical Excision

The primary approach for PPTIDs continues to be extensive microsurgical removal, considered the benchmark. This approach should always be discussed in a multidisciplinary setting, involving a neuro-oncologist, a radiation specialist, and a neurosurgeon. The choice of a specific surgical approach depends on the tumor's extensions in relation to the Galen venous complex and the surgeon's experience [61].

The most frequently utilized approaches during the past two decades have been the occipital transtentorial (OTT) and infratentorial supracerebellar (ITSC) approaches [62]. The suboccipital transtentorial approach is preferable for tumors extending upward and pushing the venous complex downward. Patients are typically positioned either sitting or in a three-quarter prone position (Park Bench). This approach provides direct access to the pineal region below the Galen venous complex. However, it requires delicate handling of bridging veins and carries a risk of visual field dysfunction and other complications [63].

The infratentorial supracerebellar approach offers a direct route for tumors extending posteriorly. It is often performed with the patient in a sitting position. This approach involves sacrificing one or two bridging veins between the superior surface of the cerebellum and the tentorium; this usually does not entail risks as these are expendable veins that do not drain the brainstem, although there is a minimal risk of cerebellar hemorrhage [64].

Various other surgical approaches are possible depending on the tumor's lateral or anterior extension within the third ventricle, each with its associated risks and benefits. However, these approaches should be carefully considered based on each patient's unique case.

5. Radiotherapy

Radiotherapy represents a cornerstone treatment in the multidisciplinary management of pineal parenchymal tumors. However, the rarity of the disease makes it difficult to define a standard treatment. Most of the evidence, especially in the adult population, derives from retrospective studies or small case series (Table 1).

Table 1. Studies involving PPTIDs and radiotherapy treatment. Type of radiotherapy treatment, the administered dose, and radiation-related toxicity are reported. Abbreviations: BT: brachitherapy; CSI: craniospinal irradiation; IMRT: intensity-modulated radiation therapy; SRS: stereotactic radiosurgery; WBI: whole brain irradiation; WVI: whole ventricular irradiation.

Article	RT	Technique	Dose	Radiotherapy Toxicity
Balossier et al. [65]	curative	SRS	SRS: 15.5 Gy (isodose 50%)	no
Kumar et al. [66]	adjuvant	1 CSI, 3 WBI	IMRT: 54 Gy, CSI: 36 Gy	no
Park et al. [67]	curative	2 SRS, 3 IMRT	SRS: 13.3 Gy (isodose 50%), IMRT 30 Gy/5 fr (isodose 80%)	not reported for PPTID
Hasegawa et al. [68]	salvage	1 SRS	mean marginal dose 14 Gy. maximum marginal doses 28 Gy	not reported for PPTID
Kunigelis et al. [44]	adjuvant, salvage	IMRT, SRS, CSI	not reported	not reported
Ito et al. [25]	adjuvant, salvage	4 IMRT, 1 CSI.	IMRT: 50 Gy/25 fr, CSI: 54.4/28 fr	1 decline in activities of daily living by radionecrosis
Watanabe et al. [69]	adjuvant, salvage	IMRT, CSI	IMRT: 54 Gy;CSI 36 Gy +18 Gy WVI	2 neurocognitive disorder, 2 hypopituitarism
Lu et al. [70]	adjuvant	IMRT	IMRT: 54 Gy	not reported
Iorio-Morin et al. [71]	curative, salvage	SRS	median marginal dose 17 Gy (isodose 50%), median maximum dose 34 Gy	focal neurological deficit 9%, parinaud syndrome 7%, hydrocephalus 3%
Raleigh et al. [72]	adjuvant, salvage	2 IMRT, 12 CSI	CSI: 36 Gy + 55.8 Gy boost on pineal gland or local RT on pineal region	Growth defects, endocrine dysfunction, infertility, cognitive deficits
Stoiber et al. [73]	adjuvant	IMRT	IMRT: 54 Gy	no
Lutterbach et al. [29]	adjuvant, curative	IMRT, SRS, I125BT	IMRT: 54 Gy.	not reported

Table 1. Cont.

Article	RT	Technique	Dose	Radiotherapy Toxicity
Choque-Velasquez et al. [74]	adjuvant, salvage	1 I125BTafter biopsy, 1 SRS, 6 IMRT, 2 unknown	IMRT: 54 Gy; SRS: 14 Gy	mild neuropsychologic deficits, depression, double vision
Nam et al. [75]	adjuvant	12 CSI (5 proton, 7 IMRT), 3 local RT (1proton, 2 SRS).	not reported	not reported
Chatterjee et al. [76]	adjuvant, salvage	IMRT	IMRT: 50–54 Gy, CSI: 36 Gy	not reported
Low, J.T. et al. [77]	adjuvant	IMRT	IMRT: 55.8–59.4 Gy/1.8 Gy: WVI 25.2 Gy + bed SRS boost 25.2 Gy + residual SRS boost 5.4–9 Gy	5 fatigue, 1 nausea, 1 alopecia, 1 hyponatriemia
Fauchon et al. [17]	adjuvant, curative	12 CSI, 8 WBI, 18 IMRT, 6 SRS	CSI: 31 Gy + boost, WBI 32.4 Gy + boost, IMRT: 78.8 Gy Gr. 2 and 53 Gy Gr. 3	1 radionecrosis in the talamus after SRS, 1 encephalitis after WBI

The spectrum of radiation therapy recommendations is quite broad, ranging from focal treatment to craniospinal irradiation, based on histology. Modern radiation techniques (radiosurgery or stereotactic radiotherapy, VMAT) offer the opportunity to tailor radiation dose to the tumor volume, sparing normal brain tissue with a deeper gradient dose between the target and surrounding organs at risk. Similarly, the wider spread of proton therapy might reduce radiation-induced toxicity, especially in craniospinal irradiation.

Historically, in well-differentiated pineocytomas, radiation therapy was used as focal treatment in recurrent disease. Recent studies using SRS as part of multimodal treatment or as salvage therapy with the administration of marginal doses ranging from 14 to 16 Gy show high local tumor control ranging from 80% to 100%, with PFS of 80–100% at 5 years (Table 2).

Table 2. Disease progression, recurrence, and survival outcomes in PPT patients. Abbreviations: CR: complete response; LC: local control; LR: local recurrence; OS: overall survival; PD: progression disease; PR: partial response; SD: stable disease.

Article	Patient Number	Median Follow Up Time (Months)	Local Control and Recurrence	Progression Free Surivival	Overall Survival
Balossier et al. [65]	12 (6 PPTID Gr. 2)	24	100% SD	not reported	not reported for PPTID
Kumar et al. [66]	14 (4 PPTID)	21.5	50% CR, 50% PR	not reported for PPTID	100% OS rate at reported follow up
Park et al. [67]	9 (5 PPTID)	78.6	40% CR, 60% PR	not reported	100% OS rate at reported follow up
Hasegawa et al. [68]	16 (2 PPTID)	61	33.3% CR, 16.67% PR, 16.67% SD	not reported	100% OS rate at reported follow up
Kunigelis et al. [44]	9 PPTID: 5 Gr. 2, 4 Gr. 3	95.3	22.2%LC (60% Gr. 2—100% Gr. 3 recurrence)	50.5 months	100% OS rate at 5 years follow up
Ito et al. [25]	6 PPTID	41	66.7% CR, 16.7% PD	50% after mean 3 years	83.33% OS rate at reported follow up
Watanabe et al. [69]	5 PPTID	not reported	60% CR, 40% PR, 40% PD	72.9 months	median OS 94.1 months
Lu et al. [70]	103 PPTID: 63 Gr. 2, 40 Gr. 3	49–75	not reported	not reported	OS rate at 1–2–5 year: 70%–58%–54%,
Iorio-Morin et al. [71]	70 (7 PPTID)	47	50% LC	34 months	OS rate at 5 years follow up: 56%

Table 2. Cont.

Article	Patient Number	Median Follow Up Time (Months)	Local Control and Recurrence	Progression Free Surivival	Overall Survival
Raleigh et al. [72]	75 (18 PPTID: 10 Gr. 2, 8 Gr. 3)	49	16.67% recurrence: 10% Gr. 2, 25% Gr. 3	82% and 65% after 5 and 10 years	OS rate at 5–10 years: 76% and 61%
Stoiber et al. [73]	14 (1PPTID)	84	100% LC	PPTID free from relapse after 84mo	100% OS rate at reported follow up
Lutterbach et al. [29]	101 (37 PPTID)	38	3–5–10 years LC 86%–79%–53%. 3–5–10 years Spinal control 93%–92%–81%	93 months	median OS 165 months
Choque-Velasquez et al. [74]	15 PPTID	39-248	66.7% CR, 20% PR	33.3% at last follow up	OS rate at 5–10 years: 92% and 71%
Nam et al. [75]	17 PPTID	62.6	43.75% recurrence	20.9 months	OS rate at 5 years follow up: 64.7%
Chatterjee et al. [76]	16 PPTID: 6 Gr. 2, 10 Gr. 3	12–127	Gr. 3: 20% LR, 10% Spinal recurrence. Gr. 2 LC 100%	3–127 months	81.25% OS at reported follow up (100% Gr. 2, 70% Gr. 3)
Low, J.T. et al. [77]	5 PPTID Gr. 3	min 36	60% PD	not reported	60% OS rate at reported follow up
Fauchon et al. [17]	76 (28 PPTID, 27 Gr. 2, 20 Gr. 3)	85	Gr. 2–Gr. 3: 26%–56% recurrence	51 months	OS rate at 5 years follow up: 74% Gr. 2, 39% Gr. 3

Mori et al. [78] reported in six pineocytoma patients treated with SRS a PFS of 80% at 5 years; Lekovic et al. [79] achieved 100% local tumor control in eight patients with a mean follow up ranging from 2 to 56 months. In the series by Wilson et al. [80], five patients with subtotally resected pineocytoma underwent SRS as adjuvant therapy in three cases and as curative treatment in two cases with local tumor control at 65 months, without any toxicity. A multicentric retrospective large series on pineal tumors reported a local control rate of 80% at 20 years for 26 pineocytomas [71].

On the other hand, in aggressive pineoblastomas, due to the high risk of cerebrospinal dissemination, craniospinal irradiation represents the standard adjuvant treatment in combination with chemotherapy, with a total dose of 24–36 Gy to the entire craniospinal axis and a tumor boost to 54–55.8 Gy in 1.8–2 Gy fractions.

Recently, a cohort analysis on 201 adult patients with pineoblastoma from the SEER database (1975–2016) was published [81], showing that radiation treatment improves 5-year OS regardless of surgical treatment (5-year OS of 77.3% in the radiotherapy group versus 63.2% in the no-radiotherapy group). In this context, adjuvant radiotherapy improves local tumor control and overall survival.

The role of radiation therapy remains unclear in the management of the subgroup of pineal tumors of intermediate differentiation (PPTID), due to the lack of evidence and heterogeneous biological behavior in grade 2–3 tumors. Table 1 summarizes the most relevant clinical series on PPTID patients.

Some reports tried to collect individual patient data from the literature to show clinical characteristics, patterns of care, survival outcomes connected to treatment strategy, and finally to find out prognostic factors to guide clinicians in clinical practice.

Mallick et al. in 2016 [51] published an individual patient data analysis, based on 29 retrospective studies involving 127 patients. Information regarding radiation treatment was available for 65 cases; adjuvant radiation therapy was employed in 46 cases. Most of the patients received local irradiation (32.6% of cases), 14 patients received craniospinal irradiation, 2 patients received whole ventricular irradiation, and 1 patient received whole brain irradiation. Radiosurgery was employed in four patients. Twenty-four patients had recurrence, including nine local and fifteen leptomeningeal. The 3-year PFS was 63.4%, and the 5-year PFS was 52.2%. Median overall survival was 14 years, with 3- and 5-year

OS values of 91% and 84.1%, respectively. In univariate analysis, female sex and adjuvant radiation were associated with better overall survival ($p = 0.009$), with a median OS of 252 months in irradiated patients versus 168 months in the untreated group.

In summary, the management of PPTID varies widely in the literature, including heterogeneous radiation treatment modalities concerning volume and doses, depending on local practices and physician preferences. Radiotherapy is commonly recommended for subtotally removed PPTID or as adjuvant therapy in grade 3 tumors.

Concerning the optimal treatment volume, a prevalent approach involves focal irradiation covering the surgical bed, residual disease, and all areas of suspected infiltration, utilizing modern high-gradient techniques. The total dose typically ranges from 54 to 59.4 Gy in conventional fractionation. Whole ventricle irradiation has been explored to reduce the risk of spinal metastases while mitigating the adverse effects associated with craniospinal irradiation (CSI), considering PPTID's malignancy level between pineocytoma and pineoblastoma.

Justin T. Low et al. [77] treated five adult patients with grade 3 PPTID using adjuvant radiotherapy after resection, incorporating whole ventricle irradiation up to 25.2 Gy in 1.8 Gy daily fractions delivered with IMRT. This was followed by a stereotactic boost to the resection bed of 25.2 Gy and a second boost to the residual tumor of 5.5–9 Gy, reaching a total dose of 55.8 Gy–59.4 Gy. Three of the five patients experienced favorable outcomes, while three had progressive disease, resulting in two deaths. These findings suggest the feasibility of reduced-dose ventricular irradiation for treating PPTIDs.

According to Tsubasa Watanabe et al. [69], whole ventricle irradiation (WVI) might also have a role in association with CSI in PPTIDs with spinal dissemination. Two of five patients in their retrospective review had cerebrospinal dissemination at diagnosis and underwent biopsy-only surgery followed by 36 Gy of CSI + 18 Gy of WVI. Although the median relapse-free and overall survival were 72.9 and 94.1 months, respectively (three complete responses, two partial responses and two recurrences after treatment), some patients experienced cerebral white matter abnormalities and cognitive disturbance due to the association with CSI.

6. Conclusions

Surgical removal, when feasible, remains the primary treatment for PPTIDs, providing the potential for a curative outcome. However, due to the complexity of these tumors and their anatomical location, these procedures necessitate skilled surgeons and meticulous preoperative planning to optimize outcomes. In cases where complete excision is not achievable, a biopsy approach, whether stereotactic or otherwise, becomes essential to consider a radiation treatment plan. Radiation therapy assumes a pivotal role, especially in higher-grade lesions. The evolution of modern techniques, such as stereotactic radiosurgery and proton therapy, offers tailored approaches to optimize efficacy while minimizing collateral damage.

Author Contributions: Conceptualization, A.B. and C.M.; methodology, B.L.Z.; investigation, A.D.T., B.L.Z. and F.P.; writing—original draft preparation, A.D.T., B.L.Z. and F.P.; writing—review and editing, A.B., L.B. and C.M.; supervision, F.C., D.G., P.C. and U.R. All authors have read and agreed to the published version of the manuscript.

Funding: This research received no external funding.

Institutional Review Board Statement: Not applicable.

Informed Consent Statement: Not applicable.

Data Availability Statement: No new data were generated in this study.

Conflicts of Interest: The authors declare no conflicts of interest.

References

1. Louis, D.N.; Perry, A.; Wesseling, P.; Brat, D.J.; Cree, I.A.; Figarella-Branger, D.; Hawkins, C.; Ng, H.K.; Pfister, S.M.; Reifenberger, G.; et al. The 2021 WHO Classification of Tumors of the Central Nervous System: A summary. *Neuro-Oncology* **2021**, *23*, 1231–1251. [CrossRef]
2. Jouvet, A.; Derrington, E.; Pialat, J.; Lapras, C.; Fèvre-Montagne, M.; Besançon, R.; Belin, M.F.; Saint-Pierre, G. Structural and ultrastructural characteristics of human pineal gland, and pineal parenchymal tumors. *Acta Neuropathol.* **1994**, *88*, 334–348. [CrossRef] [PubMed]
3. Gras, E.; Catasus, L.; Argü, R.; Moreno-Bueno, G.; Palacios, J.; Gamallo, C.; Matias-Guiu, X.; Prat, J. Pineal Parenchymal Tumors Clinical, Pathologic, and Therapeutic Aspects. *Cancer* **1993**, *72*, 870–880. [CrossRef]
4. Rahmanzade, R.; Pfaff, E.; Banan, R.; Sievers, P.; Suwala, A.K.; Hinz, F.; Bogumil, H.; Cherkezov, A.; Kaan, A.F.; Schrimpf, D. Genetical and epigenetical profiling identifies two subgroups of pineal parenchymal tumors of intermediate differentiation (PPTID) with distinct molecular, histological and clinical characteristics. *Acta Neuropathol.* **2023**, *146*, 853–856. [CrossRef] [PubMed]
5. Borit, A.; Blackwood, W.; Mair, W.G.P. The Separation of Pineocytoma from Pineoblastoma. *Cancer* **1980**, *45*, 1408–1418. [CrossRef] [PubMed]
6. Scheithauer, B.W. Pathobiology of the pineal gland with emphasis on parenchymal tumors. *Brain Tumor Pathol.* **1999**, *16*, 1–9. [CrossRef] [PubMed]
7. Chiechi, M.V.; Smirniotopoulos, J.G.; Mena, H. Pineal Parenchymal Tumors. *J. Comput. Assist. Tomogr.* **1995**, *19*, 509–517. [CrossRef] [PubMed]
8. Schild, S.E.; Scheithauer, B.W.; Haddock, M.G.; Wong, W.W.; Lyons, M.K.; Marks, L.B.; Norman, M.G.; Burger, P.C. Histologically confirmed pineal tumors and other germ cell tumors of the brain. *Cancer* **1996**, *78*, 2564–2571. [CrossRef]
9. Jouvet, A.; Saint-Pierre, G.; Fauchon, F.; Privat, K.; Bouffet, E.; Ruchoux, M.; Chauveinc, L.; Fèvre-Montagne, M. Pineal Parenchymal Tumors: A Correlation of Histological Features with Prognosis in 66 Cases. *Brain Pathol.* **2000**, *10*, 49–60. [CrossRef]
10. Fèvre-Montagne, M.; Szathmari, A.; Champier, J.; Mokhtari, K.; Chrétien, F.; Coulon, A.; Figarella-Branger, D.; Polivka, M.; Varlet, P.; Uro-Coste, E.; et al. Pineocytoma and Pineal Parenchymal Tumors of Intermediate Differentiation Presenting Cytologic Pleomorphism: A Multicenter Study. *Brain Pathol.* **2008**, *18*, 354–359. [CrossRef]
11. Kanno, H.; Nishihara, H.; Oikawa, M.; Ozaki, Y.; Murata, J.; Sawamura, Y.; Kato, M.; Kubota, K.; Tanino, M.; Kimura, T.; et al. Expression of O^6-methylguanine DNA methyltransferase (MGMT) and immunohistochemical analysis of 12 pineal parenchymal tumors. *Neuropathology* **2012**, *32*, 647–653. [CrossRef]
12. Fauchon, F. Utility of Ki67 immunostaining in the grading of pineal parenchymal tumours: A multicentre study. *Neuropathol. Appl. Neurobiol.* **2012**, *38*, 87–94.
13. Arivazhagan, A.; Anandh, B.; Santosh, V.; Chandramouli, B. Pineal parenchymal tumors—Utility of immunohistochemical markers in prognostication. *Clin. Neuropathol.* **2008**, *27*, 325–333. [CrossRef] [PubMed]
14. Kuchelmeister, K.; Gullotta, F.; von Borcke, I.M.; Klein, H.; Bergmann, M. Pleomorphic pineocytoma with extensive neuronal differentiation: Report of two cases. *Acta Neuropathol.* **1994**, *88*, 448–453. [CrossRef] [PubMed]
15. Numoto, R.T. Pineal parenchymal tumors: Cell differentiation and prognosis. *J. Cancer Res. Clin. Oncol.* **1994**, *120*, 683–690. [CrossRef] [PubMed]
16. Yamane, Y.; Mena, H.; Nakazato, Y. Immunohistochemical characterization of pineal parenchymal tumors using novel monoclonal antibodies to the pineal body. *Neuropathology* **2002**, *22*, 66–76. [CrossRef] [PubMed]
17. Fauchon, F.; Jouvet, A.; Paquis, P.; Saint-Pierre, G.; Mottolese, C.; Ben Hassel, M.; Chauveinc, L.; Sichez, J.-P.; Philippon, J.; Schlienger, M.; et al. Parenchymal pineal tumors: A clinicopathological study of 76 cases. *Endocrine* **2000**, *46*, 959–968. [CrossRef]
18. Clark, A.J.; Sughrue, M.E.; Ivan, M.E.; Aranda, D.; Rutkowski, M.J.; Kane, A.J.; Chang, S.; Parsa, A.T. Factors influencing overall survival rates for patients with pineocytoma. *J. Neuro-Oncol.* **2010**, *100*, 255–260. [CrossRef] [PubMed]
19. Santagata, S.; Maire, C.L.; Idbaih, A.; Geffers, L.; Correll, M.; Holton, K.; Quackenbush, J.; Ligon, K.L. CRX Is a Diagnostic Marker of Retinal and Pineal Lineage Tumors. *PLoS ONE* **2009**, *4*, e7932. [CrossRef] [PubMed]
20. Manila, A.; Mariangela, N.; Libero, L.; Francesca, G.; Romana, B.F.; Felice, G. Is CRX Protein a Useful Marker in Differential Diagnosis of Tumors of the Pineal Region? *Pediatr. Dev. Pathol.* **2014**, *17*, 85–88. [CrossRef]
21. Fukuda, T.; Akiyama, N.; Ikegami, M.; Takahashi, H.; Sasaki, A.; Oka, H.; Komori, T.; Tanaka, Y.; Nakazato, Y.; Akimoto, J.; et al. Expression of Hydroxyindole-O-Methyltransferase Enzyme in the Human Central Nervous System and in Pineal Parenchymal Cell Tumors. *J. Neuropathol. Exp. Neurol.* **2010**, *69*, 498–510. [CrossRef] [PubMed]
22. Rickert, C.H.; Simon, R.; Bergmann, M.; Dockhorn-Dworniczak, B.; Paulus, W. Comparative genomic hybridization in pineal germ cell tumors. *J. Neuropathol. Exp. Neurol.* **2000**, *59*, 815–821. [CrossRef] [PubMed]
23. Bello, M.; Rey, J.A.; de Campos, J.M.; Kusak, M. Chromosomal abnormalities in a pineocytoma. *Cancer Genet. Cytogenet.* **1993**, *71*, 185–186. [CrossRef] [PubMed]
24. Pfaff, E.; Aichmüller, C.; Sill, M.; Stichel, D.; Snuderl, M.; Karajannis, M.A.; Schuhmann, M.U.; Schittenhelm, J.; Hasselblatt, M.; Thomas, C.; et al. Molecular subgrouping of primary pineal parenchymal tumors reveals distinct subtypes correlated with clinical parameters and genetic alterations. *Acta Neuropathol.* **2020**, *139*, 243–257. [CrossRef] [PubMed]

25. Ito, T.; Kanno, H.; Sato, K.-I.; Oikawa, M.; Ozaki, Y.; Nakamura, H.; Terasaka, S.; Kobayashi, H.; Houkin, K.; Hatanaka, K.; et al. Clinicopathologic Study of Pineal Parenchymal Tumors of Intermediate Differentiation. *World Neurosurg.* **2014**, *81*, 783–789. [CrossRef] [PubMed]
26. Tsumanuma, I.; Tanaka, R.; Washiyama, K. Clinicopathological study of pineal parenchymal tumors: Correlation between histopathological features, proliferative potential, and prognosis. *Brain Tumor Pathol.* **1999**, *16*, 61–68. [CrossRef]
27. Yu, T.; Sun, X.; Wang, J.; Ren, X.; Lin, N.; Lin, S. Twenty-seven cases of pineal parenchymal tumours of intermediate differentiation: Mitotic count, Ki-67 labelling index and extent of resection predict prognosis. *J. Neurol. Neurosurg. Psychiatry* **2016**, *87*, 386–395. [CrossRef]
28. Zhu, L.; Ren, G.; Li, K.; Liang, Z.; Tang, W.; Ji, Y.; Li, Y.; Cheng, H.; Geng, D. Pineal Parenchymal Tumours: Minimum Apparent Diffusion Coefficient in Prediction of Tumour Grading. *J. Int. Med. Res.* **2011**, *39*, 1456–1463. [CrossRef]
29. Lutterbach, J.; Fauchon, F.; Schild, S.E.; Chang, S.M.; Pagenstecher, A.; Volk, B.; Ostertag, C.; Momm, F.; Jouvet, A. Malignant Pineal Parenchymal Tumors in Adult Patients: Patterns of Care and Prognostic Factors. *Neurosurgery* **2002**, *51*, 44–56. [CrossRef]
30. Lee, J.C.; Mazor, T.; Lao, R.; Wan, E.; Diallo, A.B.; Hill, N.S.; Thangaraj, N.; Wendelsdorf, K.; Samuel, D.; Kline, C.N.; et al. Recurrent KBTBD4 small in-frame insertions and absence of DROSHA deletion or DICER1 mutation differentiate pineal parenchymal tumor of intermediate differentiation (PPTID) from pineoblastoma. *Acta Neuropathol.* **2019**, *137*, 851–854. [CrossRef]
31. Mena, H.; Rushing, E.J.; Ribas, J.L.; Delahunt, B.; Mccarthy, W.F. Tumors of pineal parenchymal cells: A correlation of histological features, including nucleolar organizer regions, with survival in 35 cases. *Hum. Pathol.* **1995**, *26*, 20–30. [CrossRef]
32. Miller, S.; Ward, J.H.; Rogers, H.A.; Lowe, J.; Grundy, R.G. Loss of INI1 Protein Expression Defines a Subgroup of Aggressive Central Nervous System Primitive Neuroectodermal Tumors. *Brain Pathol.* **2013**, *23*, 19–27. [CrossRef]
33. Herrick, M.K.; Rubinstein, L.J. The cytological differentiating potential of pineal parenchymal neoplasms (true pinealomas). A clinicopathological study of 28 tumours. *Brain* **1979**, *102*, 289–320. [CrossRef]
34. Garibotto, F.; Pavanello, M.; Milanaccio, C.; Gaggero, G.; Fiaschi, P. Management of hydrocephalus related to diffuse leptomeningeal glioneuronal tumour: A multifaceted condition. *Child's Nerv. Syst.* **2021**, *37*, 1039–1040. [CrossRef]
35. Jakacki, R.I.; Burger, P.C.; Kocak, M.; Boyett, J.M.; Goldwein, J.; Mehta, M.; Packer, R.J.; Tarbell, N.J.; Pollack, I.F. Outcome and prognostic factors for children with supratentorial primitive neuroectodermal tumors treated with carboplatin during radiotherapy: A report from the Children's Oncology Group. *Pediatr. Blood Cancer* **2015**, *62*, 776–783. [CrossRef]
36. Farnia, B.; Allen, P.K.; Brown, P.D.; Khatua, S.; Levine, N.B.; Li, J.; Penas-Prado, M.; Mahajan, A.; Ghia, A.J. Clinical Outcomes and Patterns of Failure in Pineoblastoma: A 30-Year, Single-Institution Retrospective Review. *World Neurosurg.* **2014**, *82*, 1232–1241. [CrossRef]
37. Tate, M.; Sughrue, M.E.; Rutkowski, M.J.; Kane, A.J.; Aranda, D.; McClinton, L.; Barani, I.J.; Parsa, A.T. The long-term postsurgical prognosis of patients with pineoblastoma. *Cancer* **2012**, *118*, 173–179. [CrossRef] [PubMed]
38. Brown, A.E.; Leibundgut, K.; Niggli, F.K.; Betts, D.R. Cytogenetics of pineoblastoma: Four new cases and a literature review. *Cancer Genet. Cytogenet.* **2006**, *170*, 175–179. [CrossRef] [PubMed]
39. Miller, S.; Rogers, H.A.; Lyon, P.; Rand, V.; Adamowicz-Brice, M.; Clifford, S.C.; Hayden, J.T.; Dyer, S.; Pfister, S.; Korshunov, A.; et al. Genome-wide molecular characterization of central nervous system primitive neuroectodermal tumor and pineoblastoma. *Neuro-Oncology* **2011**, *13*, 866–879. [CrossRef] [PubMed]
40. de Kock, L.; Sabbaghian, N.; Druker, H.; Weber, E.; Hamel, N.; Miller, S.; Choong, C.S.; Gottardo, N.G.; Kees, U.R.; Rednam, S.P.; et al. Germ-line and somatic DICER1 mutations in pineoblastoma. *Acta Neuropathol.* **2014**, *128*, 583–595. [CrossRef] [PubMed]
41. Snuderl, M.; Kannan, K.; Pfaff, E.; Wang, S.; Stafford, J.M.; Serrano, J.; Heguy, A.; Ray, K.; Faustin, A.; Aminova, O.; et al. Recurrent homozygous deletion of DROSHA and microduplication of PDE4DIP in pineoblastoma. *Nat. Commun.* **2018**, *9*, 2868. [CrossRef]
42. Li, B.K.; Vasiljevic, A.; Dufour, C.; Yao, F.; Ho, B.L.B.; Lu, M.; Hwang, E.I.; Gururangan, S.; Hansford, J.R.; Fouladi, M.; et al. Pineoblastoma segregates into molecular sub-groups with distinct clinico-pathologic features: A Rare Brain Tumor Consortium registry study. *Acta Neuropathol.* **2020**, *139*, 223–241. [CrossRef] [PubMed]
43. Liu, A.P.Y.; Gudenas, B.; Lin, T.; Orr, B.A.; Klimo, P.; Kumar, R.; Bouffet, E.; Gururangan, S.; Crawford, J.R.; Kellie, S.J.; et al. Risk-adapted therapy and biological heterogeneity in pineoblastoma: Integrated clinico-pathological analysis from the prospective, multi-center SJMB03 and SJYC07 trials. *Acta Neuropathol.* **2020**, *139*, 259–271. [CrossRef]
44. Kunigelis, K.E.; Kleinschmidt-DeMasters, B.; Youssef, A.S.; Lillehei, K.O.; Ormond, D.R. Clinical Features of Pineal Parenchymal Tumors of Intermediate Differentiation (PPTID): A Single-Institution Series. *World Neurosurg.* **2021**, *155*, e229–e235. [CrossRef]
45. Fakhran, S.; Escott, E. Pineocytoma Mimicking a Pineal Cyst on Imaging: True Diagnostic Dilemma or a Case of Incomplete Imaging? *Am. J. Neuroradiol.* **2008**, *29*, 159–163. [CrossRef] [PubMed]
46. Banks, K.P.; Brown, S.J. AJR Teaching File: Solid Masses of the Pineal Region. *Am. J. Roentgenol.* **2006**, *186*, S233–S235. [CrossRef] [PubMed]
47. Korogi, Y.; Takahashi, M.; Ushio, Y. MRI of pineal region tumors. *J. Neuro-Oncol.* **2001**, *54*, 251–261. [CrossRef]
48. Tamrazi, B.; Nelson, M.; Blüml, S. Pineal Region Masses in Pediatric Patients. *Neuroimaging Clin. N. Am.* **2017**, *27*, 85–97. [CrossRef]
49. Morello, A.; Bianconi, A.; Cogoni, M.; Borgarello, S.; Garbossa, D.; Micon, B.M. Bilateral idiopathic optic nerve sheath meningocele: A case report and literature review. *J. Neurosci. Rural. Pr.* **2022**, *13*, 781–784. [CrossRef]

60. MWebb, M.; Johnson, D.R.; Mahajan, A.; Brown, P.; Neth, B.; Kizilbash, S.H.; Sener, U. Clinical experience and outcomes in patients with pineal parenchymal tumor of intermediate differentiation (PPTID): A single-institution analysis. *J. Neuro-Oncol.* **2022**, *160*, 527–534. [CrossRef]
61. Mallick, S.; Benson, R.; Rath, G. Patterns of care and survival outcomes in patients with pineal parenchymal tumor of intermediate differentiation: An individual patient data analysis. *Radiother. Oncol.* **2016**, *121*, 204–208. [CrossRef] [PubMed]
62. Aruta, G.; Fiaschi, P.; Ceraudo, M.; Piatelli, G.; Capra, V.; Bianconi, A.; Rossi, A.; Secci, F.; Pavanello, M. Practical Algorithm for the Management of Multisutural Craniosynostosis with Associated Chiari Malformation and/or Hydrocephalus. *Pediatr. Neurosurg.* **2023**, *58*, 67–79. [CrossRef]
63. Roth, J.; Constantini, S. Combined rigid and flexible endoscopy for tumors in the posterior third ventricle. *J. Neurosurg.* **2015**, *122*, 1341–1346. [CrossRef] [PubMed]
64. Morgenstern, P.F.; Souweidane, M.M. Pineal Region Tumors: Simultaneous Endoscopic Third Ventriculostomy and Tumor Biopsy. *World Neurosurg.* **2013**, *79*, S18.e9–S18.e13. [CrossRef] [PubMed]
65. Abbassy, M.; Aref, K.; Farhoud, A.; Hekal, A. Outcome of single-trajectory rigid endoscopic third ventriculostomy and biopsy in the management algorithm of pineal region tumors: A case series and review of the literature. *Child's Nerv. Syst.* **2018**, *34*, 1335–1344. [CrossRef]
66. Hua, W.; Xu, H.; Zhang, X.; Yu, G.; Wang, X.; Zhang, J.; Pan, Z.; Zhu, W. Pure endoscopic resection of pineal region tumors through supracerebellar infratentorial approach with 'head-up' park-bench position. *Neurol. Res.* **2023**, *45*, 354–362. [CrossRef] [PubMed]
67. Malara, N.; Guzzi, G.; Mignogna, C.; Trunzo, V.; Camastra, C.; Della Torre, A.; Di Vito, A.; Lavecchia, A.M.; Gliozzi, M.; Ceccotti, C.; et al. Non-invasive real-time biopsy of intracranial lesions using short time expanded circulating tumor cells on glass slide: Report of two cases. *BMC Neurol.* **2016**, *16*, 127. [CrossRef] [PubMed]
68. De Marco, R.; Pesaresi, A.; Bianconi, A.; Zotta, M.; Deandreis, D.; Morana, G.; Zeppa, P.; Melcarne, A.; Garbossa, D.; Cofano, F. A Systematic Review of Amino Acid PET Imaging in Adult-Type High-Grade Glioma Surgery: A Neurosurgeon's Perspective. *Cancers* **2022**, *15*, 90. [CrossRef]
69. Bianconi, A.; Bonada, M.; Zeppa, P.; Colonna, S.; Tartara, F.; Melcarne, A.; Garbossa, D.; Cofano, F. How Reliable Is Fluorescence-Guided Surgery in Low-Grade Gliomas? A Systematic Review Concerning Different Fluorophores. *Cancers* **2023**, *15*, 4130. [CrossRef]
70. Gaab, M.R.; Schroeder, H.W.S. Neuroendoscopic approach to intraventricular lesions. *J. Neurosurg.* **1998**, *88*, 496–505. [CrossRef]
71. Tomita, T.; Alden, T.D.; Dipatri, A.J. Pediatric pineal region tumors: Institutional experience of surgical managements with posterior interhemispheric transtentorial approach. *Child's Nerv. Syst.* **2023**, *39*, 2293–2305. [CrossRef]
72. Little, K.M.; Friedman, A.H.; Fukushima, T. Surgical approaches to pineal region tumors. *J. Neuro-Oncol.* **2001**, *54*, 287–299. [CrossRef]
73. Shepard, M.J.; Haider, A.S.; Prabhu, S.S.; Sawaya, R.; DeMonte, F.; McCutcheon, I.E.; Weinberg, J.S.; Ferguson, S.D.; Suki, D.; Fuller, G.N.; et al. Long term outcomes following surgery for pineal region tumors. *J. Neuro-Oncol.* **2022**, *156*, 491–498. [CrossRef]
74. Cavalheiro, S.; Valsechi, L.C.; Dastoli, P.A.; Nicácio, J.M.; Cappellano, A.M.; da Silva, N.S.; da Costa, M.D.S. Outcomes and surgical approaches for pineal region tumors in children: 30 years' experience. *J. Neurosurg. Pediatr.* **2023**, *32*, 184–193. [CrossRef]
75. Balossier, A.; Blond, S.; Touzet, G.; Sarrazin, T.; Lartigau, E.; Reyns, N. Role of radiosurgery in the management of pineal region tumours: Indications, method, outcome. *Neurochirurgie* **2015**, *61*, 216–222. [CrossRef] [PubMed]
76. Kumar, N.; Srinivasa, G.Y.; Madan, R.; Salunke, P. Role of radiotherapy in residual pineal parenchymal tumors. *Clin. Neurol. Neurosurg.* **2018**, *166*, 91–98. [CrossRef]
77. Park, J.H.; Kim, J.H.; Kwon, D.H.; Kim, C.J.; Khang, S.K.; Cho, Y.H. Upfront Stereotactic Radiosurgery for Pineal Parenchymal Tumors in Adults. *J. Korean Neurosurg. Soc.* **2015**, *58*, 334–340. [CrossRef] [PubMed]
78. Hasegawa, T.; Kondziolka, D.; Hadjipanayis, C.G.; Flickinger, J.C.; Lunsford, L.D. The Role of Radiosurgery for the Treatment of Pineal Parenchymal Tumors. *Neurosurgery* **2002**, *51*, 880–889. [CrossRef] [PubMed]
79. Watanabe, T.; Mizowaki, T.; Arakawa, Y.; Iizuka, Y.; Ogura, K.; Sakanaka, K.; Miyamoto, S.; Hiraoka, M. Pineal parenchymal tumor of intermediate differentiation: Treatment outcomes of five cases. *Mol. Clin. Oncol.* **2014**, *2*, 197–202. [CrossRef] [PubMed]
70. Lu, V.M.; Luther, E.M.; Eichberg, D.G.; Morell, A.A.; Shah, A.H.; Komotar, R.J.; Ivan, M.E. Prognosticating survival of pineal parenchymal tumors of intermediate differentiation (PPTID) by grade. *J. Neuro-Oncology* **2021**, *155*, 165–172. [CrossRef] [PubMed]
71. Iorio-Morin, C.; Kano, H.; Huang, M.; Lunsford, L.D.; Simonová, G.; Liscak, R.; Cohen-Inbar, O.; Sheehan, J.; Lee, C.-C.; Wu, H.-M.; et al. Histology-Stratified Tumor Control and Patient Survival After Stereotactic Radiosurgery for Pineal Region Tumors: A Report From the International Gamma Knife Research Foundation. *World Neurosurg.* **2017**, *107*, 974–982. [CrossRef]
72. Raleigh, D.R.; Solomon, D.A.; Lloyd, S.A.; Lazar, A.; Garcia, M.A.; Sneed, P.K.; Clarke, J.L.; McDermott, M.W.; Berger, M.S.; Tihan, T.; et al. Histopathologic review of pineal parenchymal tumors identifies novel morphologic subtypes and prognostic factors for outcome. *Neuro-Oncology* **2017**, *19*, 78–88. [CrossRef]
73. Stoiber, E.M.; Schaible, B.; Herfarth, K.; Schulz-Ertner, D.; E Huber, P.; Debus, J.; Oertel, S. Long term outcome of adolescent and adult patients with pineal parenchymal tumors treated with fractionated radiotherapy between 1982 and 2003—A single institution's experience. *Radiat. Oncol.* **2010**, *5*, 122. [CrossRef]

74. Choque-Velasquez, J.; Resendiz-Nieves, J.C.; Jahromi, B.R.; Colasanti, R.; Raj, R.; Tynninen, O.; Collan, J.; Hernesniemi, J. Pineal Parenchymal Tumors of Intermediate Differentiation: A long-Term Follow-Up Study in Helsinki Neurosurgery. *World Neurosurg.* **2019**, *122*, e729–e739. [CrossRef]
75. Nam, J.Y.; Gilbert, A.; Cachia, D.; Mandel, J.; Fuller, G.N.; Penas-Prado, M.; de Groot, J.; Kamiya-Matsuoka, C. Pineal parenchymal tumor of intermediate differentiation: A single-institution experience. *Neuro-Oncology Pr.* **2020**, *7*, 613–619. [CrossRef] [PubMed]
76. Chatterjee, D.; Lath, K.; Singla, N.; Kumar, N.; Radotra, B.D. Pathologic Prognostic Factors of Pineal Parenchymal Tumor of Intermediate Differentiation. *Appl. Immunohistochem. Mol. Morphol.* **2019**, *27*, 210–215. [CrossRef]
77. Low, J.T.; Kirkpatrick, J.P.; Peters, K.B. Pineal Parenchymal Tumors of Intermediate Differentiation Treated With Ventricular Radiation and Temozolomide. *Adv. Radiat. Oncol.* **2022**, *7*, 100814. [CrossRef]
78. Mori, Y.; Kobayashi, T.; Hasegawa, T.; Yoshida, K.; Kida, Y. Stereotactic radiosurgery for pineal and related tumors. *Prog. Neurol. Surg.* **2009**, *23*, 106–118. [CrossRef]
79. Lekovic, G.P.; Gonzalez, L.F.; Shetter, A.G.; Porter, R.W.; Smith, K.A.; Brachman, D.; Spetzler, R.F. Role of Gamma Knife surgery in the management of pineal region tumors. *Neurosurg. Focus* **2007**, *23*, E11. [CrossRef]
80. Wilson, D.A.; Awad, A.-W.; Brachman, D.; Coons, S.W.; McBride, H.; Youssef, E.; Nakaji, P.; Shetter, A.G.; Smith, K.A.; Spetzler, R.F.; et al. Long-term radiosurgical control of subtotally resected adult pineocytomas. *J. Neurosurg.* **2012**, *117*, 212–217. [CrossRef]
81. Mehkri, Y.; Gendreau, J.L.; Fox, K.; Hameed, N.F.; Jimenez, M.A.; Mukherjee, D. Radiotherapy Is Associated with Improved Overall Survival in Adult Pineoblastoma: A SEER Database Analysis. *World Neurosurg.* **2023**, *172*, e312–e318. [CrossRef] [PubMed]

Disclaimer/Publisher's Note: The statements, opinions and data contained in all publications are solely those of the individual author(s) and contributor(s) and not of MDPI and/or the editor(s). MDPI and/or the editor(s) disclaim responsibility for any injury to people or property resulting from any ideas, methods, instructions or products referred to in the content.

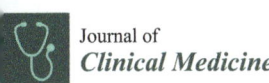

Review

Primary Intracranial Gliosarcoma: Is It Really a Variant of Glioblastoma? An Update of the Clinical, Radiological, and Biomolecular Characteristics

Domenico La Torre [1,*], Attilio Della Torre [1], Erica Lo Turco [1,*], Prospero Longo [1], Dorotea Pugliese [2], Paola Lacroce [1], Giuseppe Raudino [2], Alberto Romano [2], Angelo Lavano [1] and Francesco Tomasello [2]

[1] Department of Medical and Surgery Sciences, School of Medicine, AOU "Renato Dulbecco", University of Catanzaro, 88100 Catanzaro, Italy; a.dellatorre@unicz.it (A.D.T.); lngpsp97b07a225j@studenti.unime.it (P.L.); paola.lacroce@studenti.unime.it (P.L.); lavano@unicz.it (A.L.)

[2] Humanitas, Istituto Clinico Catanese, 95045 Catania, Italy; dorotea.pugliese@humanitascatania.it (D.P.); giuraudino@hotmail.it (G.R.); alberto.romano@ccocatania.it (A.R.); ftomasel@unime.it (F.T.)

* Correspondence: dlatorre@unicz.it (D.L.T.); ltrrce93h55c616t@studenti.unime.it (E.L.T.); Tel.: +39-0961-3647206 (D.L.T.)

Abstract: Gliosarcomas (GS) are sporadic malignant tumors classified as a Glioblastoma (GBM) variant with IDH-wild type phenotype. It appears as a well-circumscribed lesion with a biphasic, glial, and metaplastic mesenchymal component. The current knowledge about GS comes from the limited literature. Furthermore, recent studies describe peculiar characteristics of GS, such as hypothesizing that it could be a clinical–pathological entity different from GBM. Here, we review radiological, biomolecular, and clinical data to describe the peculiar characteristics of PGS, treatment options, and outcomes in light of the most recent literature. A comprehensive literature review of PubMed and Web of Science databases was conducted for articles written in English focused on gliosarcoma until 2023. We include relevant data from a few case series and only a single meta-analysis. Recent evidence describes peculiar characteristics of PGS, suggesting that it might be a specific clinical–pathological entity different from GBM. This review facilitates our understanding of this rare malignant brain tumor. However, in the future we recommend multi-center studies and large-scale metanalyses to clarify the biomolecular pathways of PGS to develop new specific therapeutic protocols, different from conventional GBM therapy in light of the new therapeutic opportunities.

Keywords: primary gliosarcoma; overall survival; glioblastoma; IDH; MGMT; hTERT

Citation: La Torre, D.; Della Torre, A.; Lo Turco, E.; Longo, P.; Pugliese, D.; Lacroce, P.; Raudino, G.; Romano, A.; Lavano, A.; Tomasello, F. Primary Intracranial Gliosarcoma: Is It Really a Variant of Glioblastoma? An Update of the Clinical, Radiological, and Biomolecular Characteristics. *J. Clin. Med.* **2024**, *13*, 83. https://doi.org/10.3390/jcm13010083

Academic Editor: Chunsheng Kang

Received: 22 October 2023
Revised: 14 December 2023
Accepted: 18 December 2023
Published: 22 December 2023

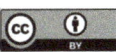

Copyright: © 2023 by the authors. Licensee MDPI, Basel, Switzerland. This article is an open access article distributed under the terms and conditions of the Creative Commons Attribution (CC BY) license (https://creativecommons.org/licenses/by/4.0/).

1. Introduction

Gliosarcoma (GS) was first described by Ströebe in 1895, but its acceptance and complete understanding developed later thanks to the detailed description provided by Feigen and Gross in 1955. They were the first to recognize three malignant brain tumors composed of two different tissues: one of glial origin, similar to Glioblastoma, and the other of mesenchymal origin, with characteristics reminiscent of spindle cell sarcomas [1–3]. In the 2000 World Health Organization (WHO) Classification, GS was first recognized as a variant of GBM [4]. In 2016 and 2021, WHO successfully classified GS as a variant of GBM with IDH-wild type phenotype [5,6]. Effectively, the radiological, biomolecular, and clinical features reported in the literature about GS are similar to those of GBM. GS is described as a rare form of neoplasm with an inferior prognosis [7]. Its incidence varies between 1% and 8% of all malignant gliomas, representing only 0.48% of all brain tumors and from 1.8% to 2.8% of cases of GBM [2,7–9]. GS are most common in adults, with a median age of diagnosis of 60 years, with a male predilection (M:F 1.8:1). In pediatric individuals, it is scarce. With regard to ethnicity, it is more frequent in the white and non-Hispanic races [1,2,8,10,11]. This type of cancer can occur in both primary and secondary forms, with the latter thought of arising from previously treated GBM. From a therapeutic point of view, the commonly used strategy is the same adopted for GBM, or the Stupp protocol, which involves the administration of TMZ concomitantly with RT [2,12,13]. Nevertheless, without any treatment, the prognosis of GS is inferior, with a median survival of approximately four months [9]. While with standard treatments, survival for GS remains still poor, with a median survival of 9 months, compared to other forms of GBM associated with an average of 15 months survival [9,14,15]. Moreover, the most recent literature suggests that GS may have neuroradiological, histological, and biomolecular characteristics that differ from GBM [8,11,16]. Given ongoing debate and uncertainty, we conducted an updated systematic review of the relevant literature to evaluate the possibility that GS may be a distinct entity from GBM, with its own peculiar radiological, biomolecular, and clinical patterns, to push research to develop more specific and effective treatments able to improve overall survival (OS).

2. Materials and Methods

2.1. Protocol, Search Strategy, and Study Selection

The systematic review was performed per the Preferred Reporting Items for Systematic Reviews and Meta-Analysis (PRISMA) guidelines. At first, a comprehensive literature review of the databases PubMed and Web of Science was conducted over the past 20 years (2013–2023) using search terms relevant to the different topics: "(high-grade glioma [MeSH Terms])", "(gliosarcoma [MeSH Terms]) or (genetic alterations [MeSH Terms])" combined with "globlastoma [MeSH Terms])", including articles focused on gliosarcoma until 2023. Subsequently, given the small number of articles published in GS and the relatively few cases reported per study, all manuscripts published between 1988 and 2023 were considered. Therefore, we identified 1023 manuscripts. Among these, after reading the title and abstract, we assessed the eligibility of 41 studies. One of these documents was later excluded because it was written in Chinese. Ultimately, we included 40 relevant studies, all written in English. (Figure 1) Summary of all the studies included in the systematic literature review are shown in Table 1.

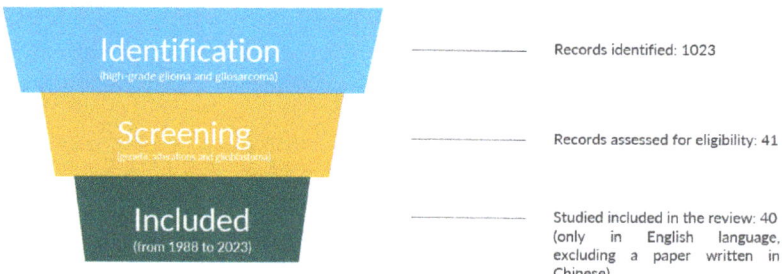

Figure 1. PRISMA flow diagram of included studies.

Table 1. Summary of studies included in the systematic literature review.

No.	Author, Journal, Year	Title	Type of Study	Study Period	Sample Size	Area of Interest
1	Oh et al. 2016 [17]	Genetic Alterations in Gliosarcoma and Giant Cell Glioblastoma.	Case series	N/A	55	Biomolecular
2	Saadeh et al. 2019 [9]	Prognosis and management of gliosarcoma patients: A review of literature.	Review	Up to 2019	N/A	Characteristic, prognosis and management

Table 1. Cont.

No.	Author, Journal, Year	Title	Type of Study	Study Period	Sample Size	Area of Interest
3	Tauziède-Espariat et al. 2018 [18]	Cerebellar high-grade gliomas do not present the same molecular alterations as supratentorial high-grade gliomas and may show histone H3 gene mutations.	Retrospective study	1982–2016	19	Biomolecular
4	Li et al. 2021 [19]	Genetic alteration and clonal evolution of primary glioblastoma into secondary gliosarcoma.	Case Report	2016	1	Biomolecular
5	Esteban-Rodríguez et al. 2023 [20]	Cytological features of diffuse and circumscribed gliomas.	Review	N/A	N/A	Biomolecular
6	Sahu et al. 2022 [21]	Rat and Mouse Brain Tumor Models for Experimental Neuro-Oncology Research.	Review	N/A	N/A	Characteristics and biomolecular
7	Zaki et al. 2021 [2]	Genomic landscape of gliosarcoma: distinguishing features and targetable alterations.	Scientific Reports	N/A	30	Biomolecular
8	Kleihues et al. 2000 [22]	Phenotype vs. genotype in the evolution of astrocytic brain tumors.	Case series	N/A	N/A	Genetics and biomolecular
9	Wang et al. 2017 [23]	Gliosarcomas with the BRAFV600E mutation: a report of two cases and review of the literature.	Case report	N/A	2	Biomolecular
10	Bax et al. 2009 [24]	EGFRvIII deletion mutations in pediatric high-grade glioma and response to targeted therapy in pediatric glioma cell lines.	Retrospective study	N/A	90	Biomolecular
11	Reis et al. 2000 [25]	Genetic profile of gliosarcomas.	Short communication	N/A	19	Genetics and biomolecular
12	Cheng et al. 2022 [26]	Gliosarcoma: The Distinct Genomic Alterations Identified by Comprehensive Analysis of Copy Number Variations.	Retrospective study	2016–2019	36	Genetics and biomolecular
13	Lowder et al. 2019 [27]	Gliosarcoma: distinct molecular pathways and genomic alterations identified by DNA copy number/SNP microarray analysis.	Metanalysis	2014–2015	18	Genetics and biomolecular
14	Codispoti et al. 2014 [28]	Genetic and pathologic evolution of early secondary gliosarcoma.	Case report	N/A	1	Genetics and biomolecular
15	Anderson et al. 2020 [29]	Molecular and clonal evolution in recurrent metastatic gliosarcoma.	Case report	N/A	1	Characteristics and biomolecular
16	Garber et al. 2016 [30]	Immune checkpoint blockade as a potential therapeutic target: surveying CNS malignancies.	Retrospective analysis	2009–2016	347	Biomolecular and prognosis

Table 1. Cont.

No.	Author, Journal, Year	Title	Type of Study	Study Period	Sample Size	Area of Interest
17	Pierscianek et al. 2021 [31]	Demographic, radiographic, molecular and clinical characteristics of primary gliosarcoma and differences to glioblastoma.	Retrospective cohort study	2001–2018	56	Clinical, prognosis and neuroradiological features
18	Walker et al. 2001 [32]	Characterisation of molecular alterations in microdissected archival gliomas.	Retrospective analysis	N/A	47	Genetics and biomolecular
19	Hiniker et al. 2013 [33]	Gliosarcoma arising from an oligodendroglioma (oligosarcoma).	Case report	N/A	1	Biomolecular, clinical
20	Dejonckheere et al. 2022 [34]	Chasing a rarity: a retrospective single-center evaluation of prognostic factors in primary gliosarcoma.	Retrospective study	1995–2021	26	Clinical features, treatment and prognosis
21	Chen et al. 2022 [35]	Gliosarcoma with osteosarcomatous component: A case report and short review illustration.	Case report+ Review	1950–2022	13	Biomolecular, neuroradiology, treatment and prognosis
22	Nagaishi et al. 2012 [36]	Amplification of the STOML3, FREM2, and LHFP genes is associated with mesenchymal differentiation in gliosarcoma.	Case series	N/A	74	Biomolecular
23	Boerman et al. 1996 [37]	The glial and mesenchymal elements of gliosarcomas share similar genetic alterations.	Case series	N/A	5	Genetics and biomolecular
24	Schwetye et al. 2016 [38]	Gliosarcomas lack BRAFV600E mutation, but a subset exhibit β-catenin nuclear localization.	Case series	N/A	48	Biomolecular
25	Cho et al. 2017 [39]	High prevalence of TP53 mutations is associated with poor survival and an EMT signature in gliosarcoma patients.	Comparative analyses	N/A	103	Biomolecular
26	Actor et al. 2002 [40]	Comprehensive analysis of genomic alterations in gliosarcoma and its two tissue components.	Comprehensive analysis	N/A	38	Genetics and biomolecular
27	Sargen et al. 2023 [41]	Estimated Prevalence, Tumor Spectrum, and Neurofibromatosis Type 1-Like Phenotype of CDKN2A-Related Melanoma-Astrocytoma Syndrome.	Retrospective cohort study	1976–2020	640 292	Genetics and biomolecular
28	Gondim et al. 2019 [42]	Determining IDH-Mutational Status in Gliomas Using IDH1-R132H Antibody and Polymerase Chain Reaction.	Case series	N/A	62	Biomolecular
29	Reis et al. 2005 [43]	Molecular characterization of PDGFR-alpha/PDGF-A and c-KIT/SCF in gliosarcomas.	Case series	N/A	160	Biomolecular
30	Tabbarah et al. 2012 [44]	Identification of t(1;19) (q12;p13) and ploidy changes in an ependymosarcoma: a cytogenetic evaluation.	Case report	N/A	1	Genetics and biomolecular

Table 1. Cont.

No.	Author, Journal, Year	Title	Type of Study	Study Period	Sample Size	Area of Interest
31	Knobbe et al. 2003 [45]	Genetic alterations and aberrant expression of genes related to the phosphatidyl-inositol-3′-kinase/protein kinase B (Akt) signal transduction pathway in glioblastomas.	Comparative Study	N/A	103	Genetics and biomolecular
32	Bigner et al. 1988 [46]	Specific chromosomal abnormalities in malignant human gliomas.	Case series	1981–1986	54	Genetics and biomolecular
33	Jimenez et al. 2011 [47]	Sarcoma arising as a distinct nodule within glioblastoma: a morphological and molecular perspective on gliosarcoma.	Case report	N/A	1	Biomolecular
34	Albrecht et al. 1993 [48]	Distribution of p53 protein expression in gliosarcomas: an immunohistochemical study.	Case series	N/A	8	Biomolecular
35	Lusis et al. 2010 [49]	Glioblastomas with giant cell and sarcomatous features in patients with Turcot syndrome type 1: a clinicopathological study of 3 cases.	Case report	1996–2010	3	Biomolecular
36	Visani et al. 2017 [50]	Non-canonical IDH1 and IDH2 mutations: a clonal and relevant event in an Italian cohort of gliomas classified according to the 2016 World Health Organization (WHO) criteria.	Multicenter study	N/A	288	Genetics and biomolecular
37	Barnett et al. 2004 [51]	Intra-arterial delivery of endostatin gene to brain tumors prolongs survival and alters tumor vessel ultrastructure.	Prospective study	N/A	344	Genetics, treatment and prognosis
38	Bigner et al. 1988 [52]	Gene amplification in malignant human gliomas: clinical and histopathologic aspects. J Neuropathol Exp Neurol.	Retrospective study	N/A	64	Genetics, biomolecular and clinical features
39	Koelsche et al. 2013 [53]	Distribution of TERT promoter mutations in pediatric and adult tumors of the nervous system.	Systematic analysis	N/A	1515	Genetics and biomolecular
40	Venkatraj et al. 1998 [54]	Genomic changes in glioblastoma cell lines detected by comparative genomic hybridization.	Comparative Study	N/A	5	Biomolecular

2.2. Data Collection and Analysis

After screening and reviewing the studies, we searched and extracted the following information: author, country, journal, title, and year of publication; design and period in which the population was collected; sample size, mean, and age range; genetic and biomolecular data; clinical features, including mild symptoms to more severe conditions; number and percentages of metastases, radiological features, treatment options including surgery, adjuvant radiation therapy (RT), chemotherapy, and other adjuvant therapies; follow-up period; and prognosis and outcome.

3. Radiological Features: GS vs. GBM

GS may have some radiological characteristics that can help to distinguish it from GBM. These features include well-demarcated margins, solid-cystic components, the salt and pepper (S–P) sign (a crescent-shaped area of enhancement at the junction of the solid and cystic components), an uneven rim- and a ring-like or paliform enhancement (P-E) patterns enhancement, intra-tumoral strip enhancement, involvement of deep structures such as the thalamus, brainstem, and spinal cord. In addition, GS may also present with other radiological findings, such as midline shift, mass effect, and calcifications [3,11]. However, although they are typical radiological features of GS, similar radiological features can also be observed in several brain tumors, including GBM and high-grade gliomas (HGG) [3,11,55,56].

Yi et al. [55], in their radiological analysis, found that the degree of tumor wall thickening tends to be more significant in GS compared to GBM. Moreover, GS, unlike GBM, seems to have a higher rate of bleeding, S–P signs, an eccentric cystic portion (ECP), and a P-E pattern. In their 48 patients, they found that GS tumors are typically larger than GBM tumors, with more areas of enhancement. Unlike GBM, GS tumors are more likely to involve the brain's cortex and are less likely to have necrosis, invade the ependyma, and cause edema that crosses the brain's midline [55]. Moreover, a higher percentage of eccentric tumor cysts in GS was found (19/48, 39.6%) [12].

Zhang et al. [11], in their retrospective single-center study focused on 103 GS, found that 67 tumors were single lesions, and 31 were cystic, solid lesions. All GS showed marked enhancement, and most tumors showed it in functional areas. Notably, 35, 4, 15, 13, and 22 patients showed a pattern of enhancement in the thalamus, brainstem, motor available cortex, sensory functional cortex, and the ependyma of the lateral ventricle, respectively. On T2WI MRI sequences, the average edema diameter was calculated at 7.90 cm (range, 3.55–12.88 cm), and the median tumor diameter evaluated by contrast-enhanced T1WI was 4.84 cm (range, 1.58–8.73 cm) [11]. Tumors involved the frontal, parietal, temporal, or multiple lobes in 18, 6, 29, and 40 patients. While only in 5 patients, the tumors were located in different areas (thalamus, ventricle, brainstem, and spinal cord). Similar results have been reported by Xi et al. [55]. In their series of 48 patients, GS was mainly located in the temporal lobe (27%), frontal lobe (17%), and ventricles (10%), while more rarely in the parieto-occipital lobes (2%), brainstem, and cerebellum (2%). Regarding the laterality, the right hemisphere is mainly affected [55].

Aya Fukuda et al. [57], in their report of three patients, described that at the CT scan, GS typically appears as an expansive lesion with well-delimited and irregular contours, associated with perilesional edema with a frequent hyperattenuating sign of the solid part. Regarding MRI on the T1- and T2-weighted sequences of MRI, GS were characterized as uneven, heterogeneous tumors correlated with bleeding at distinct stages with a hypo-isointense on T1 and as hypo/iso/hyperintense on T2 of the solid part. Similarly, the necrotic part was described as hypointense on T1 and hyperintense on T2. Inhomogeneous enhancement of the solid components occurred after the injection of gadolinium. The SWI or T2* sequence supplied other information; the variable magnetic susceptibility (high heterogeneity) areas showed hypointensity within the tumor due to bleeding or newly formed vessels/flow voids. On DWI/ADC mapping sequences, GSM has previously been associated with hyperintensity on DWI and hypointensity in the solid component on the ADC map (compatible with restricted diffusion) [57].

Han et al. [58]. classified two different subgroups of patients: one with tumors that resembled the characteristics of meningioma (meningioma-like) and the other that mimicked the appearance of GBM (GBM-like). The meningioma-like tumors displayed significant rim enhancement on MRI, and more of them demonstrated homogeneous enhancement compared to the GBM-like sub-group [58]. However, these findings were not found to be statistically significant [58]. Results are summarized in Table 2.

Table 2. Common radiological features in Gliosarcoma (GS) vs. Glioblastoma (GBM).

Radiological Features	Study	Result
Larger wall thickening GS > GBM.	Yi et al. (2018) [55]	Confirmed
Higher rate of bleeding, and S–P sign, presence of eccentric cystic portion (ECP) and a P-E pattern. GS > GBM.	Yi et al. (2018) [55]	Confirmed
Larger tumors with more areas of enhancement. GS > GBM	Yi et al. (2018) [55]	Confirmed
More likely to involve the brain's cortex. Less likely to have necrosis, to invade the ependyma and to cause edema that crosses the brain's midline. GS > GBM	Yi et al. (2018) [55]	Confirmed
Higher percentage of eccentric tumor cysts. GS > GBM	Yi et al. (2018) [55]	Confirmed
Marked enhancement, and most of tumors showing it in functional areas. GS > GBM	Zhang et al. (2021) [11]	Confirmed
GS: mainly located in temporal lobe (27%), frontal lobe (17%) and ventricles (10%); while more rarely in the parieto-occipital lobes (2%), brainstem and cerebellum (2%).	Zhang et al. (2021) [11]	Confirmed
Appearance as an expansive lesion with well-delimited and irregular contours, associated with perilesional edema with a frequent hyperattenuating sign of the solid part. GS > GBM	Aya Fukuda et al. (2020) [57]	Confirmed
Association with hyperintensity on DWI and hypointensity in the solid component on the ADC map (compatible with restricted diffusion). GS > GBM	Aya Fukuda et al. (2020) [57]	Confirmed

4. Genetics and Biomolecular Patters: GS vs. GBM

It has been observed that the monoclonal origin of GS would be associated with the p53 mutation, found in 23% of GS compared to 11% of primary GBM, and the deletion of p16. Epidermal Growth Factor Receptor (EGFR) amplification was only seen in 4% of GS compared to 35% of GBM [2,3,59,60].

There were slight differences between GBM and GS in Phosphatase and Tensin homolog (PTEN) mutations and Cyclin-dependent kinase (CDK) amplification found in both glial and sarcomatous components [61]. In addition, less than 12% of GS have methylation of the O6-methylguanine-DNA methyltransferase gene promoter (pMGMT), which is associated with a good prognosis [11].

From a biomolecular point of view, GS has mutations in common with soft tissue sarcoma due to involvement in the promoter of the Telomerase reverse transcriptase gene (pTERT), Tumor Protein 53 (TP53), Neurofibromin 1 (NF1), Cyclin-dependent kinase inhibitor 2A (CDKN2A), Cyclin-dependent kinase inhibitor 2B (CDKN2B) and Retinoblastoma associated Protein Type 1 (RB1) [60,62]. Similarly, to GBM, GS shows mutations in PTEN, EGFR, Stromal Antigen 2 (STAG2), and Protein Tyrosine Phosphatase Non-Receptor Type 11 (PTPN11) [7,9,11].

Sarcomatous-predominant GS has several features similar to meningioma. It is characterized by positivity to reticulin and the absence of GFAP expression, while predominant gliomatous GS has characteristics reminiscent of GBM, such as necrosis, lack of reticulin production, and GFAP positivity [8].

Zaki et al., in their study, compared common gene alteration, greater than 5%, in GS, GBM, and soft tissue sarcoma. Among these, GS shared only four genes with GBM, none with sarcomas, while nine common genes were found unique for GS amongst the 5% threshold for each respective tumor type [2]. They concluded that most of these mutations overlap with GBM and other cancers; nevertheless, GS has its own genetic mutations, such as MutS Homolog 6 (MSH6), B-Raf proto-oncogene serine/threonine kinase (BRAF), Suppressor of Zeste 12 (SUZ12), Sex Determining Region Y Box Transcription Factor 2 (SOX2), and Box and WD Repeat Domain Containing 7 (FBXW7) [2,7,11,16,60].

Nevertheless, it has been previously reported that, BRAF V600E mutation, SOX2 amplifications, and MSH6 mutation are present approximately in 3%, 10% and 20% of GBMs, respectively [16,63]. Results are summarized in Table 3.

Table 3. Common biomolecular markers in Gliosarcoma (GS) vs. Glioblastoma (GBM).

Biomolecular Markers	GS	GBM	Study
p53 mutation	23%	11%	Saadeh et al. (2019) [9] Wojtas et al. (2019) [60]
p16 deletion	37%	No	Saadeh et al. (2019) [9] Zaki et al. (2021) [2]
EGFR amplification	4%	35%	Romero et al. (2013) [3]
EGFR mutation	No	Yes	Zaki et al. (2021) [2]
PTEN mutation	(37%)	Yes	Saadeh et al. (2019) [9]
CDK amplification	Yes	Yes	Dardis et al. (2021) [16]
pMGMT methylation	<12%	Yes	Smith et al. (2018) [10]
pTERT mutation	Yes	Yes	Zaki et al. (2021) [2]
NF1 mutation	Yes	Yes	Zaki et al. (2021) [2]
CDKN2A/B mutation	Yes	Yes	Wojtas et al. (2019) [60]
RB1 mutation	Yes	Less common (~20%)	Wojtas et al. (2019) [60]
STAG2 mutation	Yes	Yes	Wojtas et al. (2019) [60]
PTPN11 mutation	Yes	Yes	Saadeh et al. (2019) [9]
Reticulin positivity	Sarcomatous-predominant GS	No	Han et al. (2010) [58]
GFAP expression	Gliomatosus-predominant GS	Yes	Han et al. (2010) [58]
MSH6 mutation L1244dup, T1133A	Yes	No	Zaki et al. (2021) [2]
BRAF mutation	10%	3%	Zaki et al. (2021) [2]
BRAF mutations (all alteration types)	10%	0%	Zaki et al. (2021) [2]
SUZ12 mutation	Yes	No	Zaki et al. (2021) [2]
SOX2 mutation	Yes	No	Zaki et al. (2021) [2]
FBXW7 mutation	Yes	No	Zaki et al. (2021) [2]

5. Clinical Features and Behavior

5.1. Clinical Characteristics

Han et al. [58] observed that clinical manifestations of GS are not specific. Still, it can manifest with intracranial hypertension syndrome characterized by symptoms ranging from headache, projectile vomiting, and hemiparesis up to more severe conditions such as the state of drowsiness and, finally, coma [58]. This symptomatology is due to the mass effect given by the tumor and the extensive peri-lesional edema or acute, intra-lesional, or more rarely peri-lesional symptomatic intracranial bleeding [11,58]. Other symptoms are asthenia, personality disorders, and mental confusion [10,58]. Moreover, depending on the site in which the tumor occurs, it can lead to different neurological deficits: language disorder (dysphasia, aphasia), sensory alterations, paresis of a part of the body, decreased visual acuity, and campimetric deficit [1,10].

5.2. Metastases

Saadeh et al. [9] observed that extracranial metastases from GS tend to be more frequent than from GBM and other malignant brain tumors, in which they are sporadic. Indeed, extracranial metastases were reported in 11% (range 0–16%) of GS, mainly including the lungs, liver, and lymph nodes, 72%, 41%, and 18%, respectively. While, more rarely, metastases occur in the spleen, adrenal glands, kidneys, oral mucosa, skin, bone marrow, skull, ribs, and spine [1,9,58,64].

Other organs affected may be the thyroid, pericardium, myocardium, diaphragm, pancreas, and stomach [1,9,58].

Moreover, it has been reported that metastatic foci of GS may have both gliomatous and sarcomatous components [9]. However, recent studies reported that the sarcomatous component was mainly represented. These findings may suggest that the sarcomatous component of GS is more likely to metastasize and disseminate by the hematogenous route than its gliomatous counterpart [9,10,58].

The development of metastasis from GS is established through numerous case reports, and the rate of metastasis found in the literature is about 11%. Despite the rarity of

PGS, these reports support the clinical experience that GS may have a more significant potential for metastasis than GBM [9,65]. Indeed, it has been suggested that due to the higher resistance of GS to current treatment compared to GBM, malignant cells that are not destroyed might become more aggressive, metaplastic, and, thus, angio-invasive [9,66].

6. Treatment and Prognosis

6.1. Surgical Strategy

The prognosis of GS is inferior, with a median survival of approximately four months without any treatment [9,14].

To date, no specific treatment for GS has been developed. Currently, standard GBM treatment is adopted for GS patients with good Karnofsky Performance Status (KPS) [16,67,68]. However, the most recent literature shows that GS presents different response patterns to therapies than GBM, thus hypothesizing that GS might be a different clinical–pathological entity [8,16,66].

Indeed, a Maximal Safe Resection (MSR) associated with a concomitant Radio- and Adjuvant Chemotherapy (CCRT) reduces the mortality rate in both cancers. Still, the response to treatments seems to be different in GS [12,13]. The peculiar biphasic, glial, and metaplastic mesenchymal components of GS might explain it.

Gross Total Resection (GTR) or Subtotal Resection (STR) when resection involves >90% but <100% of tumor tissue or biopsy are standard surgical treatments for GS [12,13]. GTR should be the option of choice. Nevertheless, GTR is almost always possible only in meningioma-like forms, while STR is often performed for GBM-like forms due to its invasive and infiltrative nature. In some cases, due to the location and extent of the lesion, the only viable strategy is stereotactic biopsy [9,12].

Therefore, the higher survival rate of meningioma-like tumors can be attributed to the higher GTR rate in this subtype, which correlates with OS. Due to its characteristics that mimic meningiomas, Sarcomatous GS appears well-delimited to the brain parenchyma; therefore, radical surgical resection is often possible. On the contrary, gliomatous GS, which usually infiltrates, even extensively, the surrounding parenchyma, makes radical excision much more challenging, so it is mainly treated with a STR surgery or biopsy [9].

Unlike GBM, 5-ALA (5-aminolevulinic acid) staining during fluorescence-guided surgery (FGS) in GS tends to assume a heterogenic fluorescence pattern, probably due to its biphasic component [12,16]. However, its role is still being studied [13].

Postoperative complications in GS surgery are similar to those of GBM, including transient or permanent neurological deficits, CSF fistula, surgical focus bleeding, seizure, stroke, and meningitis [12,58,66,69].

6.2. Radiotherapy

Only a few studies have evaluated radiotherapy's (RT) effectiveness in treating patients with GS [12,66]. A significant increase in OS has been observed with surgery followed by RT, which offers a higher outcome (8–15 weeks longer) than surgery alone [12]. Perry et al. confirmed this finding because, in their analysis, 25/32 patients treated with adjuvant radiotherapy had a higher survival rate (46 vs. 13 weeks; $p = 0.025$) [70]. Similar results were found in a study conducted by Castelli et al. [14]. Radiation therapy includes adjuvant external beam radiation therapy (EBRT) and Gamma Knife adjuvant radiosurgery [71]. The standard dose administered is 60 Gray (Gy) in 30 fractions, or another option may be hypofractionated radiation at 40 Gray (Gy) in 15 fractions [13,14,67]. Kozak et al. [7]. investigated the efficacy of radiotherapy in a large cohort of GS patients. In their study, the authors demonstrated that age, extent of resection, and adjuvant radiotherapy (RT) were the most significant predictors of OS. However, the metastatic potential of heavily irradiated tumors needs still to be further investigated. Finally, although the addition of chemotherapeutic agents does not appear to increase OS, it has been theorized that a higher dosage of chemotherapy could still increase survival in patients with GS compared to radiotherapy and surgery alone [14].

6.3. Bevacizumab

Bevacizumab, a recombinant monoclonal antibody targeting VEGF receptors on endothelial cells, has demonstrated significant anti-tumor activity in various colon, breast, pancreas, and prostate cancers [72]. Its potential in GBM, a highly vascularized tumor known to produce pro-angiogenic factors, was recognized [73]. Bevacizumab is thought to work by inhibiting the growth of new blood vessels that supply the tumor with oxygen and nutrients. This can lead to tumor shrinkage and a slowing of tumor growth. Bevacizumab can also reduce tumor-related edema, which can improve neurological symptoms [72]. Given the rationale that bevacizumab could hinder GBM and the progression of GS, it was administered to patients with primary gliosarcoma (PGS) and secondary gliosarcoma (SGS). PSG patients who received bevacizumab had improved progression-free survival (PFS) and OS of 4.2 and 8.4 months, respectively, at diagnosis [1]. SGS patient had a PFS of 3.8 months and an OS of 7.3 months [1]. Although the improved outcomes observed in these patients could be attributed to bevacizumab, particularly in recurrent GS, it is also possible that the study population, coming from a referral hospital and already enrolled in clinical trials, may have influenced the results.

6.4. Chemotherapy

Various chemotherapeutic agents have been used, and numerous researchers have studied the role and effectiveness of chemotherapy in treating patients with GS [12,13,59,64,74]. Although some studies have presented negative results, others could shed light on the benefits of specific chemotherapeutic agents. Over the years, various agents have been used, such as mitramycin (inhibitor of RNA synthesis), carmustine, administrated alone or together with other systemic agents such as diaziquone, mitomycin C, 6-mercaptopurine and cisplatin), and nitrosureas. These agents, whether used individually or in combination with each other or with radiotherapy, did not appear to have efficacy, either for GBM or GS.

6.5. Temozolamide (TZM)

TMZ is an effective treatment in malignant gliomas and still represents the most used chemotherapy drug to manage these tumors. However, although some studies have demonstrated the efficacy of TMZ in treating GS, its role as an effective treatment for GS is still debatable [7,9,12,13].

Indeed, while several studies have reported that TMZ may increase overall survival in patients with GS, others have documented no benefit in prognosis [9,12,14,66]. In their research, Castelli et al. recorded that TMZ, in addition to radiotherapy, effectively increases OS in GBM treatment but not in GS [14]. These findings may be due to the different MGMT methylation of GS compared to GBM. Indeed, GS has a lower rate of MGMT methylation compared to GBM, and this might explain the poor therapeutic response of GS to TMZ [14]. This hypothesis is also confirmed by Kang et al., who demonstrated that GS patients with MGMT methylation had more prolonged overall survival when treated with TMZ [75].

6.6. Immunotherapy

Immunotherapy for recurrent GBM, including patients with GS, has been addressed in a few trials. A phase II clinical trial (NCT02798496: CAPTIVE/KEYNOTE-192) evaluated the combination of DNX-2401, an oncolytic adenovirus, with the anti-PD-1 antibody pembrolizumab in patients with recurrent GBM or GS. In this trial, DNX-2401 is delivered directly inside the tumors by intravenous administration of pembrolizumab every three weeks for up to 2 years or until disease progression. Interim data from 42 patients showed a median OS of 12.3 months. This is favorable compared with the OS observed for standard-of-care agents lomustine and temozolomide, which had a median OS of 7.2 months. Four patients survived more than 23 months, and 11.9% (5/42) had durable responses. No dose-limiting toxicities were observed, and adverse events were mild to moderate and unrelated to DNX-2401 [76,77]. However, in the CAPTIVE study, 48 patients with histopathological diagnosis of GBM and only one gliosarcoma (2%) were enrolled; therefore, it is not possible to conclusively argue that there is a different therapeutic response between GBM and GS.

6.7. Combined Therapy

Summarizing the findings reported in the reviewed literature, treatment based on Gross Total Resection (GTR), followed by radio- and chemotherapy (TMZ), leads to an increased outcome compared to the single treatment (on average 8–10 months), while no improvements were seen between the dual therapy (TMZ + RT) and monotherapy (TMZ or RT) [9,10].

Castelli et al., in a large series of patients who were treated with a combination of surgery, TMZ, and radiotherapy, reported an average OS of 13 months, and 12% of patients achieved a 2-year OS [14].

Furthermore, Kozak et al. said similar results, showing a significant benefit in the prognosis of GS patients when treated with the multimodal approach. In their study, the authors demonstrated that tumor resection (not just biopsy) and adjuvant RT correlated with increased OS [7].

6.8. Prognosis and Outcome

GS owns various prognostic factors that differ from its parent tumor. Older patient age, poorer preoperative clinical status, larger tumor diameter, and tumor location in midline or infratentorial structures were independently associated with shorter OS in the GS cohort [78]. Age and clinical performance are known survival factors in both GS and GBM. The extent of resection (EOR) was not a prognostic factor in the GS cohort [79]. This finding contradicts the convincing data from GBM studies demonstrating the significant role of EOR on patient outcomes. This difference may be due to the small sample size of GS patients [11]. Furthermore, no independent association was found between combined RTX/CTX and GS prognosis. This finding may also be related to the lower MGMT promoter methylation rate in GS. Some studies have also reported lower MGMT promoter methylation rates in GS [11,64]. This difference between GS and GBM may contribute to the limited response of GS to combined treatment with CTX/RTX and TMZ. Other known outcome factors, such as age, preoperative clinical status, and RTX/CTX coadministration, were confirmed to be an independent predictor of survival [31,67].

7. Discussion

GS has long been considered a variant of GBM [4,6]. Still, according to our findings, some clinical, radiological, and biomolecular characteristics appear more frequent in GS than in GBM, thus hypothesizing the possibility of underlying differences between these two pathologies [13,16,31] (see Table 4). Analysis of the literature revealed that there were no differences between the two cancers regarding clinical characteristics, age, gender, and preoperative clinical status [31,58]. GS can be characterized by specific radiological features including well-demarcated margins, solid-cystic components, the salt and pepper sign (a crescent-shaped area of enhancement at the junction of the solid and cystic components), an uneven rim- and a ring-like or paliform enhancement (P-E) patterns enhancement, intra-tumoral strip enhancement, and involvement of deep structures such as the thalamus, brainstem, and spinal cord, but all these features may also be found in other malignant brain tumors, including GBM and high-grade gliomas [3,11,55]. Moreover, an eccentric cyst seems to be independently associated with the diagnosis of GS [12]. These typical radiological characteristics of GS may help to distinguish it from GBM.

Interestingly, recent data concerning biomolecular characteristics of GS documented that, although GS has a genetic profile that overlaps with GBM and other neoplasms, it is also true that GS has its genetic mutations, such as MSH6, BRAF, SUZ12, SOX2, and FBXW7 [2,3,10,11,16,80].

Table 4. Summary of common features in Gliosarcoma (GS) vs. Glioblastoma (GBM).

Feature	GS	GBM
Clinical presentation	Non-specific; can manifest with intracranial hypertension syndrome	Non-specific; can manifest with intracranial hypertension syndrome
Radiological features	Well-demarcated margins, solid-cystic components, salt and pepper sign, uneven rim- and ring-like enhancement patterns	Irregular margins, necrosis and peritumoral edema
Genetic profile	More likely to have p53 mutations and p16 deletions, less likely to have EGFR amplification and pMGMT methylation	p53 mutations, p16 deletions, PTEN mutations, CDK amplification, EGFR amplification, STAG2 mutations and PTPN11 mutations
Extracranial metastatic potential	More frequent (11%)	Extremely rare
Sites of metastases	Lungs (72%), liver (41%), lymph nodes (18%), spleen, adrenal glands, kidneys, oral mucosa, skin, bone marrow, skull, ribs and spine	N/A
Treatment	Maximum safe surgical resection followed by CCRT	Maximum safe surgical resection followed by CCRT
Prognosis	Worse than GBM	Poor

CCRT: chemo-radiotherapy.

Nevertheless, as reported in the literature, BRAF V600E mutation is present in 10% of GSs, compared to 3% of GBMs, while amplifications of the SOX2 gene and MSH6 mutation are present approximately in 10% and 20% of GBMs, respectively [16,63]. However, Zaki et al., in their recent study, reported that BRAF mutations (G32_A33duo, G466E, V600E protein alteration), MSH6 mutations (L1244dup, T1133A protein alteration), and SOX2 amplification (11% alteration frequency), are unique to GS [2].

This apparent contradiction could be due to the fact that in their study, Zaki et al. considered as common genetic alterations only those genes that were altered in more than 5% of the samples analyzed for each tumor type, with a minimum of genetic alteration in >2 samples. Therefore, although with some concerns, these specific biomolecular mutations could partially explain the different biological behavior, response to therapy, and prognosis of GS compared to GBM [9,14].

Previous studies have vaguely reported survival rates in patients with GBM and GS. While some studies did not find a significant difference in survival between the two tumors, others found a worse prognosis in patients with GS [14,15]. To some extent, heterogeneous landscapes with different distributions of genetic alterations in GBM and GS could explain these discrepant previous findings. In a multivariate analysis, histological diagnosis of GS was associated with a worse prognosis, independent of age, preoperative KPS, EOR, and postoperative treatment. This association is due to lower MGMT promoter methylation rates and lower frequency of IDH1 mutations in the GS cohort [7,13,81]. Indeed, after including only IDH1 wild-type patients in the analysis and MGMT promoter methylation, it was found that the histological diagnosis of GS was no longer associated with worse outcomes [9]. Furthermore, lower levels of GFAP and higher levels of TP53 staining predicted GS diagnosis [3,7,10].

Unlike GBM, GS appears to have a greater propensity to metastasize outside the central nervous system. Based on older studies, until 2007, it has been estimated that the frequency of metastases varies between 0.4% and 2.0%. However, the only two systematic reviews summarizing results published up to 2008 are partly conflicting; therefore, many relevant questions remained unanswered, including the rate of extracranial metastases. On the other hand, the available literature on this issue mainly reported that GSs are more prone to extracranial metastasis than GBM [1,9,58,64]. Furthermore, a recent meta-analysis including ten studies published between 2008 and 2018 said that extracranial metastases in GS were up to 11% and significantly higher than in GBM (11% versus 0.2–4.0%, respectively) [12].

Nevertheless, considering data reported in the available literature, the percentages of extracranial metastasis ranged from 0 to 16%.

From a therapeutic point of view, the literature data are speculative and inconclusive. Currently, the Stupp protocol is widely recommended for GS patients in clinical settings, involving radiotherapy and chemotherapy following surgery GBM. However, in GS, the response to the therapy is variable and different if compared to those of GBM. Radiotherapy has been proposed to enhance patient outcomes, as it can extend overall survival by 2–4 months [9,15,78,79]. TMZ still represents the most effective drug for malignant gliomas [67]. Despite this, there is an ongoing debate about the therapeutic benefits of RT and TMZ in GS, as there is no prospective or large scale analysis. It should stimulate further research into GS-targeted therapies.

8. Conclusions and Future Directions

Overall, the present review supports the hypothesis that GS is a rare yet devastating tumor with specific imaging, immunohistochemical, and clinical features that are more likely to occur when compared to GBM. This raises the possibility of distinguishing this disease from other malignant brain neoplasms. To date, the standard treatment for GS is similar to that most used to treat GBM, which involves surgery associated with adjuvant therapy, including RT, chemotherapy alone or in combination. It has been shown that maximum safe resection followed by radio and chemotherapy (TMZ) leads to a better outcome than a single treatment.

GTR (when possible) should be the option of choice among other surgical procedures, including subtotal resection (STR) or biopsy. On the other hand, different published studies documented that EOR was not a prognostic factor in GS patients. On the contrary, credible data from GBM studies demonstrate the significant role of EOR on patient outcomes. We believe that, similarly to other malignant brain tumors, GTR reduces the mortality rate in GS. But, due to the small sample size of patients, the peculiar biphasic, glial, and metaplastic mesenchymal, which sometimes makes it challenging to achieve a GTR, and the different response to treatments of GS compared to GBM may explain this apparent contradiction. Nevertheless, GS's prognosis is poorer than GBM's, and the optimal treatment for this rare neoplasm remains speculative. Moreover, we need more extensive prospective studies to evaluate new specific treatment regimens. It should stimulate further research into GS-targeted therapies. The results of the CAPTIVE/KEYNOTE-192 trial are promising but not definitive. However, it could open up possible future scenarios for developing effective and safe treatments for GS [76,77]. With some limitations, mainly due to the scarcity of data and the rarity of this tumor, which limits the relevant literature on the topic, this review could represent a valid background for designing future studies better to describe the characteristics of this rare and dismal malignancy. Therefore, we recommend multi-center studies and large-scale metanalyses to better elucidate typical features of GS, thus hypothesizing specific treatment regimens.

Funding: This research received no external funding.

Data Availability Statement: Not applicable.

Conflicts of Interest: The authors declare no conflict of interest.

References

1. Cachia, D.; Kamiya-Matsuoka, C.; Mandel, J.J.; Olar, A.; Cykowski, M.D.; Armstrong, T.S.; Fuller, G.N.; Gilbert, M.R.; De Groot, J.F. Primary and secondary gliosarcomas: Clinical, molecular and survival characteristics. *J. Neurooncol.* **2015**, *125*, 401–410. [CrossRef] [PubMed]
2. Zaki, M.M.; Mashouf, L.A.; Woodward, E.; Langat, P.; Gupta, S.; Dunn, I.F.; Wen, P.Y.; Nahed, B.V.; Bi, W.L. Genomic landscape of gliosarcoma: Distinguishing features and targetable alterations. *Sci. Rep.* **2021**, *11*, 18009. [CrossRef] [PubMed]
3. Romero-Rojas, A.E.; Diaz-Perez, J.A.; Ariza-Serrano, L.M.; Amaro, D.; Lozano-Castillo, A. Primary Gliosarcoma of the Brain: Radiologic and Histopathologic Features. *Neuroradiol. J.* **2013**, *26*, 639–648. [CrossRef] [PubMed]

4. Kleihues, P.; Louis, D.N.; Scheithauer, B.W.; Rorke, L.B.; Reifenberger, G.; Burger, P.C.; Cavenee, W.K. The WHO classification of tumors of the nervous system. *J. Neuropathol. Exp. Neurol.* **2002**, *61*, 215–225. [CrossRef] [PubMed]
5. Osborn, A.G.; Louis, D.N.; Poussaint, T.Y.; Linscott, L.L.; Salzman, K.L. The 2021 World Health Organization Classification of Tumors of the Central Nervous System: What Neuroradiologists Need to Know. *AJNR Am. J. Neuroradiol.* **2022**, *43*, 928–937. [CrossRef] [PubMed]
6. Wesseling, P.; Capper, D. WHO 2016 Classification of gliomas. *Neuropathol. Appl. Neurobiol.* **2018**, *44*, 139–150. [CrossRef]
7. Kozak, K.R.; Mahadevan, A.; Moody, J.S. Adult gliosarcoma: Epidemiology, natural history, and factors associated with outcome. *Neuro Oncol.* **2009**, *11*, 183–191. [CrossRef]
8. Han, S.J.; Yang, I.; Tihan, T.; Prados, M.D.; Parsa, A.T. Primary gliosarcoma: Key clinical and pathologic distinctions from glioblastoma with implications as a unique oncologic entity. *J. Neurooncol.* **2010**, *96*, 313–320. [CrossRef]
9. Saadeh, F.; El Iskandarani, S.; Najjar, M.; Assi, H.I. Prognosis and management of gliosarcoma patients: A review of the literature. *Clin. Neurol. Neurosurg.* **2019**, *182*, 98–103. [CrossRef]
10. Smith, D.R.; Wu, C.C.; Saadatmand, H.J.; Isaacson, S.R.; Cheng, S.K.; Sisti, M.B.; Bruce, J.N.; Sheth, S.A.; Lassman, A.B.; Iwamoto, F.M.; et al. Clinical and molecular characteristics of gliosarcoma and modern prognostic significance relative to conventional glioblastoma. *J. Neurooncol.* **2018**, *137*, 303–311. [CrossRef]
11. Zhang, Y.; Ma, J.P.; Weng, J.C.; Wang, L.; Wu, Z.; Li, D.; Zhang, J.-T. The clinical, radiological, and immunohistochemical characteristics and outcomes of primary intracranial gliosarcoma: A retrospective single-center study. *Neurosurg. Rev.* **2021**, *44*, 1003–1015. [CrossRef] [PubMed]
12. Wang, X.; Jiang, J.; Liu, M.; You, C. Treatments of gliosarcoma of the brain: A systematic review and meta-analysis. *Acta Neurol. Belg.* **2021**, *121*, 1789–1797. [CrossRef] [PubMed]
13. Hong, B.; Lalk, M.; Wiese, B.; Merten, R.; Heissler, H.E.; Raab, P.; Hartmann, C.; Krauss, J.K. Primary and secondary gliosarcoma: Differences in treatment and outcome. *Br. J. Neurosurg.* **2021**. [CrossRef] [PubMed]
14. Castelli, J.; Feuvret, L.; Haoming, Q.C.; Biau, J.; Jouglar, E.; Berger, A.; Truc, G.; Gutierrez, F.L.; Morandi, X.; Le Reste, P.J.; et al. Prognostic and therapeutic factors of gliosarcoma from a multi-institutional series. *J. Neurooncol.* **2016**, *129*, 85–92. [CrossRef] [PubMed]
15. Yu, Z.; Zhou, Z.; Xu, M.; Song, K.; Shen, J.; Zhu, W.; Wei, L.; Xu, H. Prognostic Factors of Gliosarcoma in the Real World: A Retrospective Cohort Study. *Comput. Math. Methods Med.* **2023**, *2023*, 1553408. [CrossRef] [PubMed]
16. Dardis, C.; Donner, D.; Sanai, N.; Xiu, J.; Mittal, S.; Michelhaugh, S.K.; Pandey, M.; Kesari, S.; Heimberger, A.B.; Gatalica, Z.; et al. Gliosarcoma vs. glioblastoma: A retrospective case series using molecular profiling. *BMC Neurol.* **2021**, *21*, 231. [CrossRef]
17. Oh, J.E.; Ohta, T.; Nonoguchi, N.; Satomi, K.; Capper, D.; Pierscianek, D.; Sure, U.; Vital, A.; Paulus, W.; Mittelbronn, M.; et al. Genetic Alterations in Gliosarcoma and Giant Cell Glioblastoma. *Brain Pathol.* **2016**, *26*, 517–522. [CrossRef] [PubMed]
18. Tauziède-Espariat, A.; Saffroy, R.; Pagès, M.; Pallud, J.; Legrand, L.; Besnard, A.; Lacombe, J.; Lot, G.; Borha, A.; Tazi, S.; et al. Cerebellar high-grade gliomas do not present the same molecularalterations as supratentorial high-grade gliomas and may show histone H3 genemutations. *Clin. Neuropathol.* **2018**, *37*, 209–216. [CrossRef]
19. Li, J.; Zhao, Y.H.; Tian, S.F.; Xu, C.S.; Cai, Y.X.; Li, K.; Cheng, Y.B.; Wang, Z.F.; Li, Z.Q. Genetic alteration and clonal evolution of primary glioblastoma into secondarygliosarcoma. *CNS Neurosci. Ther.* **2021**, *27*, 1483–1492. [CrossRef]
20. Esteban-Rodríguez, I.; López-Muñoz, S.; Blasco-Santana, L.; Mejías-Bielsa, J.; Gordillo, C.H.; Jiménez-Heffernan, J.A. Cytological features of diffuse andcircumscribed gliomas. *Cytopathology* **2023**. [CrossRef]
21. Sahu, U.; Barth, R.F.; Otani, Y.; McCormack, R.; Kaur, B. Rat and Mouse Brain Tumor Models for Experimental Neuro-Oncology Research. *J. Neuropathol. Exp. Neurol.* **2022**, *81*, 312–329. [CrossRef] [PubMed]
22. Kleihues, P.; Ohgaki, H. Phenotype vs genotype in the evolution of astrocytic brain tumors. *Toxicol. Pathol.* **2000**, *28*, 164–170. [CrossRef] [PubMed]
23. Wang, L.; Sun, J.; Li, Z.; Chen, L.; Fu, Y.; Zhao, L.; Liu, L.; Wei, Y.; Teng, L.; Lu, D. Gliosarcomas with the BRAFV600E mutation: A report of two cases and review of the literature. *J. Clin. Pathol.* **2017**, *70*, 1079–1083. [CrossRef] [PubMed]
24. Bax, D.A.; Gaspar, N.; Little, S.E.; Marshall, L.; Perryman, L.; Regairaz, M.; Viana-Pereira, M.; Vuononvirta, R.; Sharp, S.Y.; Reis-Filho, J.S.; et al. EGFRvIII deletion mutations in pediatric high-grade glioma and response to targeted therapy in pediatric glioma cell lines. *Clin. Cancer Res.* **2009**, *15*, 5753–5761. [CrossRef] [PubMed]
25. Reis, R.M.; Könü-Leblebicioglu, D.; Lopes, J.M.; Kleihues, P.; Ohgaki, H. Genetic profile of gliosarcomas. *Am. J. Pathol.* **2000**, *156*, 425–432. [CrossRef] [PubMed]
26. Cheng, C.D.; Chen, C.; Wang, L.; Dong, Y.F.; Yang, Y.; Chen, Y.N.; Niu, W.X.; Wang, W.C.; Liu, Q.S.; Niu, C.S. Gliosarcoma: The Distinct Genomic Alterations Identified by Comprehensive Analysis of Copy Number Variations. *Anal. Cell. Pathol.* **2022**, *2022*, 2376288. [CrossRef] [PubMed]
27. Lowder, L.; Hauenstein, J.; Woods, A.; Chen, H.R.; Rupji, M.; Kowalski, J.; Olson, J.J.; Saxe, D.; Schniederjan, M.; Neill, S.; et al. Gliosarcoma: Distinct molecular pathways and genomic alterations identified by DNA copy number/SNP microarray analysis. *J. Neurooncol.* **2019**, *143*, 381–392. [CrossRef] [PubMed]
28. Codispoti, K.E.; Mosier, S.; Ramsey, R.; Lin, M.T.; Rodriguez, F.J. Genetic and pathologic evolution of early secondary gliosarcoma. *Brain Tumor Pathol.* **2014**, *31*, 40–46. [CrossRef]
29. Anderson, K.J.; Tan, A.C.; Parkinson, J.; Back, M.; Kastelan, M.; Newey, A.; Brewer, J.; Wheeler, H.; Hudson, A.L.; Amin, S.B.; et al. Molecular and clonal evolution in recurrent metastatic gliosarcoma. *Cold Spring Harb. Mol. Case Stud.* **2020**, *6*, a004671. [CrossRef]

30. Garber, S.T.; Hashimoto, Y.; Weathers, S.P.; Xiu, J.; Gatalica, Z.; Verhaak, R.G.; Zhou, S.; Fuller, G.N.; Khasraw, M.; de Groot, J.; et al. Immune checkpoint blockade as a potential therapeutic target: Surveying CNS malignancies. *Neuro Oncol.* **2016**, *18*, 1357–1366. [CrossRef]
31. Pierscianek, D.; Ahmadipour, Y.; Michel, A.; Rauschenbach, L.; Oppong, M.D.; Deuschl, C.; Kebir, S.; Wrede, K.H.; Glas, M.; Stuschke, M.; et al. Demographic, radiographic, molecular, and clinical characteristics of primary gliosarcoma and differences to glioblastoma. *Clin. Neurol. Neurosurg.* **2021**, *200*, 106348. [CrossRef] [PubMed]
32. Walker, C.; Joyce, K.A.; Thompson-Hehir, J.; Davies, M.P.; Gibbs, F.E.; Halliwell, N.; Lloyd, B.H.; Machell, Y.; Roebuck, M.M.; Salisbury, J.; et al. Characterisation of molecular alterations in microdissected archival gliomas. *Acta Neuropathol.* **2001**, *101*, 321–333. [CrossRef] [PubMed]
33. Hiniker, A.; Hagenkord, J.M.; Powers, M.P.; Aghi, M.K.; Prados, M.D.; Perry, A. Gliosarcoma arising from an oligodendroglioma (oligosarcoma). *Clin. Neuropathol.* **2013**, *32*, 165–170. [CrossRef] [PubMed]
34. Dejonckheere, C.S.; Böhner, A.M.C.; Koch, D.; Schmeel, L.C.; Herrlinger, U.; Vatter, H.; Schneider, M.; Schuss, P.; Giordano, F.A.; Köksal, M.A. Chasing a rarity: A retrospective single-center evaluation of prognostic factors in primary gliosarcoma. *Strahlenther. Onkol.* **2022**, *198*, 468–474. [CrossRef] [PubMed]
35. Chen, Y.; Zhou, S.; Zhou, X.; Dai, X.; Wang, L.; Chen, P.; Zhao, S.; Shi, C.; Xiao, S.; Dong, J. Gliosarcoma with osteosarcomatous component: A case report and short review illustration. *Pathol. Res. Pract.* **2022**, *232*, 153837. [CrossRef]
36. Nagaishi, M.; Kim, Y.H.; Mittelbronn, M.; Giangaspero, F.; Paulus, W.; Brokinkel, B.; Vital, A.; Tanaka, Y.; Nakazato, Y.; Legras-Lachuer, C.; et al. Amplification of the STOML3, FREM2, and LHFP genes is associated with mesenchymal differentiation in gliosarcoma. *Am. J. Pathol.* **2012**, *180*, 1816–1823. [CrossRef]
37. Boerman, R.H.; Anderl, K.; Herath, J.; Borell, T.; Johnson, N.; Schaeffer-Klein, J.; Kirchhof, A.; Raap, A.K.; Scheithauer, B.W.; Jenkins, R.B. The glial and mesenchymal elements of gliosarcomas share similar genetic alterations. *J. Neuropathol. Exp. Neurol.* **1996**, *55*, 973–981. [CrossRef]
38. Schwetye, K.E.; Joseph, N.M.; Al-Kateb, H.; Rich, K.M.; Schmidt, R.E.; Perry, A.; Gutmann, D.H.; Dahiya, S. Gliosarcomas lack BRAF V600E mutation, but a subset exhibit β-catenin nuclear localization. *Neuropathology* **2016**, *36*, 448–455. [CrossRef]
39. Cho, S.Y.; Park, C.; Na, D.; Han, J.Y.; Lee, J.; Park, O.K.; Zhang, C.; Sung, C.O.; Moon, H.E.; Kim, Y.; et al. High prevalence of TP53 mutations is associated with poor survival and an EMT signature in gliosarcoma patients. *Exp. Mol. Med.* **2017**, *49*, e317. [CrossRef]
40. Actor, B.; Cobbers, J.M.; Büschges, R.; Wolter, M.; Knobbe, C.B.; Lichter, P.; Reifenberger, G.; Weber, R.G. Comprehensive analysis of genomic alterations in gliosarcoma and its two tissue components. *Genes Chromosomes Cancer* **2002**, *34*, 416–427. [CrossRef]
41. Sargen, M.R.; Kim, J.; Potjer, T.P.; Velthuizen, M.E.; Martir-Negron, A.E.; Odia, Y.; Helgadottir, H.; Hatton, J.N.; Haley, J.S.; Thone, G.; et al. Estimated Prevalence, Tumor Spectrum, and Neurofibromatosis Type 1-Like Phenotype of CDKN2A-Related Melanoma-Astrocytoma Syndrome. *JAMA Dermatol.* **2023**, *159*, 1112–1118. [CrossRef] [PubMed]
42. Gondim, D.D.; Gener, M.A.; Curless, K.L.; Cohen-Gadol, A.A.; Hattab, E.M.; Cheng, L. Determining IDH-Mutational Status in Gliomas Using IDH1-R132H Antibody and Polymerase Chain Reaction. *Appl. Immunohistochem. Mol. Morphol.* **2019**, *27*, 722–725. [CrossRef] [PubMed]
43. Reis, R.M.; Martins, A.; Ribeiro, S.A.; Basto, D.; Longatto-Filho, A.; Schmitt, F.C.; Lopes, J.M. Molecular characterization of PDGFR-alpha/PDGF-A and c-KIT/SCF in gliosarcomas. *Cell Oncol.* **2005**, *27*, 319–326. [CrossRef] [PubMed]
44. Tabbarah, A.Z.; Carlson, A.W.; Oviedo, A.; Ketterling, R.P.; Rodriguez, F.J. Identification of t(1;19)(q12;p13) and ploidy changes in an ependymosarcoma: A cytogenetic evaluation. *Clin. Neuropathol.* **2012**, *31*, 142–145. [CrossRef] [PubMed]
45. Knobbe, C.B.; Reifenberger, G. Genetic alterations and aberrant expression of genes related to the phosphatidyl-inositol-3'-kinase/protein kinase B (Akt) signal transduction pathway in glioblastomas. *Brain Pathol.* **2003**, *13*, 507–518. [CrossRef]
46. Bigner, S.H.; Mark, J.; Burger, P.C.; Mahaley, M.S., Jr.; Bullard, D.E.; Muhlbaier, L.H.; Bigner, D.D. Specific chromosomal abnormalities in malignant human gliomas. *Cancer Res.* **1988**, *48*, 405–411.
47. Jimenez, C.; Powers, M.; Parsa, A.T.; Glastonbury, C.; Hagenkord, J.M.; Tihan, T. Sarcoma arising as a distinct nodule within glioblastoma: A morphological and molecular perspective on gliosarcoma. *J. Neurooncol.* **2011**, *105*, 317–323. [CrossRef]
48. Albrecht, S.; Connelly, J.H.; Bruner, J.M. Distribution of p53 protein expression in gliosarcomas: An immunohistochemical study. *Acta Neuropathol.* **1993**, *85*, 222–226. [CrossRef]
49. Lusis, E.A.; Travers, S.; Jost, S.C.; Perry, A. Glioblastomas with giant cell and sarcomatous features in patients with Turcot syndrome type 1: A clinicopathological study of 3 cases. *Neurosurgery* **2010**, *67*, 811–817. [CrossRef]
50. Visani, M.; Acquaviva, G.; Marucci, G.; Paccapelo, A.; Mura, A.; Franceschi, E.; Grifoni, D.; Pession, A.; Tallini, G.; Brandes, A.A.; et al. Non-canonical IDH1 and IDH2 mutations: A clonal and relevant event in an Italian cohort of gliomas classified according to the 2016 World Health Organization (WHO) criteria. *J. Neurooncol.* **2017**, *135*, 245–254. [CrossRef]
51. Barnett, F.H.; Scharer-Schuksz, M.; Wood, M.; Yu, X.; Wagner, T.E.; Friedlander, M. Intra-arterial delivery of endostatin gene to brain tumors prolongs survival and alters tumor vessel ultrastructure. *Gene Ther.* **2004**, *11*, 1283–1289. [CrossRef] [PubMed]
52. Bigner, S.H.; Burger, P.C.; Wong, A.J.; Werner, M.H.; Hamilton, S.R.; Muhlbaier, L.H.; Vogelstein, B.; Bigner, D.D. Gene amplification in malignant human gliomas: Clinical and histopathologic aspects. *J. Neuropathol. Exp. Neurol.* **1988**, *47*, 191–205. [CrossRef] [PubMed]

53. Koelsche, C.; Sahm, F.; Capper, D.; Reuss, D.; Sturm, D.; Jones, D.T.; Kool, M.; Northcott, P.A.; Wiestler, B.; Böhmer, K.; et al. Distribution of TERT promoter mutations in pediatric and adult tumors of the nervous system. *Acta Neuropathol.* **2013**, *126*, 907–915. [CrossRef]
54. Venkatraj, V.S.; Begemann, M.; Sobrino, A.; Bruce, J.N.; Weinstein, I.B.; Warburton, D. Genomic changes in glioblastoma cell lines detected by comparative genomic hybridization. *J. Neurooncol.* **1998**, *36*, 141–148. [CrossRef] [PubMed]
55. Yi, X.; Cao, H.; Tang, H.; Gong, G.; Hu, Z.; Liao, W.; Sun, L.; Chen, B.T.; Li, X. Gliosarcoma: A clinical and radiological analysis of 48 cases. *Eur. Radiol.* **2019**, *29*, 429–438. [CrossRef] [PubMed]
56. Qian, Z.; Zhang, L.; Hu, J.; Chen, S.; Chen, H.; Shen, H.; Zheng, F.; Zang, Y.; Chen, X. Machine Learning-Based Analysis of Magnetic Resonance Radiomics for the Classification of Gliosarcoma and Glioblastoma. *Front. Oncol.* **2021**, *11*, 699789. [CrossRef]
57. Fukuda, A.; de Queiroz, L.S.; Reis, F. Gliosarcomas: Magnetic resonance imaging findings. *Arq. Neuropsiquiatr.* **2020**, *78*, 112–120. [CrossRef]
58. Han, S.J.; Yang, I.; Ahn, B.J.; Otero, J.J.; Tihan, T.; McDermott, M.W.; Berger, M.S.; Prados, M.D.; Parsa, A.T. Clinical characteristics and outcomes for a modern series of primary gliosarcoma patients. *Cancer* **2010**, *116*, 1358–1366. [CrossRef]
59. Patel, D.M.; Foreman, P.M.; Nabors, L.B.; Riley, K.O.; Gillespie, G.Y.; Markert, J.M. Design of a Phase I Clinical Trial to Evaluate M032, a Genetically Engineered HSV-1 Expressing IL-12, in Patients with Recurrent/Progressive Glioblastoma Multiforme, Anaplastic Astrocytoma, or Gliosarcoma. *Hum. Gene Ther. Clin. Dev.* **2016**, *27*, 69–78. [CrossRef]
60. Wojtas, B.; Gielniewski, B.; Wojnicki, K.; Maleszewska, M.; Mondal, S.S.; Nauman, P.; Grajkowska, W.; Glass, R.; Schüller, U.; Herold-Mende, C.; et al. Gliosarcoma Is Driven by Alterations in PI3K/Akt, RAS/MAPK Pathways and Characterized by Collagen Gene Expression Signature. *Cancers* **2019**, *11*, 284. [CrossRef]
61. Romeo, S.G.; Conti, A.; Polito, F.; Tomasello, C.; Barresi, V.; La Torre, D.; Cucinotta, M.; Angileri, F.; Bartolotta, M.; Di Giorgio, R.M.; et al. miRNA regulation of Sirtuin-1 expression in human astrocytoma. *Oncol. Lett.* **2016**, *12*, 2992–2998. [CrossRef] [PubMed]
62. Torregrossa, F.; Aguennouz, M.; La Torre, D.; Sfacteria, A.; Grasso, G. Role of Erythropoietin in Cerebral Glioma: An Innovative Target in Neuro-Oncology. *World Neurosurg.* **2019**, *131*, 346–355. [CrossRef] [PubMed]
63. Alonso, M.M.; Diez-Valle, R.; Manterola, L.; Rubio, A.; Liu, D.; Cortes-Santiago, N.; Urquiza, L.; Jauregi, P.; de Munain, A.L.; Sampron, N.; et al. Genetic and epigenetic modifications of Sox2 contribute to the invasive phenotype of malignant gliomas. *PLoS ONE* **2011**, *6*, e26740. [CrossRef] [PubMed]
64. Frandsen, S.; Broholm, H.; Larsen, V.A.; Grunnet, K.; Møller, S.; Poulsen, H.S.; Michaelsen, S.R. Clinical Characteristics of Gliosarcoma and Outcomes from Standardized Treatment Relative to Conventional Glioblastoma. *Front. Oncol.* **2019**, *9*, 1425. [CrossRef] [PubMed]
65. Beaumont, T.L.; Kupsky, W.J.; Barger, G.R.; Sloan, A.E. Gliosarcoma with multiple extracranial metastases: Case report and review of the literature. *J. Neurooncol.* **2007**, *83*, 39–46. [CrossRef] [PubMed]
66. Jin, M.C.; Liu, E.K.; Shi, S.; Gibbs, I.C.; Thomas, R.; Recht, L.; Soltys, S.G.; Pollom, E.L.; Chang, S.D.; Gephart, M.H.; et al. Evaluating Surgical Resection Extent and Adjuvant Therapy in the Management of Gliosarcoma. *Front. Oncol.* **2020**, *10*, 337. [CrossRef]
67. Stupp, R.; Mason, W.P.; van den Bent, M.J.; Weller, M.; Fisher, B.; Taphoorn, M.J.B.; Belanger, K.; Brandes, A.A.; Marosi, C.; Bogdahn, U.; et al. Radiotherapy plus concomitant and adjuvant temozolomide for glioblastoma. *N. Engl. J. Med.* **2005**, *352*, 987–996. [CrossRef]
68. Tomasello, F.; Conti, A.; La Torre, D. 3D printing in Neurosurgery. *World Neurosurg.* **2016**, *91*, 633–634. [CrossRef]
69. Singh, G.; Das, K.; Sharma, P.; Guruprasad, B.; Jaiswal, S.; Mehrotra, A.; Srivastava, A.; Sahu, R.; Jaiswal, A.; Behari, S. Cerebral gliosarcoma: Analysis of 16 patients and review of literature. *Asian J. Neurosurg.* **2015**, *10*, 195–202. [CrossRef]
70. Perry, J.R.; Ang, L.C.; Bilbao, J.M.; Muller, P.J. Clinicopathologic features of primary and postirradiation cerebral gliosarcoma. *Cancer* **1995**, *75*, 2910–2918. [CrossRef]
71. Conti, A.; Pontoriero, A.; Iatì, G.; Marino, D.; La Torre, D.; Vinci, S.; Germanò, A.; Pergolizzi, S.; Francesco, T. 3D-Printing in Neurosurgery. of Arteriovenous Malformations for Radiosurgical Treatment: Pushing Anatomy Understanding to Real Boundaries. *Cureus* **2016**, *8*, e594. [CrossRef] [PubMed]
72. Gil-Gil, M.J.; Mesia, C.; Rey, M.; Bruna, J. Bevacizumab for the Treatment of Glioblastoma. *Clin. Med. Insights Oncol.* **2013**, *7*. Available online: https://journals.sagepub.com/doi/10.4137/CMO.S8503 (accessed on 22 October 2023). [CrossRef] [PubMed]
73. Angiogenesis in Brain Tumors | Nature Reviews Neuroscience. Available online: https://www.nature.com/articles/nrn2175 (accessed on 22 October 2023).
74. Pinheiro, L.; Perdomo-Pantoja, A.; Casaos, J.; Huq, S.; Paldor, I.; Vigilar, V.; Mangraviti, A.; Wang, Y.; Witham, T.F.; Brem, H.; et al. Captopril inhibits Matrix Metalloproteinase-2 and extends survival as a temozolomide adjuvant in an intracranial gliosarcoma model. *Clin. Neurol. Neurosurg.* **2021**, *207*, 106771. [CrossRef] [PubMed]
75. Kang, S.H.; Park, K.J.; Kim, C.Y.; Yu, M.O.; Park, C.-K.; Park, S.-H.; Chung, Y.-G. O6-methylguanine DNA methyltransferase status determined by promoter methylation and immunohistochemistry in gliosarcoma and their clinical implications. *J. Neurooncol.* **2011**, *101*, 477–486. [CrossRef] [PubMed]
76. Mahmoud, A.B.; Ajina, R.; Aref, S.; Darwish, M.; Alsayb, M.; Taher, M.; AlSharif, S.A.; Hashem, A.M.; Alkayyal, A.A. Advances in immunotherapy for glioblastoma multiforme. *Front. Immunol.* **2022**, *13*, 944452. Available online: https://www.frontiersin.org/articles/10.3389/fimmu.2022.944452 (accessed on 22 October 2023). [CrossRef] [PubMed]

77. Wang, E.J.; Chen, J.S.; Jain, S.; Morshed, R.A.; Haddad, A.F.; Gill, S.; Beniwal, A.S.; Aghi, M.K. Immunotherapy Resistance in Glioblastoma. *Front. Genet.* **2021**, *12*, 750675. [CrossRef] [PubMed]
78. Gittleman, H.; Lim, D.; Kattan, M.W.; Chakravarti, A.; Gilbert, M.R.; Lassman, A.B.; Lo, S.S.; Machtay, M.; Sloan, A.E.; Sulman, E.P.; et al. An independently validated nomogram for individualized survival estimation among patients with newly diagnosed glioblastoma: NRG Oncology RTOG 0525 and 0825. *Neuro Oncol.* **2017**, *19*, 669–677. [CrossRef] [PubMed]
79. Li, Y.M.; Suki, D.; Hess, K.; Sawaya, R. The influence of maximum safe resection of glioblastoma on survival in 1229 patients: Can we do better than gross-total resection? *J. Neurosurg.* **2016**, *124*, 977–988. [CrossRef]
80. Kröger, S.; Niehoff, A.C.; Jeibmann, A.; Sperling, M.; Paulus, W.; Stummer, W.; Karst, U. Complementary Molecular and Elemental Mass-Spectrometric Imaging of Human Brain Tumors Resected by Fluorescence-Guided Surgery. *Anal. Chem.* **2018**, *90*, 12253–12260. [CrossRef]
81. Huang, Q.; Li, F.; Chen, Y.; Hong, F.; Wang, H.; Chen, J. Prognostic factors and clinical outcomes in adult primary gliosarcoma patients: A Surveillance, Epidemiology, and End Results (SEER) analysis from 2004 to 2015. *Br. J. Neurosurg.* **2020**, *34*, 161–167. [CrossRef]

Disclaimer/Publisher's Note: The statements, opinions and data contained in all publications are solely those of the individual author(s) and contributor(s) and not of MDPI and/or the editor(s). MDPI and/or the editor(s) disclaim responsibility for any injury to people or property resulting from any ideas, methods, instructions or products referred to in the content.

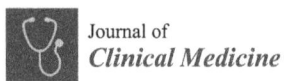

Review

Primary Anaplastic-Lymphoma-Kinase-Positive Large-Cell Lymphoma of the Central Nervous System: Comprehensive Review of the Literature

Antonio Colamaria [1,†], Augusto Leone [2,3,†], Francesco Carbone [2], Yasser Andres Dallos Laguado [4], Nicola Pio Fochi [5,*], Matteo Sacco [6], Cinzia Fesce [7], Francesca Sanguedolce [8], Guido Giordano [9], Giorgio Iaconetta [10], Uwe Spetzger [2], Luigi Coppola [10], Elena De Santis [11], Giulia Coppola [12,‡] and Matteo De Notaris [13,‡]

1. Division of Neurosurgery, Policlinico "Riuniti", 71122 Foggia, Italy; colamariaa@gmail.com
2. Department of Neurosurgery, Städtisches Klinikum Karlsruhe, 76133 Karlsruhe, Germany; augustoleone96@gmail.com (A.L.); francesco.carbone615@gmail.com (F.C.); uwe.spetzger@klinikum-karlsruhe.com (U.S.)
3. Faculty of Human Medicine, Charité Universitätsmedizin Berlin, 10117 Berlin, Germany
4. Faculty of Medicine and Surgery, University of Foggia, 71122 Foggia, Italy; yasserdallos@gmail.com
5. Division of Neurosurgery, University of Foggia, 71122 Foggia, Italy
6. Division of Neurosurgery, "Casa Sollievo della Sofferenza", 71013 San Giovanni Rotondo, Italy; matteosacco88@gmail.com
7. Hematology Unit, University Hospital, 71122 Foggia, Italy; cinzia.fesce@libero.it
8. Pathology Unit, Ospedali Riuniti di Foggia, 71122 Foggia, Italy; francesca.sanguedolce@unifg.it
9. Unit of Medical Oncology and Biomolecular Therapy, Department of Medical and Surgical Sciences, University of Foggia, 71122 Foggia, Italy; guido.giordano@unifg.it
10. Unit of Anatomy, Pathological Histology and Diagnostic Cytology, Department of Diagnostic and Pharma-Ceutical Services, Sandro Pertini Hospital, 00157 Rome, Italy; giaconetta@unisa.it (G.I.); luigi.coppola@aslroma2.it (L.C.)
11. Department of Anatomical, Histological, Forensic Medicine and Orthopedic sciences, La Sapienza University, 00185 Roma, Italy; elena.desantis@uniroma1.it
12. Department of Radiological, Oncological and Pathological Sciences, La Sapienza University, 00185 Roma, Italy; coppola1537902@studenti.uniroma1.it
13. Department of Neurosurgery, University of Salerno, 84084 Salerno, Italy; matteodenotaris@gmail.com
* Correspondence: fochinicola98@gmail.com
† These authors contributed equally to this work as co first authors.
‡ These authors contributed equally to this work as co last authors.

Citation: Colamaria, A.; Leone, A.; Carbone, F.; Dallos Laguado, Y.A.; Fochi, N.P.; Sacco, M.; Fesce, C.; Sanguedolce, F.; Giordano, G.; Iaconetta, G.; et al. Primary Anaplastic-Lymphoma-Kinase-Positive Large-Cell Lymphoma of the Central Nervous System: Comprehensive Review of the Literature. *J. Clin. Med.* **2023**, *12*, 7516. https://doi.org/10.3390/jcm12247516

Academic Editors: Morgan Broggi, Marco Zeppieri, Tamara Ius, Filippo Flavio Angileri, Antonio Pontoriero and Alessandro Tel

Received: 9 October 2023
Revised: 27 November 2023
Accepted: 4 December 2023
Published: 5 December 2023

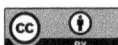

Copyright: © 2023 by the authors. Licensee MDPI, Basel, Switzerland. This article is an open access article distributed under the terms and conditions of the Creative Commons Attribution (CC BY) license (https://creativecommons.org/licenses/by/4.0/).

Abstract: Background: Primary anaplastic-lymphoma-kinase (ALK)-positive large-cell lymphoma of the central nervous system (PCNS ALK-positive ALCL) is a rare entity, with a limited consensus reached regarding its management. While this pathology often presents as solitary lesions, the occurrence of multiple tumors within the brain is not uncommon. The lack of distinctive radiological features poses a diagnostic challenge, leading to delays in initiating targeted therapy. Methods: We conducted a comprehensive literature search, identifying seventeen publications for qualitative analysis. Results: The management options and reported patient outcomes in the literature varied significantly, emphasizing the need for a patient-specific approach. The emergence of ALK-specific inhibitors represents a new frontier in this field, demonstrating promising results. Conclusion: PCNS ALK-positive ALCL necessitates a comprehensive understanding and optimized management strategies. A tailored therapeutic approach, integrating surgical intervention with radiotherapy and chemotherapy, appears pivotal in addressing this pathology. The implementation of a therapeutic protocol is anticipated for further advancement in this field.

Keywords: primary central nervous system lymphoma; anaplastic large-cell lymphoma; ALK; Ki-1; CD-30

1. Introduction

Primary central nervous system lymphomas (PCNSLs) are a rare entity, constituting less than 1.5% of all intracranial malignancies [1], with an estimated incidence of 1 in 100.000 individuals [2]. Notably, while PNCSLs predominantly affect immunocompromised subjects [3], there has been a recent increase in the incidence among immunocompetent patients [4,5]. B-cell lymphomas are more frequent than their T-cell counterparts, with T-cell lymphomas, including anaplastic large-cell lymphoma (ALCL), accounting for approximately 8.5% of all PCNSLs [1,6]. A subvariant of the T-form is referred to as anaplastic large-cell lymphoma (ALCL), characterized by large pleomorphic immunohistochemical positivity for the CD30 marker [6]. ALCL is an exceptional manifestation in the central nervous system (CNS), typically presenting as a nodal and extranodal disease [1,7] constituting 5% of all human non-Hodgkin lymphomas [4].

The 5th Edition of the World Health Organization's classification of hematolymphoid tumors delineates two subvariants of ALCL: ALK-positive and ALK-negative forms [8]. Up to 85% of systemic ALCLs exhibit the t(2;5) translocation, where the ALK1 gene on chromosome 2 fuses with the nucleoplasmin (NPM) gene on chromosome 5, resulting in the encoding of the p80 protein, which is strongly implicated in neoplastic degeneration [9]. ALK1 positivity is associated with a younger age at diagnosis and is considered a significant positive prognostic factor [10]. However, despite a generally favorable prognosis, ALK-positive ALCLs can exhibit a rapidly deteriorating clinical course [11].

PCNS ALK-positive ALCLs often manifest as solitary lesions, although multiple brain manifestations are not uncommon. Despite a higher tendency to affect the leptomeninges compared to more common B-cell PCNSLs [12], the absence of pathognomonic radiological features complicates diagnosis, leading to delays in targeted therapy initiation [11].

To date, there is no consensus on treatment protocols for PCNS ALK-positive ALCLs, and management is predominantly empirical, relying on individual institution standards of care [7]. Various therapeutic strategies, including surgical techniques, single or combined chemotherapeutic agents (such as CHOP [7] or the DeAngelis Protocol [13]), and focal or whole-brain radiotherapy, have been reported, with varying efficacies and toxicities [11]. However, diagnostic challenges, the rapid and unpredictable evolution of this malignancy, and the absence of a unified therapeutic protocol [7] contribute to often-unsatisfactory outcomes [4,10,14].

For this article, we conducted a comprehensive review of the literature to compile and critically summarize essential evidence on the clinical manifestations, treatment options, and efficacy rates for PCNS ALK-positive ALCLs.

2. Materials and Methods

2.1. Search Strategy and Selection Criteria

A comprehensive search of the literature was performed in compliance with the updated Preferred Reporting Items for Systematic Reviews and Meta-Analyses (PRISMA) 2020 guidelines, as shown in Figure 1 [15]. Article inquiry was operated via the electronic databases MEDLINE/PubMed for manuscripts reporting PCNS ALK-positive ALCLs. Human studies in English published between 1997 and April 2023 were considered for inclusion. Primary search terms included "Central Nervous System Neoplasms", "Lymphoma, T-Cell", "CD30+ Anaplastic Large Cell Lymphoma", and "Ki-1 Lymphoma" in the article titles and abstracts in various MeSH combinations. Inclusion criteria were: (1) PCNS ALCL T-cell lymphomas demonstrating immunohistochemical positivity for the AKL1 marker and (2) availability of sufficient patient-specific clinical, histological, and surgical information. Publications describing meningeal and spinal cord forms were excluded. A total of 1083 records were identified. The extracted citations were then checked for duplicates, and citations of the examined manuscripts were also screened for the purpose of this review. A total of 859 were assessed for eligibility, and 842 were excluded for not complying with the abovementioned criteria through an automated system (Covidence,

Veritas Health Innovation, Melbourne, Australia) [16]. One publication was not retrieved with its full text. Finally, seventeen publications were included in the qualitative analysis.

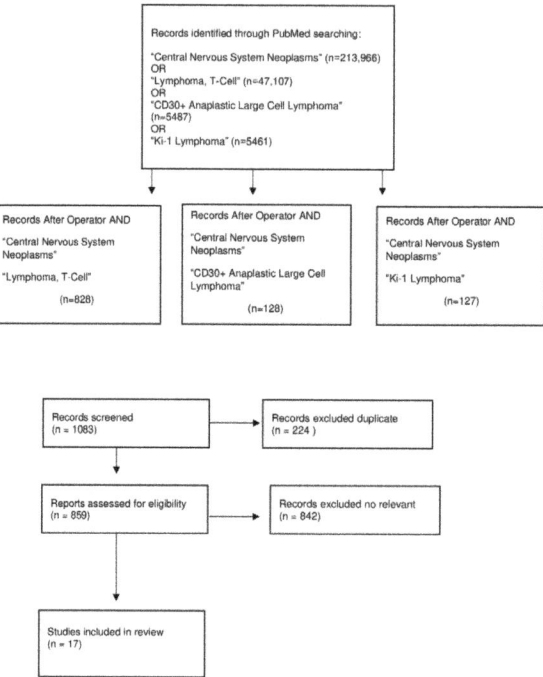

Figure 1. Preferred Reporting Items for Systematic Reviews and Meta-Analyses protocol used for the systematic review, adapted from [15].

2.2. Data Extraction

Two authors (A.Y.D. and F.C.) independently reviewed all abstracts to recognize articles that required full-text review. They investigated abstracts against predefined eligible criteria, and all included studies were discussed with a third author (N.P.F.). The following information was obtained: the author's name, patient's age and gender, site of the tumor, clinical presentation, radiological aspects on MRI, liquor characteristics, pathological findings, immunohistochemistry-positive markers, immunohistochemistry-negative markers, ALK gene mutation, treatment, and status at follow-up. Gathered data were stored in a centralized database (Microsoft Excel, Version 16.79.2, Redmond, WA, USA).

2.3. Data Analysis

A descriptive analysis of data was performed using mean, median, percentages, and maximum and minimum values. Continuous variables were represented by mean and range values, except in cases otherwise specified. Data were analyzed and processed with SPSS version 24.0.1.1 (14) (IBM, Armonk, NY, USA) and Microsoft Excel (Version 16.79.2, Redmond, WA, USA). Statistical significance was considered for p-value < 0.05. Two independent reviewers (A.L. and A.Y.D.) performed the statistical analysis.

3. Literature Review

3.1. Demographics and Tumor Characteristics

Seventeen cases of ALK-1 positive T-cell brain lymphomas have hitherto been reported (Tables 1 and 2). The data show a predominantly male prevalence (82.3%, n = 14/17). The median age at diagnosis was 15.9 years, range 2–38. A total of 12 (70.5%) patients presented single lesions, and 5 (29.4%) had multiple foci. Only one tumor affected primarily the cerebellum, one case involved the brainstem (together with the occipital lobe), and one further lesion (5.8%) was located adjacent to the planum sphenoidale; the remaining 14 cases (82.3%) affected exclusively the cerebral hemispheres. Even in the absence of a specific radiological pattern, these lesions tend to show some typically recurring characteristics. For instance, ten cases demonstrated an important contrast uptake—sometimes resulting in a non-homogeneous pattern in T1-weighted images. Among these cases, six lesions demonstrated enhancement in the leptomeninges. In nine cases, a significant perilesional edema was disclosed. Lastly, two lesions showed a peculiar cystic degeneration, and one further caused the erosion of the immediately adjacent bone component.

Table 1. Demographic, topographical, clinical, and radiological characteristics of PCNS ALK-1 positive ALCLs. George et al. [9] reviewed data from 12 previously published cases and investigated tissue samples of five of these which have been made available to the author for further immunopathologic study. Clinical histories and presentations, radiologic imaging, details of treatment, and outcomes were obtained via contact with clinicians and/or the submitting pathologists. M: male. F: female. GE: gadolinium enhancement. CT: computed tomography.

Case Number	Reference	Age/Gender	Site	Symptoms	Radiological Aspect of MRI
1	Ponzoni, M. et al. [17]	29/M	Single Cortical–subcortical fronto-temporal lobe left	Fever, cephalgia, epileptic activity	Lesional, pial, and subarachnoid GE. T2 hypo-isointense. Perilesional edema (on admission)
2	Nomura, M. et al. [6]	20/M	Single Left frontal lobe	Epileptic activity (generalized seizures)	Lesional GE. High-intensity signal on T2. Edema and midline shift
3	Geetha, N. et al. [10]	19/M	Single Right cerebellar hemisphere	Cephalgia, emesis, obstructive hydrocephalus	Well-defined lesion. T1 hypointense. T2 iso-hyperintense. Perilesional edema
4	Kuntegowdenahalli, L. et al. [3]	18/M	Single Left parieto-occipital lobe	Fever, cephalgia, epileptic activity (seizures)	Hyperintense on T2-Flair. Midline shift
5	Splavski, B. et al. [2]	26/M	Single Partial intraventricular, frontal horn of the left lateral ventricle	Incidentaloma	GE. Partial cystic degeneration. Perifocal edema. Subependimal intra-axial spread. Iso-iperintense on T2-images
6	Liu, Q. et al. [14]	12/M	Single Right occipital lobe and falx cerebrum	Cephalgia, emesis	GE. Partial cystic degeneration. Perilesional edema. Midline shift
7	Abdulkader, I. et al. [4] Reviewed by George, D. H. et al. [9]	13/M	Multiple Right parietal lobe and right frontal lobe	Cephalgia, emesis	T1 hypointense, T2 hyperintense signal. Perilesional and leptomeningeal GE
8	George, D. H. et al. [9]	18/F	Single Left temporal lobe and surrounding dura	NA	NA
9	Karikari, I. O. et al. [12]	4/M	Multiple Bilateral frontal lobe and pineal region	Epileptic activity (tonic–clonic seizures), Fever, cephalgia, emesis, nuchal rigidity	Leptomeningeal and lesional GE. T1 hypointense and T2 hyperintense
10	Ozkaynak, M. F. et al. [18]	9/M	Multiple Bilateral frontal lesions extended into the superior frontal gyri	Fever, epileptic activity (focal seizures)	Meningeal GE. MR spectroscopy: elevated choline, decrease N-acetilaspartate, inverted lactate peak

Table 1. Cont.

Case Number	Reference	Age/Gender	Site	Symptoms	Radiological Aspect of MRI
11	Shah, A. C. et al. [5]	2/M	Single Right cerebral hemisphere and surrounding leptomeninges	Lethargy, hemiparesis, epileptic activity	Edema. Uncal herniation. Midline shift
12	Furuya, K. et al. [11]	11/M	Multiple Left parietal lobe	Cephalgia, nausea	Focal meningeal GE, edema. Midline shift
13	Rupani A. et al. [19]	17/M	Single Right fronto-parietal lobe	Cephalgia, epileptic activity, left arm paresis	Well-circumscribed lesion presenting GE. Skull bone erosion. Scalp swelling
14	Vivekanandan, S. et al. [7]	20/M	Single Right silvian fissure	Epileptic activity	Peripheric GE
15	Havlioglu, N. et al. [1] Reviewed by George, D. H. et al. [9]	4.5/F	Multiple Left occipital lobe and left brain stem	Cephalgia, nausea, emesis, nuchal rigidity, fever	Multiple densities scattered over the brain surface and brain stem. CT: lesions in the cervical and lumbar segments of the spinal cord
16	Buxton, N. et al. [20] Reviewed by George, D.H. et al. [9]	10/F	Single Right parietal lobe abutting against the falx	Leftsided sensory disturbance, hemiparesis, cephalgia	Irregular, heterogeneous mass. Minor falcine GE
17	Carmichael, M. G. et al. [13]	38/M	Single Intraparenchymal parieto-occipital right	Epileptic activity, syncope, left-sided hemiparesis, visual field deficit, ataxia	Surrounding edema. Midline shift

Table 2. The main CSF and histo-pathological features of the lesions examined are summarized here. With regard to the CSF, the parameters that were most frequently altered were the leucocyte count, glicorrachia, and protidorrachia. Histological analysis showed recurrent alterations in most of the cases. Lastly, the immunohistochemical study showed great heterogeneity in the expression of markers. GCSF: granulocyte colony-stimulating factor. LCA: leucocyte common antigen. EMA: epithelial membrane antigen. GFAP: glial fibrillary acidic protein.

Case Number	Microscopic Analysis of CSF	Pathological Findings	Immunohistochemistry-Positive Markers	Immunohistochemistry-Negative Markers	ALK Gene Mutation
1	Clear, colorless 5 lymp/mm^3 Protein 53 mg/dL No malignant cells Negative cultures	Medium-to-large lymphoid-looking cells. Kidney-shaped nuclei, prominent nucleoli, abundant cytoplasm. Few "hallmark cells". Apoptotic figures, no necrosis. Infiltrate of macrophages, granulocytes, and small lymphocytes	ALK-1, LCA, CD30, EMA, monoclonal CD3 and CD45RO	CD20, CD79a, S-100 protein, GFAP, myeloperoxidase, CD34, CD68 (KP-1)	NA
2	NA	Large, atypical lymphocytes containing scattered horseshoe-shaped nuclei	ALK-1, CD3	CD20	NA
3	NA	Sheets of pleomorphic tumor cells with classical doughnut cells	ALK, LCA, CD30	CD5, CD20	NA
4	No malignant cells	Suggestive of ALCL	ALK, LCA, CD30, CD4	CD3, CD7	NA

Table 2. Cont.

Case Number	Microscopic Analysis of CSF	Pathological Findings	Immunohistochemistry-Positive Markers	Immunohistochemistry-Negative Markers	ALK Gene Mutation
5	NA	Polymorphous cells with hyperchromatic nuclei. Sporadic mitosis	ALK, Vimentin, CD45LCA, EMA, CD3, CD4, CD30, CD99, MUM-1, Ki67 75%	Cytokeratin AE1/AE3, cytokeratin MNF116, TTF-1, PLAP, HMB45, GFAP, keratin 7, keratin 20, CD20, CD10, CD8, bcl2, bcl6, NSE, Tdt	NA
6	NA	Lymphoid cells with a diffuse monotonous growth pattern with focal or sheet necrosis and starry-sky mimicking. Irregular-shaped nuclei with multiple basophilic nucleoli. Abundant pale or basophilic cytoplasm. Prominent mitosis	ALK1, CD30, Granzyme B, TIA-1, CD56, MUM-1, EMA, CD4 Ki67 95%	CD2, CD3, CD5, CD7, GFAP, PLAP, CD34, CD45, CD20, CD79a, TdT, CD99, BCL-2, BCL-6, CD10	Monoclonal TCRγ gene rearrangement Gene translocation involving ALK
7	1450 WBC/μL Glucose 34 mg/dL Protein 135 mg/dL Atypical lymphocytes with eccentric-shaped nuclei, prominent nucleoli, scant dense cytoplasm, multiple cytoplasmatic vacuoles. Binucleation. Mitotic figures	Large cells with amphophilic cytoplasm, large nuclei (often horseshoe-shaped) with prominent nucleoli. Focal necrosis, lymphoplasmacytic infiltrate. High mitotic rate. Atypical mitotic figures	ALK1, CD30, LCA, UCHL1, P80, EMA CD3, CD45RO (by George, D. H. et al. [9])	Cytokeratins, KP-1, B-cell markers	NA
8	NA	Necrosis absent	ALK1, CD45RO	B-cell markers	NA
9	Elevated WBC Glucose: low Protein levels: increased	Large, atypical cells with irregular nuclei with a moderate amount of eosinophilic and basophilic cytoplasm. No Reed–Sternberg-type cells	ALK-1, CD30, CD7	PLAP, human chorionic gonadotropin, a-fetoprotein, keratin, NFP, NEU-N, synaptophysin, S-100 protein, CD1A	Balanced reciprocal translocation between crom. 2 and crom. 15 with breakpoints at bands 2p23 and 5q35
10	In total, 27 WBC (63% lymphocytes, 31% monocytes, 6% neutrophils) Negative Gram stain and culture Flow cytometry: abnormal CD8-positive T-cell population	Large angiocentric cells invading the parenchyma. High mitotic rate	ALK-1, LCA, CD3, CD8, CD30, Ki-67 Flow cytometry CSF: CD2, CD7	CD5, CD20, CD79a, TDT, SYN, NF, GFAP Flow cytometry CSF: loss of pan T-cell markers CD3 and CD5, CD56, CD57, TdT	NA
11	NA	Multinodular, pleomorphic large cells with dural infiltration. Large mononuclear and binuclear atypical cells. Vascular/endothelial proliferation with congestion, focal hemorrhage, and broad necrosis. Scattered mitoses	ALK-1, CD30 (Ki-1), CD43	EMA, S-100 protein, CD1a, CD3, CD20, CD15 (Leu-M1), GFAP, placental alkaline-phosphatase, muscle-specific actin, desmin	NA
12	Glucose 70 mg/dL, protein 130 mg/dL, cell count 237 cells/mm^3 with a differential count of 68% polymorphonuclear cells No malignant tumor cells (on CSF cytology)	Large, polymorphic tumor cells, diffusely infiltrate throughout the cortex. Pleomorphic nuclei, prominent nucleoli, abundant clear or eosinophilic cytoplasm. No bacteria	ALK-1, EMA, LCA, CD30 (Ki-1)	GFAP, CD3, UCHL-1 (CD45RO), CD20, CD79, KP-1 (CD68)	NA

Table 2. Cont.

Case Number	Microscopic Analysis of CSF	Pathological Findings	Immunohistochemistry-Positive Markers	Immunohistochemistry-Negative Markers	ALK Gene Mutation
13	NA	Large pleomorphic cells with abundant eosinophilic-to-amphophilic cytoplasm and prominent nucleoli. Necrosis absent	ALK1, CD30, CD43, LCA, EMA	Myeloperoxidase, chloroacetate esterase	NA
14	Unremarkable	Sheets of large cytologically atypical lymphoid blast cells interspersed with frequent neutrophil polymorphs. Vesicular nuclei and prominent nucleoli, relatively abundant amphophilic cytoplasm	ALK, CD3, CD30	NA	NA
15	Total of 90 RBC/µL, 10 WBC/µL with large, atypical lymphocytes Glucose 51 mg/dL Protein 210 mg/dL	Large cells with amphophilic cytoplasm, large nuclei with prominent nuclear membrane irregularities, and prominent nucleoli. Focal necrosis and lymphoplasmacytic infiltrate. High mitotic rate, atypical mitotic figures	CD30, EMA ALK-1 (by George, D. H. et al. [9]) CSF cytology: large, atypical lymphocytes with eccentric oval-shaped nuclei, prominent nucleoli, scant dense cytoplasm containing multiple cytoplasm vacoles. Binucleation, mitotic figures	LCA, cytokeratin, neuron-specific enolase, KP-1, B-markers, T-markers, monocyte/macrophage markers. Cytometric analysis CSF: no aberrant pan-T surface marker expression	No monoclonal rearrangement of T beta receptor, K or lambda light-chain genes, or immunoglobulin heavy-chain locus
16	NA	High mitotic rate. High level of apoptosis and an unusual pattern of spread Necrosis (by George, D. H. et al. [9])	Ki-1 AKL1, CD43, CD45RO (by George, D. H. et al. [9])	B-markers (by George, D. H. et al. [9])	NA
17	NA	Malignant cells consistent with ALCL	AKL-1, CD30, CD45,	NA	NA

3.2. Management Algorithms

Treatment options were markedly heterogeneous: for instance, 5.9% (n = 1) were treated with a chemotherapy regimen alone, 23.5% (n = 4) with a combination of chemotherapy and surgical resection, 29.4% (n = 5) with the combination of systemic therapy and radiation therapy, 41.2% (n = 7) with a combination of surgical resection, chemotherapy, and radiation and, in the remaining case, the patient died before the initiation of the treatment (Table 3). Not surprisingly, equally heterogeneous were the outcomes: 55.6% of the cases showed no recurrence of the lesion following the first line of treatment (median follow-up: 54.2 months, range: 13–96); in 29.4% (n = 5) early death (within 6 months of diagnosis) was registered, and in one case (5.9%), the patient was alive at the time of discharge; however, for this last case and two other cases (n = 2; 11.8%) no data were available on survival or the post-treatment course of the disease.

With regard to available chemotherapic options, MTX proved to be the most widely used immunosuppressant agent to be administered, alone or in combination with other drugs or locoregional therapy. It was used as the sole systemic agent in three cases, achieving no evidence of disease $\geq$ 9 months (max 96 months), while the association with other chemotherapic agents was followed in 10 cases. Other frequently used chemotherapy combinations include the DeAngelis protocol (HD-MTX—with leucovorin rescue, intrathecal MTX, vincristine, procarbazine, and dexamethasone), MATRix (MTX, idarubicin, cytarabine, and thiotepa), BFM90 (prednisone, vincristine, asparaginase, cyclophosphamide, cytarabine, daunorubicin, doxorubicin, methotrexate, and 6-mercaptopurine), CHOP/CHOD (cyclophosphamide, doxorubicin, vincristine, prednisone/dexamethasone), and the VAM Protocol (vincristine, methotrexate—with folinic acid rescue—and cytarabine).

Table 3. Here, the treatment protocols and patients' outcomes are summarized. Surgical therapy, in combination with chemotherapy and/or radiotherapy regimens, was employed in ten cases: a gross-total resection (GTR) was achieved in five of these. Radiotherapy was administered in eleven patients and, in five cases, was associated with a combination of one or more chemotherapy regimens, while, in the remaining six, radiotherapy was used in conjunction with chemotherapy and surgical intervention. Equally variable are the individual application regimens: in seven out of twelve cases, radiotherapy was applied to the whole brain (in two cases, with extension to the spinal cord, as well), and in two, it had focal administration, consistent with the site of the lesion, while in the remaining two cases, the type of administration was not specified. CHT: chemotherapy. RT: radiotherapy. GTR: gross total resection. STR: subtotal resection. HD-MTX: high-dose methotrexate. NED: no evidence of disease.

Case Number	Treatment	Status at Follow Up
1	Biopsy CHT: MATILde regimen (MTX, idarubicin, cytarabine, thiotepa) RT: Whole-brain RT	NED at 13 months (from completion of the treatment)
2	GTR CHT: HD-MTX	NED at 5 years
3	STR CHT: BFM90 ALCL Protocol	Recurrence 9 months after surgery Exitus a month later
4	GTR CHT: DeAngelis protocol (HD-MTX, leucovorin, Intrathecal—MTX via lumbar puncture, vincristine, procarbazine, Dexamethasone). Cytarabine (after RT) RT: Whole brain	On prophylactic antiepileptic medication (no further info regarding OS or PFS available)
5	GTR CHT: HD-MTX, HD-Cytarabine. GCSF, folinic acid (leucovorin) RT: Whole brain	NED at 2 years
6	Biopsy	Exitus in one month
7	Biopsy CHT: vincristine, Etoposide, MTX, cyclophosphamide, dexamethasone, cytarabine	Exitus shortly after CHT treatment
8	CHT RT (local or whole brain not specified)	NED at 5.2 years
9	Biopsy CHT: doxorubicin, prednisone, vincristine. RT: Craniospinal	Alive at discharged (for completion of chemotherapy and radiation therapy)
10	STR CHT: Dexamethasone, HD-MTX, etoposide, BCNU. Intraventricular MTX, hydrocortisone, Ara-C RT: Focal	NED at 26 months
11	STR CHT: HD-MTX	NED at 8 years (from therapy completion)
12	Methylprednisolone for ICP before diagnosis STR via biopsy CHT: HD-MTX RT: Whole brain	NED at 8 years after completion of treatment
13	Biopsy CHT: Steroids, cyclophosphamide, adriamycin, vincristine RT (not specified)	Exitus after 1 month
14	GTR CHT: CHOD (cyclophosphamide, doxorubicin, vincristine, dexamethasone, allopurinol), BCNU (carmustine), VAM (vincristine, MTX, folinic acid, cytarabine) RT: focal	NED at 8 years from initial presentation

Table 3. Cont.

Case Number	Treatment	Status at Follow Up
15	STR via Biopsy CHT: CHOP Protocol (cyclophosphamide, doxorubicin, oncovin, prednisone)	Gradually improved with supportive therapy (no further info regarding OS or PFS available)
16	Dexamethasone (before diagnosis) GTR CHT: United Kingdom Children's Cancer Study Group 9003 protocol (HD-MTX, cyclophosphamide, daunorubicin, cytosine, vincristine, prednisolone) RT: craniospinal	Exitus after 6 months
17	Biopsy HD-dexamethasone, phenytoin (before diagnosis) CHT: HD-MTX/leucovorin, vincristine, procarbazine, dexamethasone. Intrathecal MTX (Ommaya reservoir). HD-systematic cytarabine (according to the DeAngelis protocol) RT: Whole brain (before and after diagnosis)	NED at 15 months following therapy

4. Discussion

A comprehensive understanding of the physiopathological features inherent to ALK-positive PCNSL remains elusive, primarily owing to the limited number of reported cases and the consequent absence of a standardized management protocol. While diverse treatments have yielded durable complete remissions, the occurrence of intracerebral recurrence is not uncommon [21].

The current diagnostic imaging modalities exhibit insufficiencies in distinguishing PCNSL from other malignant or inflammatory processes, necessitating histology for definitive diagnosis. Despite the rarity of this pathology, it is crucial to consider it among the diagnostic possibilities. The reported data indicate a significant rate of remission, even in the absence of a standardized treatment protocol, underscoring the necessity for early diagnosis and treatment.

The prompt and accurate diagnosis of primary ALCL of the CNS is infrequent. According to a previous study [22], an average of around 40 days is required for diagnosis, hindering early identification and resulting in treatment delays that could prove fatal.

Initially, small lesions discovered along the dura are often misdiagnosed as inflammatory conditions such as meningitis or sarcoidosis. Tuberculosis is commonly considered as the probable infection, because it frequently presents with leptomeningeal enhancement [23].

Before undergoing surgical intervention, a biopsy is advised, to histologically confirm the suspect of PCNSL [24]. However, despite long-standing reports indicating that the extent of surgical removal does not impact the prognosis of this pathology [25], there might be value in attempting maximal tumor resection when symptoms of increased intracranial pressure manifest due to the mass effect of the tumor [23].

Despite sharing histologic, immunophenotypic, and clinical features with extra-CNS ALCL, PCNS ALK-positive ALCL demonstrates a more aggressive clinical behavior [14]. Favorable prognostic factors in ALCL include youth, unifocal tumor presentation, and the absence of necrosis. Conversely, older age, multifocal tumor presentation, and extensive necrosis correlate with an elevated risk of mortality [9]. Notably, the expression of CD56, a neural cell-adhesion molecule, in ALCL is associated with a poorer overall prognosis, increased recurrence, CNS involvement, and a higher likelihood of bone involvement [14,26]. Despite its rarity, CD56 positivity has been observed in only two cases in the literature.

PCNS ALK-positive ALCL is a rare entity, accounting for less than 4% of all PCNSL cases in Western countries [27,28]. Due to the scarcity of this tumor, no consensus exists on its management, and treatment approaches are typically empirical, although methotrexate (MTX) monotherapy is often associated with improved survival rates [2]. While chemotherapy has demonstrated optimal outcomes, most patients necessitate combined protocols, involving locoregional therapy [2,29]. For instance, favorable outcomes have been achieved through the combination of corticosteroid therapy and radiation [30]. Considering the uncertainty surrounding the efficacy of additional combined-modality protocols in improving survival and reducing delayed neurotoxic effects, radiation may be a rational choice in younger patients, those with residual or recurrent tumors, and those with inadequate responses to chemotherapy [21,31].

Given the infrequency of PCNS ALK-positive ALCL, the reported treatment protocols exhibit substantial prognostic variability. However, with the evolution of personalized medicine, particularly the development of ALK-specific inhibitors, the molecular mechanisms governing tumorigenesis have become targets for more effective therapeutic approaches [32]. Recent research underscores the efficacy of ALK inhibitors in relapsed or refractory ALK-positive ALCL, demonstrating reduced toxicity. While first-generation ALK inhibitors like crizotinib have limitations in CNS penetration, next-generation inhibitors such as alectinib, brigatinib, ceritinib, and lorlatinib show promise in crossing the blood–brain barrier [33]. Several studies highlight the clinical significance of these next-generation ALK inhibitors in relapsed or refractory cases [34–36]. However, further research is warranted to establish their efficacy in primary settings, considering the common adverse events of gastrointestinal toxicities, elevated liver enzymes, and fatigue [33].

5. Conclusions

The lack of consensus regarding the management of PCNS ALK-positive ALCL impedes standardized therapy for this rare tumor, potentially leading to unfavorable outcomes. The emergence of targeted monoclonal therapies is anticipated to mitigate inter-institutional differences in adopted management algorithms. Nevertheless, given the extreme paucity of similar cases, this report of experiences may facilitate a more standardized and evidence-based therapeutic approach. Further comprehensive studies are envisaged to optimize our therapeutic armamentarium in cases of PCNS ALK-positive ALCL.

Author Contributions: A.C., F.C. and M.S.: conceptualization. F.C., N.P.F., Y.A.D.L. and A.L.: methodology. C.F., F.S., A.C., G.C. and M.S.: data curation. F.C., N.P.F., Y.A.D.L. and A.L.: writing—original draft preparation, visualization, investigation. A.C., M.D.N., U.S. and L.C.: supervision. M.D.N., G.G., G.I., E.D.S., U.S. and L.C.: writing—reviewing and editing. All authors have read and agreed to the published version of the manuscript.

Funding: This research received no external funding.

Institutional Review Board Statement: Not applicable.

Informed Consent Statement: Not applicable.

Data Availability Statement: No new data were created or analyzed in this study. Data sharing is not applicable to this article.

Conflicts of Interest: The authors declare no conflict of interest.

References

1. Havlioglu, N.; Manepalli, A.; Galindo, L.; Sotelo-Avila, C.; Grosso, L. Primary Ki-1 (Anaplastic Large Cell) Lymphoma of the Brain and Spinal Cord. *Am. J. Clin. Pathol.* **1995**, *103*, 496–499. [CrossRef] [PubMed]
2. Splavski, B.; Muzevic, D.; Ladenhauser-Palijan, T.; Splavski, B., Jr. Primary Central Nervous System Anaplastic Large T-cell Lymphoma. *Med. Arh.* **2016**, *70*, 311. [CrossRef] [PubMed]
3. Kuntegowdenahalli, L.; Jacob, L.; Komaranchath, A.; Amirtham, U. A rare case of primary anaplastic large cell lymphoma of the central nervous system. *J. Can. Res. Ther.* **2015**, *11*, 943. [CrossRef]
4. Abdulkader, I.; Cameselle-Teijeiro, J.; Fraga, M.; Rodriguez-Núñez, A.; Allut, A.G.; Forteza, J. Primary anaplastic large cell lymphoma of the central nervous system. *Hum. Pathol.* **1999**, *30*, 978–981. [CrossRef] [PubMed]
5. Shah, A.C.; Kelly, D.R.; Nabors, L.B.; Oakes, W.J.; Hilliard, L.M.; Reddy, A.T. Treatment of primary CNS lymphoma with high-dose methotrexate in immunocompetent pediatric patients: Methotrexate for Pediatric CNS Lymphoma. *Pediatr. Blood Cancer* **2010**, *55*, 1227–1230. [CrossRef] [PubMed]
6. Nomura, M.; Narita, Y.; Miyakita, Y.; Ohno, M.; Fukushima, S.; Maruyama, T.; Muragaki, Y.; Shibui, S. Clinical presentation of anaplastic large-cell lymphoma in the central nervous system. *Mol. Clin. Oncol.* **2013**, *1*, 655–660. [CrossRef] [PubMed]

7. Vivekanandan, S.; Dickinson, P.; Bessell, E.; O'Connor, S. An unusual case of primary anaplastic large cell central nervous system lymphoma: An 8-year success story. *Case Rep.* **2011**, *2011*, bcr1120103550. [CrossRef]
8. Li, W. The 5th Edition of the World Health Organization Classification of Hematolymphoid Tumors. In *Leukemia*; Weijie, L., Ed.; Exon Publications: Brisbane, Australia, 2022; pp. 1–21, ISBN 978-0-645-33207-0.
9. George, D.H.; Scheithauer, B.W.; Aker, F.V.; Kurtin, P.J.; Burger, P.C.; Cameselle-Teijeiro, J.; McLendon, R.E.; Parisi, J.E.; Paulus, W.; Roggendorf, W.; et al. Primary Anaplastic Large Cell Lymphoma of the Central Nervous System: Prognostic Effect of ALK-1 Expression. *Am. J. Surg. Pathol.* **2003**, *27*, 487–493. [CrossRef]
10. Geetha, N.; Sreelesh, K.P.; Nair, R.; Mathews, A. Anaplastic large cell lymphoma presenting as a cerebellar mass. *Hematol. Oncol. Stem Cell Ther.* **2014**, *7*, 157–161. [CrossRef]
11. Furuya, K.; Takanashi, S.; Ogawa, A.; Takahashi, Y.; Nakagomi, T. High-dose methotrexate monotherapy followed by radiation for CD30-positive, anaplastic lymphoma kinase-1—Positive anaplastic large-cell lymphoma in the brain of a child: Case report. *PED* **2014**, *14*, 311–315. [CrossRef]
12. Karikari, I.O.; Thomas, K.K.; Lagoo, A.; Cummings, T.J.; George, T.M. Primary Cerebral ALK-1-Positive Anaplastic Large Cell Lymphoma in a Child. *Pediatr. Neurosurg.* **2007**, *43*, 516–521. [CrossRef] [PubMed]
13. Carmichael, M.G. Central Nervous System Anaplastic Large Cell Lymphoma in an Adult: Successful Treatment with a Combination of Radiation and Chemotherapy. *Mil. Med.* **2007**, *172*, 673–675. [CrossRef] [PubMed]
14. Liu, Q.; Chen, X.; Li, G.; Ye, Y.; Liu, W.; Zhao, S.; Zhang, W. Primary central nervous system ALK-positive anaplastic large cell lymphoma with CD56 abnormally expression in a Chinese child: Challenge in diagnostic practice. *Int. J. Immunopathol. Pharmacol.* **2020**, *34*, 205873842094175. [CrossRef] [PubMed]
15. Page, M.J.; McKenzie, J.E.; Bossuyt, P.M.; Boutron, I.; Hoffmann, T.C.; Mulrow, C.D.; Shamseer, L.; Tetzlaff, J.M.; Akl, E.A.; Brennan, S.E.; et al. The PRISMA 2020 statement: An updated guideline for reporting systematic reviews. *BMJ* **2021**, *372*, n71. [CrossRef] [PubMed]
16. Veritas Health Innovation Covidence. Systematic Review Software, Melbourne, Australia. Available online: www.covidence.org (accessed on 5 May 2022).
17. Ponzoni, M.; Terreni, M.R.; Ciceri, F.; Ferreri, A.J.M.; Gerevini, S.; Anzalone, N.; Valle, M.; Pizzolito, S.; Arrigoni, G. Primary brain CD30+ ALK1+ anaplastic large cell lymphoma ('ALKoma'): The first case with a combination of 'not common' variants. *Ann. Oncol.* **2002**, *13*, 1827–1832. [CrossRef]
18. Ozkaynak, M.F. Favorable Outcome of Primary CNS Anaplastic Large Cell Lymphoma in an Immunocompetent Patient. *J. Pediatr. Hematol. Oncol.* **2009**, *31*, 128–130. [CrossRef] [PubMed]
19. Rupani, A.; Modi, C.; Desai, S.; Rege, J. Primary anaplastic large cell lymphoma of central nervous system—A case report. *J. Postgrad. Med.* **2005**, *51*, 326–327.
20. Buxton, N.; Punt, J.; Hewitt, M. Primary Ki-1-Positive T-Cell Lymphoma of the Brain in a Child. *Pediatr. Neurosurg.* **1998**, *29*, 250–252. [CrossRef]
21. Gerstner, E.R.; Batchelor, T.T. Primary Central Nervous System Lymphoma. *Arch. Neurol.* **2010**, *67*, 291–297. [CrossRef]
22. Lannon, M.; Lu, J.-Q.; Chum, M.; Wang, B.H. ALK-negative CNS anaplastic large cell lymphoma: Case report and review of literature. *Br. J. Neurosurg.* **2023**, *37*, 1245–1250. [CrossRef]
23. Hirano, Y.; Miyawaki, S.; Tanaka, S.; Taoka, K.; Hongo, H.; Teranishi, Y.; Takami, H.; Takayanagi, S.; Kurokawa, M.; Saito, N. Clinical Features and Prognostic Factors for Primary Anaplastic Large Cell Lymphoma of the Central Nervous System: A Systematic Review. *Cancers* **2021**, *13*, 4358. [CrossRef] [PubMed]
24. Grommes, C.; Rubenstein, J.L.; DeAngelis, L.M.; Ferreri, A.J.M.; Batchelor, T.T. Comprehensive approach to diagnosis and treatment of newly diagnosed primary CNS lymphoma. *Neuro-Oncology* **2019**, *21*, 296–305. [CrossRef] [PubMed]
25. Reni, M.; Ferreri, A.J.M.; Garancini, M.P.; Villa, E. Therapeutic management of primary central nervous system lymphoma in immunocompetent patients: Results of a critical review of the literature. *Ann. Oncol.* **1997**, *8*, 227–234. [CrossRef] [PubMed]
26. Suzuki, R.; Kagami, Y.; Takeuchi, K.; Kami, M.; Okamoto, M.; Ichinohasama, R.; Mori, N.; Kojima, M.; Yoshino, T.; Yamabe, H.; et al. Prognostic significance of CD56 expression for ALK-positive and ALK-negative anaplastic large-cell lymphoma of T/null cell phenotype. *Blood* **2000**, *96*, 2993–3000. [PubMed]
27. Hayabuchi, N.; Shibamoto, Y.; Onizuka, Y. Primary central nervous system lymphoma in japan: A nationwide survey. *Int. J. Radiat. Oncol. Biol. Phys.* **1999**, *44*, 265–272. [CrossRef] [PubMed]
28. Bataille, B.; Delwail, V.; Menet, E.; Vandermarcq, P.; Ingrand, P.; Wager, M.; Guy, G.; Lapierre, F. Primary intracerebral malignant lymphoma: Report of 248 cases. *J. Neurosurg.* **2000**, *92*, 261–266. [CrossRef]
29. Pulsoni, A.; Gubitosi, G.; Rocchi, L.; Iaiani, G.; Martino, B.; Carapella, C. Vaccaro Primary T-cell lymphoma of central nervous system (PTCLCNS): A case with unusual presentation and review of the literature. *Ann. Oncol.* **1999**, *10*, 1519–1523. [CrossRef]
30. Latta, S.; Myint, Z.W.; Jallad, B.; Hamdi, T.; Alhosaini, M.N.; Kumar, D.V.; Kheir, F. Primary Central Nervous System T-Cell Lymphoma in Aids Patients: Case Report and Literature Review. *Curr. Oncol.* **2010**, *17*, 63–66. [CrossRef]
31. Gerstner, E.R.; Carson, K.A.; Grossman, S.A.; Batchelor, T.T. Long-term outcome in pcnsl patients treated with high-dose methotrexate and deferred radiation. *Neurology* **2008**, *70*, 401–402. [CrossRef]
32. Ahrendsen, J.T.; Ta, R.; Li, J.; Weinberg, O.K.; Ferry, J.A.; Hasserjian, R.P.; Meredith, D.M.; Varma, H.; Sadigh, S.; Michaels, P.D. Primary Central Nervous System Anaplastic Large Cell Lymphoma, ALK Positive. *Am. J. Clin. Pathol.* **2022**, *158*, 300–310. [CrossRef]

33. Tanaka, M.; Miura, H.; Ishimaru, S.; Furukawa, G.; Kawamura, Y.; Kozawa, K.; Yamada, S.; Ito, F.; Kudo, K.; Yoshikawa, T. Future Perspective for ALK-Positive Anaplastic Large Cell Lymphoma with Initial Central Nervous System (CNS) Involvement: Could Next-Generation ALK Inhibitors Replace Brain Radiotherapy for the Prevention of Further CNS Relapse? *Pediatr. Rep.* **2023**, *15*, 333–340. [CrossRef] [PubMed]
34. Rigaud, C.; Abbou, S.; Ducassou, S.; Simonin, M.; Le Mouel, L.; Pereira, V.; Gourdon, S.; Lambilliotte, A.; Geoerger, B.; Minard-Colin, V.; et al. Profound and sustained response with next-generation ALK inhibitors in patients with relapsed or progressive ALK-positive anaplastic large cell lymphoma with central nervous system involvement. *Haematologica* **2022**, *107*, 2255–2260. [CrossRef] [PubMed]
35. Del Baldo, G.; Abbas, R.; Woessmann, W.; Horibe, K.; Pillon, M.; Burke, A.; Beishuizen, A.; Rigaud, C.; Le Deley, M.; Lamant, L.; et al. Neuro-meningeal relapse in anaplastic large-cell lymphoma: Incidence, risk factors and prognosis—A report from the European intergroup for childhood non-Hodgkin lymphoma. *Br. J. Haematol.* **2021**, *192*, 1039–1048. [CrossRef] [PubMed]
36. Woessmann, W. Prognostic factors in paediatric anaplastic large cell lymphoma role of ALK. *Front. Biosci.* **2015**, *7*, 205–216. [CrossRef]

Disclaimer/Publisher's Note: The statements, opinions and data contained in all publications are solely those of the individual author(s) and contributor(s) and not of MDPI and/or the editor(s). MDPI and/or the editor(s) disclaim responsibility for any injury to people or property resulting from any ideas, methods, instructions or products referred to in the content.

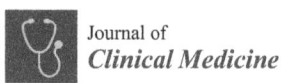

Case Report

Real-Time Neuropsychological Testing (RTNT) and Music Listening during Glioblastoma Excision in Awake Surgery: A Case Report

Grazia D'Onofrio [1,*], Nadia Icolaro [2], Elena Fazzari [2], Domenico Catapano [2], Antonello Curcio [3], Antonio Izzi [4], Aldo Manuali [4], Giuliano Bisceglia [4], Angelo Tancredi [4], Vincenzo Marchello [4], Andreaserena Recchia [4], Maria Pia Tonti [4], Luca Pazienza [5], Vincenzo Carotenuto [2], Costanzo De Bonis [2], Luciano Savarese [2], Alfredo Del Gaudio [4] and Leonardo Pio Gorgoglione [2]

[1] Clinical Psychology Service, Health Department, Fondazione IRCCS Casa Sollievo della Sofferenza, San Giovanni Rotondo, 71013 Foggia, Italy
[2] Complex Unit of Neurosurgery, Fondazione IRCCS Casa Sollievo della Sofferenza, San Giovanni Rotondo, 71013 Foggia, Italy; nadia.icolaro@gmail.com (N.I.); elena.fazzari87@gmail.com (E.F.); domenicocatapano1@gmail.com (D.C.); kino.23@virgilio.it (V.C.); costanzo.debonis@operapadrepio.it (C.D.B.); l.savarese@operapadrepio.it (L.S.); l.gorgoglione@operapadrepio.it (L.P.G.)
[3] Division of Neurosurgery, BIOMORF Department, University of Messina, 98122 Messina, Italy; antonello.curcio@gmail.com
[4] Complex Unit of Anesthesia-2, Fondazione IRCCS Casa Sollievo della Sofferenza, San Giovanni Rotondo, 71013 Foggia, Italy; antonioizzi1201@gmail.com (A.I.); a.manuali@operapadrepio.it (A.M.); giulianobisceglia@live.it (G.B.); angelotancredi2@virgilio.it (A.T.); vincenzomarchello@libero.it (V.M.); a.recchia@operapadrepio.it (A.R.); mariapiatonti@alice.it (M.P.T.); freddydelgaudio@libero.it (A.D.G.)
[5] Complex Unit of Radiology, Fondazione IRCCS Casa Sollievo della Sofferenza, San Giovanni Rotondo, 71013 Foggia, Italy; lucapazienza@libero.it
* Correspondence: g.donofrio@operapadrepio.it; Tel./Fax: +39-0882-410271

Simple Summary: In a case study, real-time neuropsychological testing (RTNT) and music listening were applied for resections in the left temporal–parietal lobe during awake surgery (AS). The preoperative, intraoperative, and postoperative neuropsychological evaluation of patients with brain tumors and those treated neurosurgically has become part of clinical protocols. It allows for the evaluation of the presence of any neuropsychological deficits and their severity, provides reliable indications regarding the patients' tolerability of an intervention in AS, and examines the cognitive and emotional motivational status of patients in the postoperative phase, thereby providing indications of the rehabilitation treatment and quality-of-life level. Moreover, we demonstrated that before/during AS and after music listening, the patient reported a decrease in depression and anxiety, in addition to an improvement in all the collected cognitive parameters. In conclusion, RTNT (also integrated with music listening) maximizes the surgical resection of lesions and minimizes the risks of post-operative neuropsychological and neurological sequelae through improving the quality of life of patients.

Abstract: In this case report, real-time neuropsychological testing (RTNT) and music listening were applied for resections in the left temporal–parietal lobe during awake surgery (AS). The case is based on a 66-year-old with glioblastoma and alterations in expressive language and memory deficit. Neuropsychological assessment was run at baseline (2–3 days before surgery), discharge from hospital (2–3 days after surgery), and follow-up (1 month and 3 months). RTNT was started before beginning the anesthetic approach (T0) and during tumor excision (T1 and T2). At T0, T1, and T2 (before performing neuropsychological tests), music listening was applied. Before AS and after music listening, the patient reported a decrease in depression and anxiety. During AS, an improvement was shown in all cognitive parameters collected at T0, T1, and T2. After the excision and music listening, the patient reported a further decrease in depression and anxiety. Three days post surgery, and at follow-ups of one month and three months, the patient reported a further improvement in cognitive aspects, the absence of depression, and a reduction in anxiety symptoms. In conclusion, RTNT has been useful in detecting cognitive function levels during tumor excision. Music listening during AS decreased the patient's anxiety and depression symptoms.

Citation: D'Onofrio, G.; Icolaro, N.; Fazzari, E.; Catapano, D.; Curcio, A.; Izzi, A.; Manuali, A.; Bisceglia, G.; Tancredi, A.; Marchello, V.; et al. Real-Time Neuropsychological Testing (RTNT) and Music Listening during Glioblastoma Excision in Awake Surgery: A Case Report. *J. Clin. Med.* **2023**, *12*, 6086. https://doi.org/10.3390/jcm12186086

Academic Editor: Morgan Broggi

Received: 21 July 2023
Revised: 1 September 2023
Accepted: 12 September 2023
Published: 20 September 2023

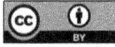

Copyright: © 2023 by the authors. Licensee MDPI, Basel, Switzerland. This article is an open access article distributed under the terms and conditions of the Creative Commons Attribution (CC BY) license (https://creativecommons.org/licenses/by/4.0/).

Keywords: awake surgery; real-time neuropsychological testing; music; glioblastoma; cognitive impairment; depression; anxiety

1. Introduction

Glioblastomas (GBMs) [1] are highly malignant tumors categorized as adult-type diffuse gliomas by the WHO in 2021. The new WHO classification system for brain tumors, published in 2021, has modified the nomenclature, creating a new family called "Adult-type diffuse gliomas", which includes the following: astrocytoma, IDH-mutant; oligodendroglioma, IDH-mutant, and 1p/19q-codeleted; glioblastoma, IDH-wildtype. For simplicity, the authors refer to this family as "GBM". GBMs are the most common adult brain tumors, with an annual incidence of approximately over 4/100,000 [1–3]. They occur predominantly between the ages of 45 and 64 years [4]. The tumor often has a rapidly progressive course (around 2–3 months). The median overall survival time is around 14.6 months, with a 5-year survival rate of only 7.2% [5,6]. The neurological signs are nonspecific as they are secondary to intracranial hypertension and/or behavioral changes and/or focal neurologic deficits [7].

The most frequent deficits detected in patients with GBM, through a pre- and post-operative cognitive assessment, were identified in executive functions, working memory, and attention [8–12]. The drastic worsening of quality of life experienced by patients who present a worsening in daily performance due to cognitive deficits is described in the literature, and it showed that cognitive rehabilitation could significantly improve performance [11–13]. Brain tumor patients often present with symptoms related to profound fatigue that prevents them from being active and reduces their social participation [12]. Therefore, the maintenance of language and cognition is essential in GBM surgery because they are fundamental features of daily life performance [13]. In a study, it was confirmed via a pre- and post-operative neuropsychological evaluation that awake surgery (AS) is associated with good cognitive and linguistic clinical outcomes in malignant tumors [14].

Moreover, detailed information provided about the cognitive status of patients during AS using a neuropsychological monitoring technique called real-time neuropsychological testing (RTNT) is considered necessary [14]. RTNT includes testing protocols based on the area where the surgery is performed and provides the surgeon with essential useful feedback on the cognitive status of patients [14].

Nevertheless, many patients report experiencing anxiety during awake craniotomy. Previous studies have evaluated the effects of music on patient anxiety during any awake medical procedures, such as nasal bone fracture reduction [15], parturition [16], transrectal prostate [17] and breast [18] biopsy, extracorporeal shock wave lithotripsy [19], colonoscopies [20], dental extractions [21], carotid endarterectomy [22], and dialysis catheter implantation [23], as well as pain and blood pressure improvement [1,6,24]. Regarding awake craniotomy, a study reported that providing music listening when patients were in the waiting room and during surgery reduced anxiety and reached the goal of improved human and perioperative care [25]. This study is supported by a previous qualitative study which reported that the effects of listening to major- and minor-key musical pieces on patients undergoing awake craniotomy could help in the design of interventions to alleviate anxiety, stress, and tension [26].

In this case report, an RTNT (preceded and followed by music listening) for resections in the left temporal–parietal lobe was performed with the following specific aims:

(1) To show a complete view of the cognitive functions of the patients and to verify how the neuropsychological status evolves during resection;
(2) To test the hypothesis that listening to music during AS decreases the patient's anxiety and agitation.

2. Materials and Methods

The present case report was conducted according to the Declaration of Helsinki, the Guidelines for Good Clinical Practice, and the Strengthening the Reporting of Observational Studies in Epidemiology (STROBE) guidelines [27], and it was approved by the local ethics committee for human experimentation (Prot. N. 1668/01DG).

2.1. Pre and Post-Operative Neuropsychological Evaluation

Neuropsychological assessment has been run at baseline (2–3 days before surgery), discharge from the hospital (2–3 days after surgery), and follow-up (1 month and 3 months). Cognitive status has been assessed using the Mini Mental State Examination (MMSE) [28], Clock Drawing Test (CDT) [29], Frontal Assessment Battery (FAB) [30], Babcock Story Recall Test (BSRT) [31], Digit Span Forward and Backward (DS-F, DS-B) [32], Attentional Matrices (AM) [33], Verbal Fluency for letters (VF-L) and for categories (VF-C) [34], Boston Naming Test (BNT) [35], Trail Making Test (TMT) parts A and B [36], Screening Test for Ideo-Motor Apraxia (STIMA) [37], Oral Apraxia (OA) [38], and Copying of Geometric Figures (CGF) [39].

The presence/absence of neuropsychiatric symptoms was evaluated with the Neuropsychiatric Inventory (NPI) [40].

2.2. Operative Setting and Procedures

The patient underwent surgery lying in the supine position with his left shoulder uplifted by a pillow. The right arm was placed laterally horizontally on a special armrest. The left arm was free and, to make the position more comfortable, resting on a pillow that the patient held to his chest. The head was only tilted to the right, and not raised or hyperextended, and held in place with a Mayfield–Kees head holder. This last procedure was adjusted with the patient awake to increase patient comfort; we slowly agreed with the patient and the head was angled to the left by about 60 degrees. Sterile drapes were positioned to allow access to the patient's face for anesthetists and the psychologist, in order to receive and respond to commands during cognitive testing.

Regarding the anesthetic management strategy for AS, the following steps were carried out:

(1) In the preoperative phase, intramuscular clonidine is administered in the evening before surgery and in the morning half an hour before, at a dosage of 2 µg/kg in order to obtain the right anxiolysis;
(2) On the day of the surgery, in the first phase, blocks of the nerves of the scalp are performed with local anesthesia to avoid not only pain during the surgical cut but above all the distress during the placement and removal of the cranial blocker, which certainly involves strong bone tension [41];
(3) The chosen strategic option for awake craniotomy has been MAC (monitored anesthesia care), which involves analgo-sedation via administering Dexmetomidine and Remifentanil in continuous intravenous infusion, allowing the patient to be sedated and in comfort, but contactable and spontaneously breathing [42].

After a wide ∩-shaped incision in the left temporo-parieto-occipital region, a 6.5 × 6.5 cm craniotomy was performed. The craniotomy shape was conducted under neuronavigation guidance in order to perform mapping in areas adjacent to the lesion as well [43,44]. The neuro-navigator defined the cortical edges of lesions and established the site of the corticectomy and the trajectory in the approach to subcortical lesions; the corticectomy in our case was performed in an area between the left angularis gyrus and left supramargina, to gain access to the deep temporo-parieto-occipital junction (Figure 1). Before removing tumor or tumor-infiltrated brain tissue, it was remembered that neurological functions can also be found in the same areas [45–48].

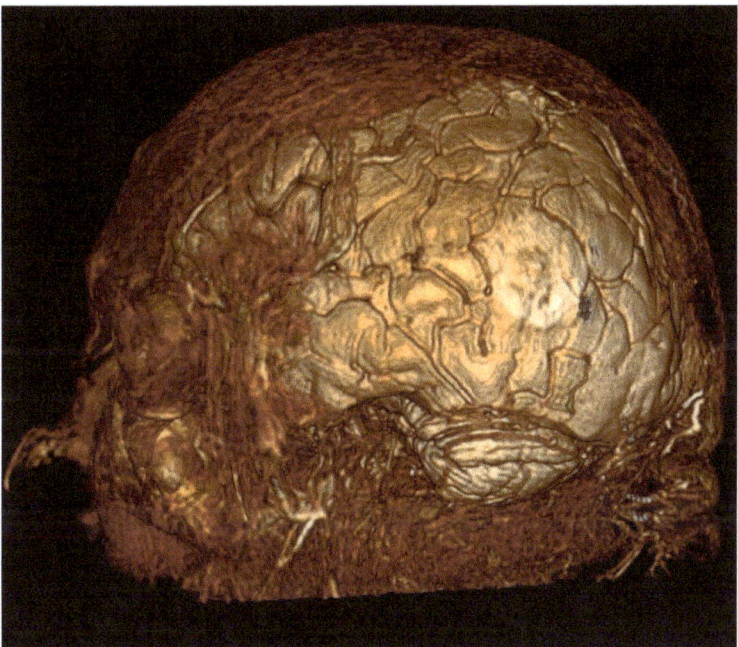

Figure 1. 3D reconstruction showing (white area) the localization of the tumor.

2.3. RTNT

The criteria we used to perform RTNT were the same as those used for AS [49]. RTNT was started at the beginning of the resection and ended at the beginning of hemostasis.

The battery of tasks included in RTNT was selected from published neuropsychological batteries available in Italian normative data. Tasks encompassing a wide range of cognitive functions have been included to have an exhaustive intraoperative neuropsychological battery. From the extensive list of tasks, a neuropsychologist selected a series of tasks according to lesion localization, magnetic resonance imaging (MRI) results, and the preoperative neuropsychological profile. The task sequence follows a fixed order with regard to an area. The sequence of tasks was repeated (presenting a different stimuli list for each sequence) until the end of the resection. In each test for a patient, the items were presented for about 30 s for each task, in a rotating manner. In this way task, assessment and task switching served as quick and dynamic methods for immediate dysfunction detection. As soon as the patient exhibited a decrement, the neurosurgeon was immediately informed and carried on with the surgical technique already described.

When this sequence was completed and if patient performance was within the normal range, we restarted testing using the first task and followed the same sequence but with different items. On the contrary, if a patient showed a decrement, we performed in-depth testing.

The following tests were performed when the patient arrived in the operating room and before starting the anesthetic approach (T0) and during tumor excision (T1 and T2): DS-F, DS-B, VF, BNT, and sensory-motor profile awake (SMP-A) [50].

2.4. Music Listening

At T0, T1, and T2 (before performing the neuropsychological tests), music listening was applied: a series of songs were chosen by the patient and followed a sensitivity linked to a music therapy approach.

The chronology of the songs was therefore studied, trying to create a sort of emotional path led by the musical melodies and songs that were part of the patient's youthful experience.

The rhythms, melodic characteristics, and the concepts expressed through the melodies and the lyrics of the songs have been taken into account.

3. Case Report

3.1. Patient Information

The present report describes the case of the second patient FS, a 66-year-old right-handed man with 8 years of education. He is a shopkeeper. His personal and medical history did not report comorbidities before the diagnosis of the tumor. No family history of epilepsy or other neurological diseases was reported.

For some months, he has been reporting alterations in expressive language and memory deficit, with more evident worsening in the last two weeks.

The patient was examined with MRI, which evidenced a lesion in the left temporo-occipital–parietal cortex of likely heteroplastic nature; the lesion (46 mm measured on the MRI image) was characterized by abundant central necrosis and a solid component with intense marginal contrast enhancement (CE), which corresponded to a significant increase in choline and the presence of lipids (Figure 2). The hypothesis of an awake surgery was considered. His neurological assessment was unremarkable regarding the sensorium, cranial nerves, motor, sensory, cerebellar, gait, reflexes, meningeal irritation, and long tract signs; only cognitive aspect results are worthy of further study using psychometric scales.

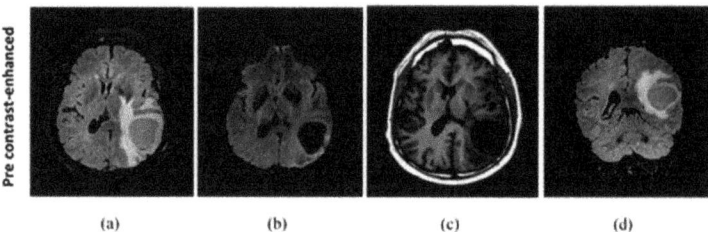

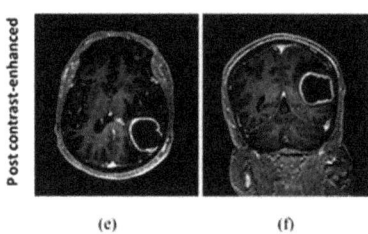

Figure 2. T1-weighted, Flair MRI images and spectroscopy acquired pre-surgery. (**a**) Pre-contrast-enhanced Flair MRI axial slice; (**b**) pre-contrast-enhanced diffusion-weighted imaging at b1000 axial slice; (**c**) pre-contrast-enhanced T1-weighted MRI axial slices; (**d**) pre-contrast-enhanced Flair MRI coronal slice; (**e**) post-contrast-enhanced T1-weighted MRI axial slices; (**f**) post-contrast-enhanced T1-weighted MRI coronal slices.

Blood samples, including routine blood count, kidney and liver function test, serum lipids, glucose level, serum lactate, lactic acid dehydrogenase, serum immunoglobulin, thyroid hormones and autoantibodies (anti-TPO), and routine autoimmunity testing (ANA, ENA, ANCA, and anti-phospholipids antibodies), were all normal.

3.2. Clinical Findings

At baseline (Table 1), the patient showed (1) a severe impairment of working memory (DS-B = 0.25), long-term memory, shifting ability (TMT-B = 482.00), and verbal fluency (VF-L = 5.00; VF-C = 15.00); (2) a mild–moderate deficit of selective attention (AM = 44.25); executive and visuospatial functions (FAB = 10.00; CDT = 3.00); lexical naming performance (BNT = 41.00); bucco-facial, ideomotor and constructive praxia (OA = 8.00; STIMA = 8.00; CGF = 9.75); (3) anxious–depressive symptoms (NPI = 17.00).

Table 1. Patient's psycho-behavioral aspects and neuropsychological performance at baseline.

	Score	Remark
Mini Mental State Examination (MMSE)	19.53	Mild cognitive impairment
Neuropsychiatric Inventory (NPI)	17	Depression, Anxiety, Insomnia
Clock Drawing Test (CDT)	3	Mild to moderate visuo-spatial disorganization
FrontalAssessmentBattery (FAB)	10	Impaired executive functions
Trail Making Test (TMT)-A	47	Mild impairment
Trail Making Test (TMT)-B	283	Severe impairment
Matrici Attentive (MA)	44.25	Mildimpairment
DigitSpan–Forward (DS-F)	6.25	No compromised
DigitSpan–Backward (DS-B)	0.25	Severe impairment
Babcock Story Recall Test (BSRT)	3.3	Severe impairment
Verbal Fluency for letter (VF-L)	5	Severe impairment
Verbal Fluency for category (VF-C)	15	Severe impairment
Boston Naming Test (BNT)	41	Mild to moderate impairment
Copying of Geometric Figures (CGF)	9.75	Moderate impairment
Screening Test for Ideo-Motor Apraxia (STIMA)	8/10	Mild impairment
OralApraxia (OA)	8/10	Mild impairment

3.3. Timeline and Intra-Operative Evaluations

As shown in Table 2, at T0, before AS and after music listening, the patient reported a decrease in depression and anxiety (NPI = 10.00).

Table 2. Patient's psycho-behavioral aspects and neuropsychological performance at different testing times: before starting the anesthetic approach (T0) and during tumor excision (T1 and T2).

Test	T0	T1	T2
Time	08:45	11:00	12:23
Neuropsychiatric Inventory (NPI)	10	10	7
DigitSpan–Forward (DS-F)	5.25	6.25	6.25
DigitSpan–Backward (DS-B)	0.25	1.25	3.25
Verbal Fluency for letter (VF-L)	5	10	14
Verbal Fluency for category (VF-C)	15	24	32
Boston Naming Test (BNT)	44	50	55
Sensory-motorprofileawake (SMP-A)	100	100	100

During AS, improvement was shown in all parameters collected, respectively, at T0, T1, and T2: DS-F (5.25 vs. 6.25 vs. 6.25), DS-B (0.25 vs. 1.25 vs. 3.25), VF-L (5.00 vs. 10.00 vs. 14.00), VF-C (15.00 vs. 24.00 vs. 32.00), and BNT (44.00 vs. 50.00 vs. 55.00). No changes turned up on the SMP-A (100.00 vs. 100.00 vs. 100.00) scale.

After excision and music listening (T2), the patient reported a further decrease in depression and anxiety (NPI = 7.00).

After the resection, histological exams confirmed the neuro-radiological suspicion of GBM.

3.4. Follow-Up and Outcomes

As shown in Table 3, at three days post surgery and at follow-up appointments after one month and three months, the patient reported only an isolated working memory (DS-B = 3.25 vs. 4.25 vs. 3.25) and praxic–constructive capacity (CGF = 10.75 vs. 10.75 vs. 11.75) impairment, the absence of depression, and a reduction in anxiety symptoms (NPI = 6.00 vs. 4.00 vs. 4.00).

Table 3. Patient's psycho-behavioral aspects and neuropsychological performance at three days post surgery and follow-up of one month and three months.

Test	3 Day Post-Surgery Score	1 Month-Follow Up Score	3 Month-Follow Up Score
Mini Mental State Examination (MMSE)	25.53	28.53	28.53
Neuropsychiatric Inventory (NPI)	0	4	4
Clock Drawing Test (CDT)	2	1	1
FrontalAssessmentBattery (FAB)	11	15	16
Trail Making Test (TMT)-A	46	32	30
Trail Making Test (TMT)-B	107	31	105
Matrici Attentive (MA)	44.25	52.25	49.25
DigitSpan–Forward (DS-F)	5.25	6.25	5.25
DigitSpan–Backward (DS-B)	3.25	4.25	3.25
Babcock Story Recall Test (BSRT)	4.3	15.7	12.6
Verbal Fluency for letter (VF-L)	14	17	18
Verbal Fluency for category (VF-C)	40	42	39
Boston Naming Test (BNT)	56	59	53
Copying of Geometric Figures (CGF)	10.75	10.75	11.75
Screening Test for Ideo-Motor Apraxia (STIMA)	10/10	10/10	10/10
OralApraxia (OA)	10/10	10/10	10/10

After a month of follow up, the MRI images (Figure 3) reported the results of left temporo-parietal craniotomy surgery for the removal of GBM with an inhomogeneous, partly hematic surgical cavity, delimited by an irregular enhancement border after the administration of CE in some points with nodular characteristics.

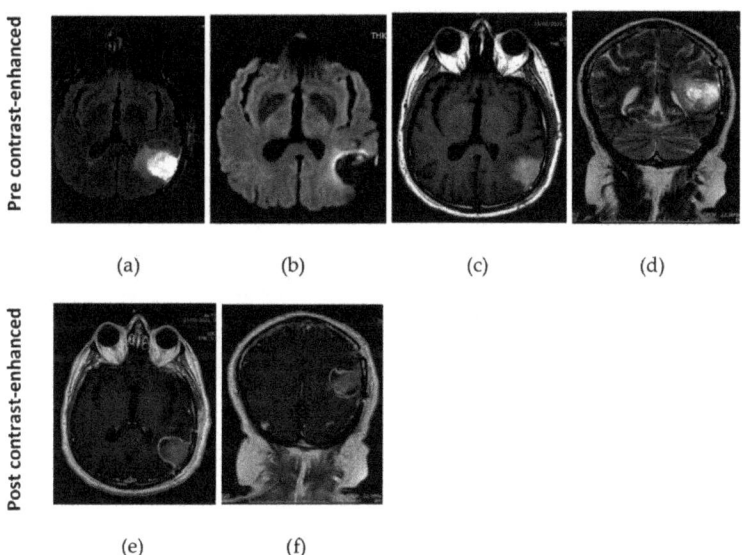

Figure 3. T1, T2-weighted, Flair MRI images acquired after a month of follow up. (**a**) Pre-contrast-enhanced Flair MRI axial slice; (**b**) pre-contrast-enhanced diffusion-weighted imaging at b1000 axial slice; (**c**) pre-contrast-enhanced T1-weighted MRI axial slices; (**d**) pre-contrast-enhanced T2-weighted coronal slice; (**e**) post-contrast-enhanced T1-weighted MRI axial slices; (**f**) post-contrast-enhanced T1-weighted MRI coronal slices.

4. Discussion

The study of cortical and cortico-axonal connectivity represents the new frontier of cognitive neuroscience for understanding the evolution of thought and mind. Furthermore, preserving cortical and axonal connectivity is the goal of brain tumor surgery in order to avoid the onset of permanent post-operative neuropsychological deficits. The surgeon can be trained to sew the surgical trajectory on the particular patient through interrupting or dislocating the fibers, minimizing injury to the neighboring fibers. White fibers can exhibit a variety of modifications, as also mentioned by Duffau [51], including morphological distortion brought on by a mass effect, tumor cell infiltration, the presence of edema, complete interruption, and occasionally functional reorganization. High-grade gliomas, on the other hand, can invade white matter tracts, leading to the displacement, rupture, and subsequent modification of the white matter signal [52]. White matter, in contrast to the cerebral cortex, shows relatively limited functional remodeling; hence, sparing fiber bundles is crucial [53].

Consequently, the preoperative, intraoperative, and postoperative neuropsychological evaluation of patients with brain tumors and those who have been treated neurosurgically has become part of clinical protocols. It allows us to evaluate the presence of any neuropsychological deficits and their severity, provides reliable indications regarding the patient's tolerability of an intervention in AS, and examines the cognitive and emotional motivational status of the patient in the postoperative phase, providing indications of the rehabilitation treatment and the quality-of-life level. It arises according to an individualized clinical–relational process aimed at exploring the interests, tastes, habits, and temperamental and personological characteristics of each patient for an adequate understanding of inter-individual differences. A complete and objective neuropsychological assessment also evaluates the functioning of a wide range of cognitive functions: language, memory, learning, working memory, visuospatial skills, attentional and executive skills, praxic skills, motivation, and emotional and behavioral regulation. Unfortunately, in the neurosurgical field, to date, much attention has been paid to language skills alone, modulating surgical resection techniques and preoperative and intraoperative mapping during awake surgery, to avoid the onset of language and aphasic deficits after surgery. However, very little has been done with respect to other cognitive functions which are equally important for an adequate level of quality of life and are seriously disabling if deficient. Many studies conducted thanks to systematic protocols of neuropsychological assessment highlight, in fact, the constant presence of cognitive problems related to functions other than language in patients suffering from brain tumors or epilepsy who are treated surgically [54,55].

In this case report, it has been shown how fundamental a complete neuropsychological profile of the patient is. The patient not only presented a language deficit but also impairment of working memory; long-term memory; shifting ability; verbal fluency; selective attention; executive and visuospatial functions; and bucco-facial, ideomotor, and constructive praxia; in addition to anxious–depressive symptoms.

Moreover, we demonstrated that before/during AS and after music listening, the patient reported a decrease in depression and anxiety in addition to the improvement of all collected cognitive parameters. These outcomes are in line with other studies that demonstrated the positive effects of music listening on patient satisfaction, anxiety, and depression [56,57]. A study showed that listening to music with headphones obtains relaxing effects comparable to those of midazolam: muscles relax, anxiety vanishes, and stress levels are lowered [58].

Through a neuropsychological evaluation performed at three days post surgery and at follow-up appointments after one month and three months, it has been possible to report the further cognitive and affective improvements of the patient. Another important factor to be taken into consideration during the neuropsychological assessment and the preoperative and intraoperative mapping of the cognitive and neurological functioning of patients with GBM is the possibility—almost systematic, as clinical practice suggests—that the brain has undergone of the reorganization of functional networks through processes of brain plasticity. This, among other things, would explain the heterogeneity of cognitive and neurological symptoms among GBM patients affecting the same brain areas.

Brain plasticity could be defined as a continuous process of remodeling and reorganizing neuronal synapses in the short, medium, and long term; during phylogenetic and ontogenetic development; and in the presence of brain lesions. It strengthens even more the modern neuroscientific conception of the brain as a complex and dynamic organ, not fixed, and emphasizes the appropriateness of the functional and neuropsychological neuro-oncological approach towards patients with GBM. The cognitive and behavioral consequences of the phenomenon of neuronal plasticity in these patients have been extensively studied [56] and justify the inhomogeneity of the preoperative and intraoperative data obtained from neurocognitive evaluations and from mapping methods. In other words, it should not be a surprise if, for example, the preoperative mapping of the linguistic functions of a patient affected by GBM who does not present linguistic deficits upon neurocognitive evaluation yields results that affect areas of the cortex not properly held responsible for linguistic and distant functions, or even contralateral to the injury. The phenomenon of neuronal plasticity is also almost systematic in patients suffering from gliomas, compared, for example, to patients affected by stroke, due to the very nature of the disease, which develops over time; over time, the glioma grows at the same time as the brain grows [59]. Cortico-subcortical reorganization can also be observed and confirmed during mapping via intraoperative stimulation induced by the presence of a brain tumor.

Plastic reorganization mechanisms are also observable in the postoperative phase [60]. Therefore, the observation of the phenomenon of the reorganization of cortical circuits through the various mapping methods and the standardized neuropsychological evaluation in neurosurgery involves different fundamental therapeutic implications for achieving the objectives that the functional neuro-oncological approach aims to achieve. It allows the surgical treatment to be extended to eloquent or near-eloquent areas, maximizes the surgical resection of the lesion, and minimizes the risks of post-operative neuropsychological and neurological sequelae through improving the quality of life of patients [61].

As usually happens, the limitations of the case report lie in the impossibility of drawing generalizations, establishing cause–effect relationships, and the danger of over-interpretation. In particular, in this case report, a control is not described; for this reason, the ability to draw conclusions is severely limited.

Cooperation with other clinicians and the use of other research methodologies are needed. An investigation of current neuropsychological approaches and working towards agreed and standardized protocols could be prospects for future research.

5. Conclusions

In conclusion, in light of what has been argued up to now, the brain of every human being is organized differently from all the others in normal conditions. This is supported by the most recent scientific research in neuroscience that suggests the existence of inter-individual differences in the organization of neuronal networks at the cortical and subcortical levels between one brain and another, significantly beyond the classic conceptions of the localization of human cognition and emotion, opening the doors to dynamic and complex approaches and models. The brains of GBM patients also undergo functional neuroplasticity phenomena that make them even more different and complex than the norm. The surgical treatment of such patients, therefore, is plausible if one uses, for the modulation of resection techniques, the data coming from the neuropsychological evaluation and from the mapping methods that do not disregard the singularity of the brain and of the patient's personality.

Author Contributions: Conceptualization, G.D. and L.P.G.; methodology, G.D.; validation, N.I., E.F., A.C. and D.C.; formal analysis, G.D.; investigation, G.D., N.I., E.F., A.C., A.M., G.B., A.T., V.M., A.R., M.P.T., D.C., V.C., C.D.B. and L.S.; resources, A.I. and L.P.; data curation, G.D.; writing—original draft preparation, G.D.; writing—review and editing, A.I., A.D.G. and L.P.G.; visualization, N.I., E.F., A.C., A.I., G.B., L.P., A.T., V.M., D.C., V.C., C.D.B. and L.S.; supervision, A.D.G. and L.P.G. All authors have read and agreed to the published version of the manuscript.

Funding: The Italian Ministry of Health (Ricerca Corrente programme 2022 2024) funded this research.

Institutional Review Board Statement: This study was conducted in accordance with the Declaration of Helsinki and approved by the Ethics Committee of Fondazione IRCCS Casa Sollievo della Sofferenza (Prot. N. 1668/01DG).

Informed Consent Statement: Informed consent was obtained from all subjects involved in the study.

Data Availability Statement: Not applicable.

Conflicts of Interest: The authors declare no conflict of interest.

References

1. WHO Classification of Tumours Editorial Board. *World Health Organization Classification of Tumours of the Central Nervous System*, 5th ed.; International Agency for Research on Cancer: Lyon, France, 2021.
2. Ho, V.K.Y.; Reijneveld, J.C.; Enting, R.H.; Bienfait, H.P.; Robe, P.; Baumert, B.G.; Visser, O.; Dutch Society for Neuro-Oncology (LWNO). Changing Incidence and Improved Survival of Gliomas. *Eur. J. Cancer* **2014**, *50*, 2309–2318. [CrossRef] [PubMed]
3. Fehr, C.M.; Auer, R.N. Simultaneous Presentation of Glioblastoma Multiforme in Divorced Spouses. *Case Rep. Oncol.* **2022**, *15*, 231–237. [CrossRef] [PubMed]
4. Tamimi, A.F.; Juweid, M. Epidemiology and Outcome of Glioblastoma. In *Glioblastoma*; De Vleeschouwer, S., Ed.; Codon Publications: Brisbane, Australia, 2017.
5. Lynes, J.P.; Nwankwo, A.K.; Sur, H.P.; Sanchez, V.E.; Sarpong, K.A.; Ariyo, O.I.; Dominah, G.A.; Nduom, E.K. Biomarkers for Immunotherapy for Treatment of Glioblastoma. *J. Immunother. Cancer* **2020**, *8*, e000348. [CrossRef] [PubMed]
6. CBTRUS Statistical Report: Primary Brain and Other Central Nervous System Tumors Diagnosed in the United States in 2013–2017—PubMed. Available online: https://pubmed.ncbi.nlm.nih.gov/33123732/ (accessed on 3 May 2023).
7. Sharma, S.; Hashmi, M.F.; Kumar, A. *Intracranial Hypertension*; StatPearls Publishing: Treasure Island, FL, USA, 2023.
8. van Loenen, I.S.; Rijnen, S.J.M.; Bruijn, J.; Rutten, G.-J.M.; Gehring, K.; Sitskoorn, M.M. Group Changes in Cognitive Performance After Surgery Mask Changes in Individual Patients with Glioblastoma. *World Neurosurg.* **2018**, *117*, e172–e179. [CrossRef]

9. Tanzilli, A.; Pace, A.; Fabi, A.; Telera, S.; Vidiri, A.; Carosi, M.; Terrenato, I.; Koudriavtseva, T.; Boccaletti, R.; Villani, V. Neurocognitive Evaluation in Older Adult Patients Affected by Glioma. *J. Geriatr. Oncol.* **2020**, *11*, 701–708. [CrossRef]
10. Early Measures of Cognitive Function Predict Survival in Patients with Newly Diagnosed Glioblastoma—PubMed. Available online: https://pubmed.ncbi.nlm.nih.gov/22508762/ (accessed on 3 May 2023).
11. Klein, M.; Postma, T.J.; Taphoorn, M.J.B.; Aaronson, N.K.; Vandertop, W.P.; Muller, M.; van der Ploeg, H.M.; Heimans, J.J. The Prognostic Value of Cognitive Functioning in the Survival of Patients with High-Grade Glioma. *Neurology* **2003**, *61*, 1796–1798. [CrossRef]
12. Noll, K.R.; Sullaway, C.M.; Wefel, J.S. Depressive Symptoms and Executive Function in Relation to Survival in Patients with Glioblastoma. *J. Neurooncol.* **2019**, *142*, 183–191. [CrossRef]
13. Bonifazi, S.; Passamonti, C.; Vecchioni, S.; Trignani, R.; Martorano, P.P.; Durazzi, V.; Lattanzi, S.; Mancini, F.; Ricciuti, R.A. Cognitive and Linguistic Outcomes after Awake Craniotomy in Patients with High-Grade Gliomas. *Clin. Neurol. Neurosurg.* **2020**, *198*, 106089. [CrossRef]
14. Tomasino, B.; Guarracino, I.; Ius, T.; Maieron, M.; Skrap, M. Real-Time Neuropsychological Testing Protocol for Left Temporal Brain Tumor Surgery: A Technical Note and Case Report. *Front. Hum. Neurosci.* **2021**, *15*, 760569. [CrossRef]
15. Ortega, A.; Gauna, F.; Munoz, D.; Oberreuter, G.; Breinbauer, H.A.; Carrasco, L. Music therapy for pain and anxiety management in nasal bone fracture reduction: Randomized controlled clinical trial. *Otolaryngol. Head Neck Surg.* **2019**, *161*, 613–619. [CrossRef]
16. Simavli, S.; Gumus, I.; Kaygusuz, I.; Yildirim, M.; Usluogullari, B.; Kafali, H. Effect of music on labor pain relief, anxiety level and postpartum analgesic requirement: A randomized controlled clinical trial. *Gynecol. Obstet. Investig.* **2014**, *78*, 244–250. [CrossRef] [PubMed]
17. Tsivian, M.; Qi, P.; Kimura, M.; Chen, V.H.; Chen, S.H.; Gan, T.J.; Polascik, T.J. The effect of noise-cancelling headphones or music on pain perception and anxiety in men undergoing transrectal prostate biopsy. *Urology* **2012**, *79*, 32–36. [CrossRef]
18. Soo, M.S.; Jarosz, J.A.; Wren, A.A.; Soo, A.E.; Mowery, Y.M.; Johnson, K.S.; Yoon, S.C.; Kim, C.; Hwang, E.S.; Keefe, F.J.; et al. Imaging-guided core-needle breast biopsy: Impact of meditation and music interventions on patient anxiety, pain, and fatigue. *J. Am. Coll. Radiol.* **2016**, *13*, 526–534. [CrossRef]
19. Karalar, M.; Keles, I.; Doğantekin, E.; Kahveci, O.K.; Sarici, H. Reduced pain and anxiety with music and noise-canceling headphones during shockwave lithotripsy. *J. Endourol.* **2016**, *30*, 674–677. [CrossRef]
20. Ko, C.H.; Chen, Y.Y.; Wu, K.T.; Wang, S.C.; Yang, J.F.; Lin, Y.Y.; Lin, C.I.; Kuo, H.J.; Dai, C.Y.; Hsieh, M.H. Effect of music on level of anxiety in patients undergoing colonoscopy without sedaion. *J. Chin. Med. Assoc.* **2017**, *80*, 154–160. [CrossRef]
21. Yamashita, K.; Kibe, T.; Ohno, S.; Kohjitani, A.; Sugimura, M. The effects of music listening during extraction of the impacted mandibular third molar on the autonomic nervous system and psychological state. *J. Oral Maxillofac. Surg.* **2019**, *77*, 1153.e1–1153.e8. [CrossRef]
22. Kavakli, A.S.; Kavrut Ozturk, N.; Yavuzel Adas, H.; Kudsioglu, S.T.; Ayoglu, R.U.; Özmen, S.; Sagdic, K.; Yapici, N. The effects of music on anxiety and pain in patients during carotid endarterectomy under regional anesthesia: A randomized controlled trial. *Complement. Ther. Med.* **2019**, *44*, 94–101. [CrossRef]
23. Jacquier, S.; Nay, M.A.; Muller, G.; Muller, L.; Mathonnet, A.; Lefèvre-Benzekri, D.; Bretagnol, A.; Barbier, F.; Kamel, T.; Runge, I.; et al. Effect of a Musical Intervention During the Implantation of a Central Venous Catheter or a Dialysis Catheter in the Intensive Care Unit: A Prospective Randomized Pilot Study. *Anesth. Analg.* **2022**, *134*, 781–790. [CrossRef]
24. Hole, J.; Hirsch, M.; Ball, E.; Meads, C. Music as an aid for postoperative recovery in adults: A systematic review and meta-analysis. *Lancet* **2015**, *386*, 1659–1671. [CrossRef] [PubMed]
25. Wu, P.Y.; Huang, M.L.; Lee, W.P.; Wang, C.; Shih, W.M. Effects of music listening on anxiety and physiological responses in patients undergoing awake craniotomy. *Complement. Ther. Med.* **2017**, *32*, 56–60. [CrossRef] [PubMed]
26. Jadavji-Mithani, R.; Venkatraghavan, L.; Bernstein, M. Music is Beneficial for Awake Craniotomy Patients: A Qualitative Study. *Can. J. Neurol. Sci.* **2015**, *42*, 7–16. [CrossRef]
27. von Elm, E.; Altman, D.G.; Egger, M.; Pocock, S.J.; Gøtzsche, P.C.; Vandenbroucke, J.P. STROBE Initiative Strengthening the Reporting of Observational Studies in Epidemiology (STROBE) Statement: Guidelines for Reporting Observational Studies. *BMJ* **2007**, *335*, 806–808. [CrossRef]
28. Folstein, M.; Folstein, S.; McHugh, P.R. Mini-mental state: A practical method for grading the cognitive state of patients for the clinician. *J. Psychiatr. Res.* **1975**, *12*, 189–198. [CrossRef] [PubMed]
29. Rouleau, I.; Salmon, D.P.; Butters, N.; Kennedy, C.; McGuire, K. Quantitative and qualitative analyses of clock drawings in Alzheimer's and Huntington's disease. *Brain Cogn.* **1992**, *18*, 70–87. [CrossRef]
30. Dubois, B.; Litvan, I. The FAB: A frontal assessment battery at bedside. *Neurology* **2000**, *55*, 1621–1626. [CrossRef]
31. Babcock, H.; Levy, L. *The Measurement of Efficiency of Mental Functioning (Revised Examination): Test and Manual of Directions*; C.H. Stoelting: Chicago, IL, USA, 1940.
32. Wechsler, D. *Wechsler Intelligence Scale for Children—III*; The Psychological Corporation: San Antonio, TX, USA, 1991.
33. Spinnler, H.; Tognoni, G. Standardizzazione e taratura italiana di test neuropsicologici. *Ital. J. Neurol. Sci.* **1987**, *8*, 21–120.
34. Lezak, M.; Howieson, D.; Bigler, E.; Tranel, D. *Neuropsychological Assessment*; Oxford University Press: New York, NY, USA, 2012.
35. Kaplan, E.; Goodglass, H.; Weintraub, S. *The Boston Naming Test*; Lea & Febiger: Philadelphia, PA, USA, 1983.
36. Reitan, R.M. Validity of the Trail Making test as an indicator of organic brain damage. *Percept. Mot. Ski.* **1958**, *8*, 271–276. [CrossRef]

37. Tessari, A.; Toraldo, A.; Lunardelli, A.; Zadini, A.; Rumiati, R.I. STIMA: A short screening test for ideo-motor apraxia, selective for action meaning and bodily district. *Neurol. Sci.* **2015**, *36*, 977–984. [CrossRef]
38. De Renzi, E.; Pieczuro, A.; Vignolo, L.A. Oral Apraxia and Aphasia. *Cortex* **1966**, *2*, 50–73. [CrossRef]
39. Arrigoni, G.; De Renzi, E. Constructional apraxia and hemispheric locus of lesion. *Cortex* **1964**, *1*, 170–197. [CrossRef]
40. Cummings, J.L.; Mega, M.; Gray, K.; Rosenberg-Thompson, S.; Carusi, D.A.; Gornbein, J. The Neuropsychiatric Inventory: Comprehensive assessment of psychopathology in dementia. *Neurology* **1994**, *44*, 2308–2314. [CrossRef]
41. Potters, J.W.; Klimek, M. Local anesthetics for brain tumor resection: Current perspectives. *Local Reg. Anesth.* **2018**, *11*, 35–44. [CrossRef]
42. Eseonu, C.I.; ReFaey, K.; Garcia, O.; John, A.; Quinones-Hinojosa, A.; Tripathi, P. Awake craniotomy anesthesia: A comparison between the monitored anesthesia care versus the asleep-awake-asleep technique. *World Neurosurg.* **2017**, *104*, 679–686. [CrossRef] [PubMed]
43. Ojemann, G.A.; Ojemann, J.; Lettich, E.; Berger, M. Cortical language localization in left, dominant hemisphere. An electrical stimulation mapping investigation in 117 patients. *J. Neurosurg.* **1989**, *71*, 316–326. [CrossRef]
44. Sanai, N.; Mirzadeh, Z.; Berger, M.S. Functional outcome after language mapping for glioma resection. *N. Engl. J. Med.* **2008**, *358*, 18–27. [CrossRef]
45. Bello, L.; Acerbi, F.; Giussani, C.; Baratta, P.; Taccone, P.; Songa, V.; Fava, M.; Stocchetti, N.; Papagno, C.; Gaini, S.M. Intraoperative language localization in multilingual patients with gliomas. *Neurosurgery* **2006**, *59*, 115–125. [CrossRef]
46. Reithmeier, T.; Krammer, M.; Gumprecht, H.H.; Gerstner, W.; Lumenta, C.B. Neuronavigation combined with electrophysiological monitoring for surgery of lesions in eloquent brain areas in 42cases: A retrospective comparison of the neurological outcome and the quality of resection with a control group withsimilar lesions. *Min-Minim. Invasive Neurosurg.* **2003**, *46*, 65–71. [CrossRef]
47. Benzagmout, M.; Gatignol, P.; Duffau, H. Resection of World Health Organization grade II gliomas involving Broca's area: Methodological and functional considerations. *Neurosurgery* **2007**, *61*, 741–752. [CrossRef] [PubMed]
48. Picht, T.; Kombos, T.; Gramm, H.; Brock, M.; Suess, O. Multimodal protocol for awake craniotomy in language cortex tumour surgery. *Acta Neurochir.* **2006**, *148*, 127–137. [CrossRef]
49. Skrap, M.; Marin, D.; Ius, T.; Fabbro, F.; Tomasino, B. Brain mapping: A novel intraoperative neuropsychological approach. *J. Neurosurg.* **2016**, *125*, 877–887. [CrossRef] [PubMed]
50. Becker, J.; Jehna, M.; Steinmann, E.; Mehdorn, H.M.; Synowitz, M.; Hartwigsen, G. The sensory-motor profile awake-A new tool for pre-, intra-, and post operative assessment of sensory-motor function. *Clin. Neurol. Neurosurg.* **2016**, *147*, 39–45. [CrossRef]
51. Duffau, H. Lessons from brain mapping in surgery for low-grade glioma: Insights into associations between tumour and brain plasticity. *Lancet Neurol.* **2005**, *4*, 476–486. [CrossRef] [PubMed]
52. Abhinav, K.; Yeh, F.C.; Mansouri, A.; Zadeh, G.; Fernandez-Miranda, J.C. High-definition fiber tractography for the evaluation of perilesional white matter tracts in high-grade glioma surgery. *Neuro-Oncology* **2015**, *17*, 1199–1209. [CrossRef] [PubMed]
53. Yogarajah, M.; Focke, N.K.; Bonelli, S.B.; Thompson, P.; Vollmar, C.; McEvoy, A.W.; Alexander, D.C.; Symms, M.R.; Koepp, M.J.; Duncan, J.S. The structural plasticity of white matter networks following anterior temporal lobe resection. *Brain J. Neurol.* **2010**, *133*, 2348–2364. [CrossRef]
54. Behrens, M.; Thakur, N.; Lortz, I.; Seifert, V.; Kell, C.A.; Forster, M.T. Neurocognitive deficits in patients suffering from glioma in speech-relevant areas of the left hemisphere. *Clin. Neurol. Neurosurg.* **2021**, *207*, 106816. [CrossRef] [PubMed]
55. van Kessel, E.; Huenges Wajer, I.M.C.; Ruis, C.; Seute, T.; Fonville, S.; De Vos, F.Y.F.L.; Verhoeff, J.J.C.; Robe, P.A.; van Zandvoort, M.J.E.; Snijders, T.J. Cognitive impairments are independently associated with shorter survival in diffuse glioma patients. *J. Neurol.* **2021**, *268*, 1434–1442. [CrossRef]
56. Tan, D.J.A.; Polascik, B.A.; Kee, H.M.; Hui Lee, A.C.; Sultana, R.; Kwan, M.; Raghunathan, K.; Belden, C.M.; Sng, B.L. The Effect of Perioperative Music Listening on Patient Satisfaction, Anxiety, and Depression: A Quasiexperimental Study. *Anesthesiol. Res. Pract.* **2020**, *2020*, 3761398. [CrossRef]
57. Pérez-Ros, P.; Cubero-Plazas, L.; Mejías-Serrano, T.; Cunha, C.; Martínez-Arnau, F.M. Preferred Music Listening Intervention in Nursing Home Residents with Cognitive Impairment: A Randomized Intervention Study. *J. Alzheimer's Dis.* **2019**, *70*, 433–442. [CrossRef]
58. Graff, V.; Cai, L.; Badiola, I.; Elkassabany, N.M. Music versus midazolam during preoperative nerve block placements: A prospective randomized controlled study. *Reg. Anesth. Pain Med.* **2019**, *44*, 796–799. [CrossRef]
59. Plaza, M.; Gatignol, P.; Leroy, M.; Duffau, H. Speaking without Broca's area after tumor resection. *Neurocase* **2009**, *15*, 294–310. [CrossRef]
60. Duffau, H. Does post-lesional subcortical plasticity exist in the human brain? *Neurosci. Res.* **2009**, *65*, 131–135. [CrossRef] [PubMed]
61. Prat-Acín, R.; Galeano-Senabre, I.; López-Ruiz, P.; García-Sánchez, D.; Ayuso-Sacido, A.; Espert-Tortajada, R. Intraoperative Brain Mapping during Awake Surgery in Symptomatic Supratentorial Cavernomas. *Neurocirugía Engl. Ed.* **2021**, *32*, 217–223. [CrossRef] [PubMed]

Disclaimer/Publisher's Note: The statements, opinions and data contained in all publications are solely those of the individual author(s) and contributor(s) and not of MDPI and/or the editor(s). MDPI and/or the editor(s) disclaim responsibility for any injury to people or property resulting from any ideas, methods, instructions or products referred to in the content.

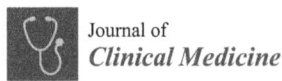

Systematic Review

Surgical Treatment of Spheno-Orbital Meningiomas: A Systematic Review and Meta-Analysis of Surgical Techniques and Outcomes

Edoardo Agosti [1], Marco Zeppieri [2,*], Lucio De Maria [1], Marcello Mangili [1], Alessandro Rapisarda [3], Tamara Ius [4], Leopoldo Spadea [5], Carlo Salati [2], Alessandro Tel [6], Antonio Pontoriero [7], Stefano Pergolizzi [7], Filippo Flavio Angileri [8], Marco Maria Fontanella [1] and Pier Paolo Panciani [1]

1. Division of Neurosurgery, Department of Surgical Specialties, Radiological Sciences and Public Health, University of Brescia, 25123 Brescia, Italy; edoardo_agosti@libero.it (E.A.)
2. Department of Ophthalmology, University Hospital of Udine, Piazzale S. Maria Della Misericordia 15, 33100 Udine, Italy
3. Department of Neurosurgery, Fondazione Policlinico Universitario Agostino Gemelli IRCSS, 00168 Rome, Italy
4. Neurosurgery Unit, Head-Neck and NeuroScience Department, University Hospital of Udine, p.le S. Maria Misericordia 15, 33100 Udine, Italy
5. Eye Clinic, Policlinico Umberto I, "Sapienza" University of Rome, 00142 Rome, Italy
6. Clinic of Maxillofacial Surgery, Head-Neck and NeuroScience Department University Hospital of Udine, p.le S. Maria Della Misericordia 15, 33100 Udine, Italy
7. Radiation Oncology Unit, Department of Biomedical, Dental Science and Morphological and Functional Images, University of Messina, 98125 Messina, Italy
8. Neurosurgery Unit, Department of Biomedical, Dental Science and Morphological and Functional Images, 98125 Messina, Italy
* Correspondence: markzeppieri@hotmail.com

Citation: Agosti, E.; Zeppieri, M.; De Maria, L.; Mangili, M.; Rapisarda, A.; Ius, T.; Spadea, L.; Salati, C.; Tel, A.; Pontoriero, A.; et al. Surgical Treatment of Spheno-Orbital Meningiomas: A Systematic Review and Meta-Analysis of Surgical Techniques and Outcomes. J. Clin. Med. 2023, 12, 5840. https://doi.org/10.3390/jcm12185840

Academic Editor: Alexandre Bozec

Received: 21 July 2023
Revised: 29 August 2023
Accepted: 5 September 2023
Published: 8 September 2023

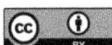

Copyright: © 2023 by the authors. Licensee MDPI, Basel, Switzerland. This article is an open access article distributed under the terms and conditions of the Creative Commons Attribution (CC BY) license (https://creativecommons.org/licenses/by/4.0/).

Abstract: Background: Spheno-orbital meningiomas (SOMs) are rare tumors arising from the meninges surrounding the sphenoid bone and orbital structures. Surgical resection is the primary treatment approach for SOMs. Several surgical approaches have been described during the decades, including microsurgical transcranial (MTAs), endoscopic endonasal (EEAs), endoscopic transorbital (ETOAs), and combined approaches, and the choice of surgical approach remains a topic of debate. Purpose: This systematic review and meta-analysis aim to compare the clinical and surgical outcomes of different surgical approaches used for the treatment of SOMs, discussing surgical techniques, outcomes, and factors influencing surgical decision making. Methods: A comprehensive literature review of the databases PubMed, Ovid MEDLINE, and Ovid EMBASE was conducted for articles published on the role of surgery for the treatment of SOMs until 2023. The systematic review was performed according to the Preferred Reporting Items for Systematic Reviews and Meta-Analysis guidelines. Meta-analysis was performed to estimate pooled event rates and assess heterogeneity. Fixed- and random-effects were used to assess 95% confidential intervals (CIs) of presenting symptoms, outcomes, and complications. Results: A total of 59 studies comprising 1903 patients were included in the systematic review and meta-analysis. Gross total resection (GTR) rates ranged from 23.5% for ETOAs to 59.8% for MTAs. Overall recurrence rate after surgery was 20.7%. Progression-free survival (PFS) rates at 5 and 10 years were 75.5% and 49.1%, respectively. Visual acuity and proptosis improvement rates were 57.5% and 79.3%, respectively. Postoperative cranial nerve (CN) focal deficits were observed in 20.6% of cases. The overall cerebro-spinal fluid (CSF) leak rate was 3.9%, and other complications occurred in 13.9% of cases. MTAs showed the highest GTR rates (59.8%, 95%CI = 49.5–70.2%; $p = 0.001$) but were associated with increased CN deficits (21.0%, 95%CI = 14.5–27.6%). ETOAs had the lowest GTR rates (23.5%, 95%CI = 0.0–52.5%; $p = 0.001$), while combined ETOA and EEA had the highest CSF leak rates (20.3%, 95%CI = 0.0–46.7%; $p = 0.551$). ETOAs were associated with better proptosis improvement (79.4%, 95%CI = 57.3–100%; $p = 0.002$), while anatomical class I lesions were associated with better visual acuity (71.5%, 95%CI = 63.7–79.4; $p = 0.003$) and proptosis (60.1%, 95%CI = 38.0–82.2; $p = 0.001$) recovery. No significant differences were found in PFS rates between surgical approaches. Conclusion: Surgical treatment of SOMs aims to preserve visual function and improve proptosis. Different surgical approaches offer varying rates of GTR, complications, and functional outcomes. A multidisciplinary approach involving a skull base team is crucial for optimizing patient outcomes.

Keywords: spheno-orbital meningiomas; systematic review; meta-analysis; surgical approaches; clinical outcomes; surgical outcomes

1. Introduction

Spheno-orbital meningiomas (SOMs) are rare tumors, accounting for 0.2% and 9% of all meningiomas, arising from the meninges surrounding the sphenoid bone and orbital structures [1,2]. These tumors pose significant challenges due to their anatomical location and proximity to critical structures, necessitating a multidisciplinary approach to management [3]. Over the years, various surgical approaches have been developed and utilized, including microsurgical transcranial (MTAs), endoscopic endonasal (EEAs), endoscopic transorbital (ETOAs), and combined approaches (Figure 1). Each approach has its unique advantages and limitations, and there is a need to comprehensively compare their clinical and surgical outcomes to guide treatment decisions [4,5].

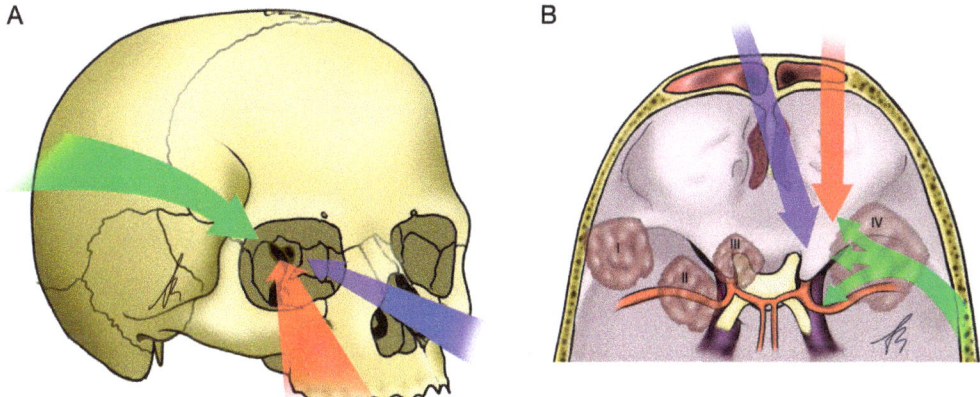

Figure 1. Graphical illustration of the surgical corridors of MTAs, EEAs, and ETOAs and anatomical classes of SOMs. (**A**) Anterolateral view of a skull: MTAs (green arrow), EEAs (blue arrow), and ETOAs (red arrow). (**B**) Supero-posterolateral view of the skull base. MTAs can provide several surgical corridors to different portion of the spheno-orbital region, including cavernous sinus, SOF and orbital apex, and anterior cranial fossa. SOMs anatomical classes are also here represented: anatomical class I (lateral or superolateral SOMs), II (medial or inferomedial SOMs), III (orbital apex SOMs), and IV (diffuse SOMs).

Surgical resection is the primary goal in the treatment of SOMs, aiming for gross total resection (GTR) to achieve optimal oncological control. However, the choice of surgical approach can have a significant impact on the extent of resection and postoperative outcomes. Additionally, postoperative complications and progression-free survival (PFS) are important outcome measures to assess the overall success of the surgical intervention [3,6].

The objective of this systematic literature review and meta-analysis is to compare the clinical and surgical outcomes among patients undergoing MTAs, EEAs, ETOAs, and combined approaches for the surgical treatment of SOMs. By examining the existing evidence, this study aims to provide clinicians with valuable insights into the advantages and limitations of each approach, and facilitate evidence-based decision making in the management of these challenging tumors.

2. Materials and Methods

2.1. Literature Search

The systematic review was performed according to the Preferred Reporting Items for Systematic Reviews and Meta-Analysis (PRISMA) guidelines [7]. A comprehensive literature search of the databases PubMed, Ovid MEDLINE, and Ovid EMBASE was designed and conducted by an experienced librarian with input from the authors. The keywords "spheno-orbital", "meningioma", and "approach", were used in "AND" and "OR" combinations. The following research string was used: "((spheno-orbital or sphenoorbital) AND (meningioma) AND (approach OR surgery OR microsurgical OR endoscopic OR endonasal OR transorbital OR combined) AND (outcome OR resection OR survival OR complication OR deficit))". The last search for articles pertinent to the topic was conducted on 1 July 2023. Other pertinent articles were retrieved through reference analysis. Two authors (E.A. and L.D.M.) independently conducted the abstract screening for eligibility. Any discordance was solved by consensus with two senior authors (M.Z. and P.P.P.). No restrictions on the date of publication were made. Exclusion criteria were as follows: studies published in languages other than English, preclinical anatomical and laboratory studies, studies which include patients with SOMs not surgically treated, meta-analysis, and literature review. Inclusion criteria: studies reporting at least a case of SOM surgically treated. The study was not registered, thus, there is no registration number.

2.2. Data Extraction

For each study, we abstracted the following baseline information: author, country, journal, title, and year of publication; design and period in which the population was collected; sample size, mean and range of age, percentage of female; histology and grade of the lesion (according to WHO classification 2021); clinical presentations, including visual acuity decrease, proptosis, cranial nerves (CNs) deficits, and other signs and symptoms; number and percentages of patient who received gross total resections, adjuvant radiotherapy (RT), other adjuvant therapies; follow-up period.

2.3. Outcomes

Outcomes were meta-analyzed based on the type of surgical approach (MTA, EEA, ETOA, or combined). The outcomes were also tested to evaluate any statistically significant differences according to the anatomical site and extension of the SOM and according to the WHO grade (grade I, II, and III, according to WHO classification 2021). Based on site, SOMs were divided into four categories, specifically, superior or superolateral, inferior or inferomedial, apex, and diffuse.

Our primary outcomes were GTR, progression-free survival at 5 years (PFS 5-y) and at 10 years (PFS 10-y), and recurrences rate. Secondary outcomes were improvement of visual acuity, improvement of proptosis, postoperative CNs deficits, postoperative cerebrospinal fluid (CSF) leak, and other complications.

2.4. Study Risk of Bias Assessment

We modified the Newcastle–Ottawa scale (NOS) to assess the methodologic quality of the studies included in our meta-analysis. This tool is designed for use in comparative studies. However, as there was no control group in our studies, we assessed their methodologic quality based on selected items from the scale, focusing on the following questions: (1) Did the study include all patients or consecutive patients vs. a selected sample? (2) Was the study retrospective or prospective? (3) Was clinical follow-up satisfactory, thus allowing ascertainment of all outcomes? (4) Were outcomes reported? (5) Were there clearly defined inclusion and exclusion criteria? (Figure 2).

MODIFIED NEWCASTLE - OTTAWA QUALITY ASSESSMENT SCALE

SELECTION

1) Representativeness of the exposed cohort
   a) Consecutive eligible participants were selected, participants were randomly selected, or all participants were invited to participate from the source population,
   b) Not satisfying requirements in part (a), or not stated.

2) Selection of the non-exposed cohort
   a) Selected from the same source population,
   b) Selected from a different source population,
   c) No description.

3) Ascertainment of exposure
   a) Medical record,
   b) Structured interview,
   c) No description.

4) Demonstration that outcome of interest was not present at the start of the study
   a) Yes,
   b) No or not explicitly stated.

COMPARABILITY

1) Were there clearly defined inclusion and exclusion criteria?
   a) Yes,
   b) No or not explicitly stated.

OUTCOME

1) Assessment of outcome
   a) Independent or blind assessment stated, or confirmation of the outcome by reference to secure records,
   b) Record linkage (e.g. identified through ICD codes on database records),
   c) Self-report with no reference to original structured injury data or imaging,
   d) No description.

2) Was follow-up long enough for outcomes to occur?
   a) Yes (≥12 months),
   b) No (<3 months).

3) Adequacy of follow up
   a) Complete follow up – all participants accounted for,
   b) Subjects lost to follow up unlikely to introduce bias (<20% lost to follow up or description provided of those lost),
   c) Follow up rate <85% and no description of those lost provided,
   d) No statement,

Figure 2. Modified Newcastle–Ottawa scale used to assess the methodologic quality of the studies included in our meta-analysis.

2.5. Statistical Analysis

Descriptive statistics were reported, including ranges and percentages. For the purpose of the meta-analysis, we estimated from each cohort the cumulative prevalence and 95% confidence interval for each outcome. Event rates were pooled across studies with a random-effects meta-analysis. Heterogeneity across studies was evaluated using the I2 statistic. An I2 value of >50% suggests substantial heterogeneity. For formal statistical comparisons and subgroup analysis, we also extracted a chi-square contingency table to calculate p values. The level of statistical significance was set to $p < 0.05$. Meta-regression was not used in this study. Statistical analyses were performed using OpenMeta Analyst http://www.cebm.brown.edu/openmeta accessed on 20 June 2023) and the R statistical package v3.4.1 http://www.r-project.org (accessed on 20 June 2023).

3. Results

3.1. Literature Review

A total of 157 papers were identified after duplicate removal. After title and abstract analysis, 94 articles were identified for full-text analysis. Eligibility was ascertained for 82 articles. The remaining 23 articles were excluded for the following reasons: (1) not relevant to the research topic (16 articles), (2) not in English (1 article), lack of method details (3 articles), systematic literature review or meta-analysis (3 articles). All studies included in the analysis had at least one or more outcome measures available for one or more of the patient groups analyzed. Figure 3 shows the flow chart according to the PRISMA statement.

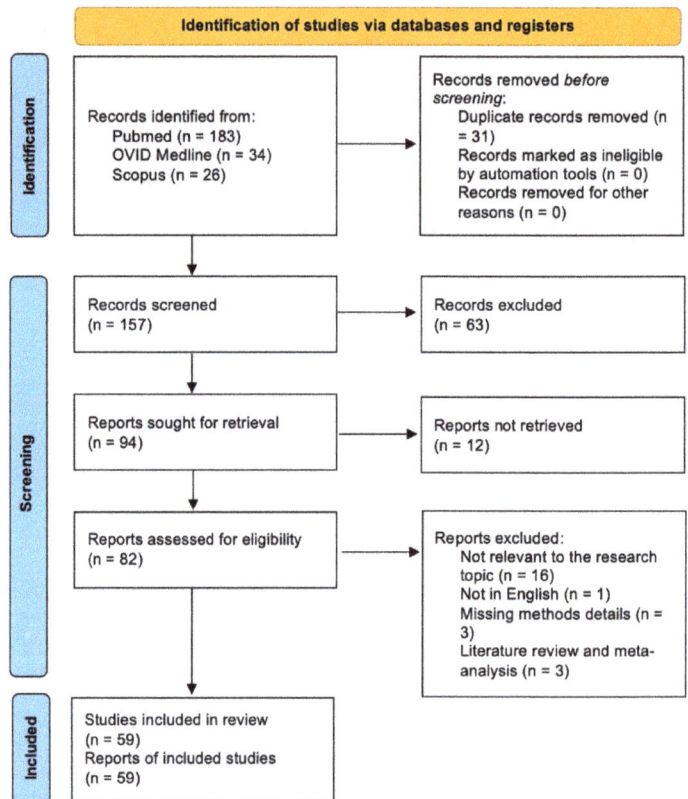

Figure 3. PRISMA flow diagram depicting the literature search process.

3.2. Baseline Data

A summary of the included studies is provided in Table 1. All studies included in our systematic review were retrospective. The study periods ranged from 1958 to 2021. A total of 1903 patients were included. The mean age at surgery ranged from 34 to 62 years. The WHO grade was reported in 31 studies (52%). At presentation, 1385/1730 patients had proptosis (80%), 920/1773 patients (52%) had a visual acuity decrease, and 191/1156 had CN deficits (13%). Regarding treatment, 875/1542 underwent GTR (57%) and 291/1420 received post-op RT (41%). The mean follow-up time ranged from 2 to 135 months.

Table 1. Summary of studies included in the systematic literature review and meta-analysis. (CN = cranial nerve; GTR = gross total resection; NA = not available; RT = radiotherapy).

No.	Study					Baseline Data				Presentation				Treatment		Mean Follow-Up Time (Months)
	Author, Journal, Year	Title	Country	Prospective /Retrospective	Study Period	Sample Size	Mean Age at Intervention (range)	F (%)	WHO Grade (No.)	Visual Acuity Decrease No. (%)	CN Deficits (III, IV, VI) No. (%)	Proptosis No. (%)	Others	No. (%) of GTR	No. (%) of Patients Receiving Post-op RT	
1	Bonnal [8], J Neurosurg, 1980	Invading Meningiomas of the Sphenoid Ridge	Belgium	Retrospective	1958–1979	21	45 (23–65)	81%	NA	8 (38%)	3 (14%)	11 (52%)	Epilepsy, hemiparesis, aphasia, headache, intracranial hypertension, visual field deficit, Foster Kennedy syndrome, deafness, 5th and 6th nerve palsy	NA	NA	NA
2	Maroon [9], J Neurosurg, 1994	Recurrent Spheno-Orbital Meningioma	USA	Retrospective	1975–1992	15	46	73%	NA	6 (40%)	2 (13%)	13 (87%)	Blindness, visual field deficit, V1 hypesthesia	9 (60%)	10 (67%)	NA
3	Gaillard [10], Plastic and Reconstructive Surgery, 1997	Strategy of Craniofacial Reconstruction After Resection of Spheno-Orbital "en Plaque" Meningiomas	France	Retrospective	1981–1993	20	NA	NA	NA	NA	2 (10%)	NA	NA	NA	NA	84
4	De Jesus [11], Surg Neurol, 2001	Surgical Management of Meningioma en Plaque of the Sphenoid Ridge	Puerto Rico	Retrospective	1990–1997	6	51 (39–64)	100%	NA	3 (50%)	NA	5 (83%)	Seizure	5 (83%)	NA	48
5	Leake [12], Arch Facial Plast Surg, 2005	Reconstruction after Resection of Sphenoid Wing Meningiomas	USA	Retrospective	1995–2004	22	53 (31–73)	77%	NA	5	NA	15 (68%)	Visual field deficit, trigeminal hypoesthesia, seizure, dysphagia	11 (50%)	4 (18%)	15

Table 1. Cont.

	Study				Baseline Data				Presentation		Treatment	Mean Follow-Up Time (Months)
6	Roser [13], Surg Neurol, 2005	Sphenoid Wing Meningiomas with Osseous Involvement	Germany	Retrospective	NA	82	53 (21–78)	77%	NA	18 (22%)	2 (2%)	31 (38%)	Headache, aphasia, trigeminal neuralgia, seizure	31 (38%)	NA	66
7	Shrivastava [14], J. Neurosurg, 2005	Spheno-Orbital Meningiomas: Surgical Limitations and Lessons Learned in Their Long-Term Management	USA	Retrospective	1991–2003	25	51 (22–76)	88%	NA	20 (80%)	5 (20%)	22 (88%)	Trigeminal hypoesthesia, scotoma	18 (70%)	2 (8%)	60
8	Sandalcioglu [15], Journal of Cranio-Maxillofacial Surgery, 2005	Spheno-orbital Meningiomas: Interdisciplinary Surgical Approach, Resectability and Long-Term Results	Germany	Retrospective	1998–2002	16	53 (3–76)	94%	I	7 (44%)	1 (6%)	14 (88%)	Diplopia	16 (100%)	2 (13%)	68
9	Schick [16], J Neurosurg, 2006	Management of Meningiomas en Plaque of the Sphenoid Wing	Germany	Retrospective	1991–2002	67	58 (32–79)	79%	I (64), II (3)	28 (42%)	11 (16%)	33 (49%)	V palsy, visual field deficit	40 (60%)	5 (7%)	46
10	Ringel [17], Operative Neurosurg, 2006	Microsurgical Technique and Results of a Series of 63 Spheno-orbital Meningiomas	Germany	Retrospective	1983–2003	63	51 (21–77)	79%	NA	28 (44%)	16 (25%)	50 (79%)	Visual field deficit, seizure, diplopia	45 (71%)	NA	54
11	Bikmaz [18], J Neurosurg, 2007	Management of Bone-Invasive, Hyperostotic Sphenoid Wing Meningiomas	USA	Retrospective	1994–2004	17	52 (36–70)	88%	NA	10 (59%)	3 (18%)	12 (71%)	Eye swelling, headache, incidental, diplopia	14 (82%)	NA	36
12	Yong [19], Chin Med J (Engl), 2009	Sphenoid Wing Meningioma en Plaque: Report of 37 Cases	China	Retrospective	1998–2009	37	46 (16–67)	59%	I (33), II (2), III (2)	26 (70%)	NA	37 (100%)	Headache, seizure	9 (24%)	10 (27%)	36

Table 1. *Cont.*

	Study				Baseline Data				Presentation			Treatment	Mean Follow-Up Time (Months)
13	Scarone [20], J Neurosurg, 2009	Long-Term Results with Exophthalmos in a Surgical Series of 30 Spheno-Orbital Meningiomas	France	Retrospective	1994–2005	30	51 (35–74)	100%	NA	6 (20%)	NA	28 (93%)	Headache, temporal swelling, visual field deficit	27 (90%)	1 (3%)	NA
14	Heufelder [21], Ophthalmic Plastic and Reconstructive Surgery, 2009	Reconstructive and Ophthalmologic Outcomes Following Resection of Spheno-Orbital Meningiomas	Germany	Retrospective	1997–2006	21	61 (47–81)	95%	I (19), II (2)	NA	NA	18 (86%)	Visual field deficit, epiphora	NA	5 (24%)	66
15	Mirone [22], Neurosurgery, 2009	En Plaque Sphenoid Wing Meningiomas: Recurrence Factors and Surgical Strategies in a Series of 71 Patients	France	Retrospective	1986–2006	71	53 (12–79)	87%	1	41 (58%)	15 (21%)	61 (86%)	Diplopia, headache, trigeminal pain, visual field deficit, chemosis, seizure	59 (83%)	1 (1%)	77
16	Cannon [5], Orbit, 2009	The Surgical Management and Outcomes for Spheno-Orbital Meningiomas: A 7-Year Review of Multi-Disciplinary Practice	UK	Retrospective	2000–2007	12	51 (34–64)	92%	I (11), II (1)	5 (42%)	1 (8%)	12 (100%)	Diplopia	NA	3 (25%)	31
17	Civit [23], Neurochirurgie, 2010	Spheno-Orbital Meningiomas	France	Retrospective	NA	41	NA	NA	NA	23 (56%)	4 (9%)	39 (95%)	V deficit, visual field deficit	NA	NA	NA

Table 1. Cont.

	Study			Baseline Data					Presentation			Treatment	Mean Follow-Up Time (Months)
18	Honig [24], Neurological research, 2010	Spheno-Orbital Meningiomas: Outcome After Microsurgical Treatment: A Clinical Review of 30 Cases	Germany	Retrospective	2001–2006	30	54 (25–74)	73%	I (26), II (3), III (1)	22 (73%)	6 (20%)	16 (53%)	Diplopia, headache, trigeminal pain, visual field deficit, chemosis, seizure	10 (33%)	8 (27%)	34
19	Oya [25], J Neurosurg, 2011	Spheno-Orbital Meningioma: Surgical Technique and Outcome	USA	Retrospective	1994–2009	39	49 (33–68)	87%	NA	21 (54%)	3 (8%)	39 (100%)	Diplopia, headache, trigeminal pain, visual field deficit	15 (38%)	4 (10%)	41
20	Luetjens [26], Clin Neurol Neurosurg, 2011	Bilateral Spheno-Orbital Hyperostotic Meningiomas with Proptosis and Visual Impairment: A Therapeutic Challenge. Report of Three Patients and Review of the Literature	Germany	Retrospective	NA	3	62 (49–70)	100%	1	3 (100%)	NA	3 (100%)	Vertigo, diplopia	2 (66%)	1 (33%)	28
21	Mariniello [27], Acta Neurochir (Wien), 2013	Surgical Unroofing of the Optic Canal and Visual Outcome in Basal Meningiomas	Italy	Retrospective	1986–2006	60	NA	NA	NA	60 (100%)	NA	NA	Visual field deficit, diplopia	NA	NA	60
22	Boari [28], British Journal of Neurosurgery, 2013	Management of Spheno-Orbital en Plaque Meningiomas: Clinical Outcome in a Consecutive Series of 40 Patients	Italy	Retrospective	2000–2010	40	53 (NA)	88%	NA	35 (88%)	2 (5%)	18 (45%)	Visual field deficit, diplopia	22 (56%)	18 (44%)	73

Table 1. Cont.

	Study						Baseline Data				Presentation			Treatment		Mean Follow-Up Time (Months)
23	Saeed [29], Br J Ophthalmol, 2011	Surgical Treatment of Spheno-Orbital Meningiomas	Netherlands	Retrospective	1980–2006	66	46 (26–68)	92%	NA	51 (77%)	NA	66 (100%)	Diplopia, headache	39 (59%)	15 (23%)	102
24	Simas [30], Surg Neurol Int, 2013	Sphenoid Wing en Plaque Meningiomas: Surgical Results and Recurrence Rates	Portugal	Retrospective	1998–2008	18	52 (27–75)	83%	I (18)	5 (28%)	1 (6%)	16 (89%)	Temporal region swelling, orbital pain, diplopia, V1, V2 hypesthesia	7 (39%)	6 (33%)	55
25	Attia [31], World Neurosurg, 2013	Combined Cranio-Nasal Surgery for Spheno-Orbital Meningiomas Invading the Paranasal Sinuses, Pterygopalatine, and Infra-Temporal Fossa	USA	Retrospective	2009–2011	3	60 (44–82)	66%	I (2), II (1)	2 (67%)	1 (33%)	2 (67%)	V palsy	1 (33%)	1 (33%)	10
26	Marcus [32], Acta Neurochir (Wien), 2013	Image-Guided Resection of Spheno-Orbital Skull-Base Meningiomas with Predominant Intra-Osseous Component	UK	Retrospective	2004–2012	19	44 (25–64)	89%	I (17), II (2)	11 (58%)	6 (32%)	12 (63%)	Temporal swelling, headache, V paresthesia, focal sensory seizures	11 (58%)	2 (11%)	60
27	Mariniello [33], Clin Neurol Neurosurg, 2013	Management of the Optic Canal Invasion and Visual Outcome in Spheno-Orbital Meningiomas	Italy	Retrospective	1986–2006	60	NA	NA	NA	36 (60%)	19 (34%)	59 (98%)	Optic disc pallor, optic disc edema	40 (67%)	5 (8%)	NA

Table 1. Cont.

#	Study	Country	Type	Years	N	Age (range)	%	Sex	Presentation			Treatment		Mean Follow-Up Time (Months)
28	Forster [34], Neurol Res, 2014 — Spheno-Orbital Meningiomas: Surgical Management and Outcome	Germany	Retrospective	2003–2013	18	50 (35–69)	100%	I (17), II (1)	7 (39%)	NA	15 (83%)	Diplopia, dizziness	13 (72%)	NA	44
29	Solmaz [35], Turk Neurosurg, 2014 — Surgical Strategies for the Removal of Spheno-Orbital Meningiomas	Turkey	Retrospective	2006–2013	13	34 (26–58)	23%	I (13)	8 (62%)	NA	10 (77%)	Facial pain, orbital pain, epilepsy	4 (31%)	0	26
30	Talacchi [36], Neurosurg Rev, 2014 — Surgical Management of Ocular Symptoms in Spheno-Orbital Meningiomas. Is Orbital Reconstruction Really Necessary?	Italy	Retrospective	1992–2012	47	57 (21–77)	56%	NA	24 (51%)	18 (32%)	46 (98%)	Periorbital and temporal swelling	24 (51%)	NA	52
31	Berhoum [37], Neurosurg Focus, 2014 — Endoscopic Endonasal Optic Nerve and Orbital Apex Decompression for Nontraumatic Optic Neuro-pathy: Surgical Nuances and Review of the Literature	France	Retrospective	2012–2014	4	58 (49–67)	75%	NA	4 (100%)	NA	NA	Visual field deficit	NA	NA	6

Table 1. Cont.

	Study				Baseline Data				Presentation		Treatment	Mean Follow-Up Time (Months)
32	Amirjamshidi [38], Surg Neurol Int, 2015	Lateral Orbitotomy Approach for Removing Hyper-ostosing en Plaque Sphenoid Wing Meningiomas. Description of Surgical Strategy and Analysis of Findings in a Series of 88 Patients with Long-Term Follow-up	Iran	Retrospective	1979–2013	88	46 (12–70)	74%	NA	65 (74%)	NA	88 (100%)	Visual field deficit, diplopia	NA	31 (35%)	135
33	Leroy [39], Acta Neurochir (Wein), 2016	Internal and External Spheno-Orbital Meningioma Varieties: Different Outcomes and Prog-noses	France	Retrospective	1995–2012	70	52 (21–80)	90%	I (60), II (5), III (5)	27 (39%)	NA	56 (80%)	Soft tissue tumefaction, headache, retrobulbar pain, whimpering, seizure, dizziness, diplopia	15 (11%)	18 (30%)	57
34	Bowers [40], J Neurosurg, 2016	Outcomes After Surgical Treatment of Meningioma-Associated Proptosis	USA	Retrospective	2002–2015	33	52 (12–76)	73%	NA	17 (52%)	NA	22 (22%)	Visual field deficit, diplopia, proptosis	31 (94%)	2 (6%)	54
35	Peron [41], Acta Neurochir Suppl, 2017	Spheno-Orbital Meningiomas: When the Endoscopic Approach is Better	Italy	Retrospective	2013–2014	30	46 (8–82)	73%	NA	1 (3%)	8 (27%)	21 (70%)	Visual field deficit, diplopia, V1 and V2 hypoesthesia	24 (80%)	NA	NA

Table 1. Cont.

	Study				Baseline Data				Presentation		Treatment	Mean Follow-Up Time (Months)
36	Terrier [42], World Neurosurgery, 2017	Spheno-Orbital Meningiomas Surgery: Multicenter Management Study for Complex Extensive Tumors	France	Retrospective	1996–2016	130	51 (28–74)	92%	I	49 (38%)	13 (10%)	123 (95%)	Retro-orbital pain, diplopia, headache	97 (75%)	2 (2%)	77
37	Freeman [4], World Neurosurgery, 2017	Spheno-Orbital Meningiomas: A 16-Year Surgical Experience	USA	Retrospective	2000–2016	25	51 (39–71)	92%	I (21), II (5)	19 (76%)	NA	22 (88%)	Diplopia, headache, seizure	NA	11 (25%)	45
38	Gonen [43], Neurosurg Rev, 2017	Spheno-Orbital Meningioma: Surgical Series and Design of an Intra-Operative Management Algorithm	Israel	Retrospective	2005–2014	27	53 (27–78)	89%	NA	10 (37%)	4 (15%)	25 (92%)	Visual field deficit, diplopia, proptosis, seizure	14 (52%)	1 (3%)	41
39	Almeida [44], J Neurosurg, 2018	Trans-Orbital Endoscopic Eyelid Approach for Resection of Spheno-Orbital Meningiomas with Predominant Hyper-ostosis: Report of 2 Cases	USA	Retrospective	NA	2	59 (53–65)	100%	I (2)	2 (100%)	NA	2 (100%)	Visual field deficit	0 (0%)	2 (100%)	2
40	Belinsky [45], Ophthalmic Plast Reconstr Surg, 2018	Spheno-Orbital Meningiomas: An Analysis Based on World Health Organization Classification and Ki-67 Proliferative Index	USA	Retrospective	2000–2016	46	56 (27–85)	58%	I (30), II (4), III (4)	15 (33%)	4 (9%)	15 (33%)	seizure, altered mental status, double vision, epiphora, headache, V1 hypoesthesia	NA	25 (66%)	63

166

Table 1. *Cont.*

	Study				Baseline Data				Presentation		Treatment	Mean Follow-Up Time (Months)
41	Dallan [46], Oper Neurosurg (Hagerstown), 2018	Endoscopic Trans-Orbital Superior Eyelid Approach for the Management of Selected Spheno-Orbital Meningiomas: Preliminary Experience	Italy	Retrospective	2012–2015	14	51 (35–73)	86%	I (14)	6 (43%)	2 (14%)	14 (100%)	Diplopia, pain, epiphora	3 (21%)	0 (0%)	25
42	Kong [47], J Neurosurg, 2018	Clinical and Ophthalmological Outcome of Endoscopic Trans-Orbital Surgery for Cranio-Orbital Tumors	Korea	Retrospective	2016–2017	12	56 (38–73)	92%	NA	7 (58%)	7 (39%)	14 (78%)	NA	4 (33%)	NA	5
43	Pace [48], Ophthalmic Plast Reconstr Surg, 2019	Orbital Reconstruction via Deformable Titanium Mesh Following Spheno-Orbital Meningioma Resection: Ophthalmic Presentation and Outcomes	USA	Retrospective	1996–2017	20	56 (19–89)	80%	NA	9 (45%)	3 (15%)	20 (100%)	Diplopia, visual field deficit	15 (75%)	4 (20%)	47
44	Nagahama [3], World Neurosurg, 2019	Spheno-Orbital Meningioma: Surgical Outcomes and Management of Recurrence	Japan	Retrospective	1996–2017	12	49 (20–71)	58%	I (15), II (2)	3 (25%)	NA	11 (92%)	Trigeminal hypoesthesia	3 (23%)	1 (8%)	74

Table 1. Cont.

	Study					Baseline Data				Presentation			Treatment	Mean Follow-Up Time (Months)
45	Endoscopic Endo- and Extra-Orbital Corridors for Spheno-Orbital Region: Anatomic Study with Illustrative Case	De Rosa [49], Acta Neurochir (Wien), 2019	Italy	Retrospective	NA	1	37	100%	NA	0	0	1 (100%)	Lateral nystagmus, hypesthesia V1	NA	NA	6
46	A Single Centre's Experience of Managing Spheno-Orbital Meningiomas: Lessons for Recurrent Tumour Surgery	Shapey [1], Acta Neurochir (Wien), 2019	London	Retrospective	2005–2016	31	49 (44–58)	65%	I (23), II (11)	13 (38%)	6 (18%)	13 (38%)	Diplopia, seizures, headaches, trigeminal pain, confusion/somnolence	29 (85%)	4 (11,8%)	52
47	Combined NeuroSurgical and Orbital Intervention for Spheno-Orbital Meningiomas—the Manchester Experience	Young [6], Orbit, 2019	UK	Retrospective	2000–2017	24	50 (NA)	92%	I (23), II (1)	17 (71%)	3 (13%)	21 (88%)	Diplopia, headache, visual field deficit	0 (0%)	7 (29%)	82
48	Spheno-Orbital Meningiomas: Optimizing Visual Outcome	Menon [50], J Neurosci Rural Pract, 2020	India	Retrospective	10 years	17	51 (17–72)	76%	I (14) e II (3)	14 (82%)	NA	14 (82%)	Headache, facial paresthesia	2 (12%)	15 (88%)	56
49	Trans-Orbital Endoscopic Surgery for Sphenoid Wing Meningioma: Long-Term Outcomes and Surgical Technique	Goncalves [51], J Neurol Surg B Skull Base, 2020	South Africa	Retrospective	2015–2019	21	48.8 (34–79)	95%	I (20), II (1)	21 (100%)	1 (5%)	20 (95%)	Headache, facial pain, diplopia, blocked nose, epiphora	NA	1 (5%)	12

Table 1. *Cont.*

	Study				Baseline Data				Presentation		Treatment	Mean Follow-Up Time (Months)
50	Park [52], World Neurosurg, 2020	Comparative Analysis of Endoscopic Trans-Orbital Approach and Extended Mini-Pterional Approach for Sphenoid Wing Meningiomas with Osseous Involvement: Preliminary Surgical Results	Republic of Korea	Retrospective	2015–2019	24	54 (24–73)	67%	NA	NA	Headache, cognitive decline, diplopia	21 (88%)	NA	20
51	Parish [53], J Neurol Surg Rep, 2020	Proptosis, Orbital Pain, and Long-Standing Monocular Vision Loss Resolved by Surgical Resection of Intra-Osseous Spheno-Orbital Meningioma: A Case Report and Literature Review	USA	Retrospective	2013	1	43	100%	NA	1 (100%)	NA	1 (100%)	Headache, periorbital pain	NA	12
52	Samadian, World Neurosurg, 2020	Surgical Outcomes of Spheno-Orbital en Plaque Meningioma: A 10-Year Experience in 57 Consecutive Cases	Iran	Retrospective	2007–2017	57	48 (22–76)	93%	NA	16 (28%)	NA	47 (83%)	Visual field deficit, diplopia	48 (84%)	6 (11%)	46

169

Table 1. Cont.

	Study				Baseline Data				Presentation			Treatment	Mean Follow-Up Time (Months)
53	Zamanipoor Najafabadi [54], Acta Neurochirurgica (Wein), 2021	Visual Outcomes Endorse Surgery of Patients with Spheno-Orbital Meningioma with Minimal Visual Impairment or Hyperostosis	Netherlands	Retrospective	2015–2019	19	47 (45–50)	95%	I	10 (53%)	NA	16 (84%)	Diplopia, headache, visual field deficit	14 (76%)	3 (16%)	46
54	In Woo [55], Graefes Arch Clin Exp Ophthalmol, 2021	Orbital Decompressive effect of Endoscopic Transorbital Surgery for Spheno-Orbital Meningioma	South Korea	Retrospective	2016–2019	18	54 (38–72)	89%	I (16), II (1)	10 (56%)	4 (22%)	17 (94%)	Visual field deficit	3 (17%)	12 (67%)	20
55	Masalha [56], Front Oncol, 2021	Progression-Free Survival, Prognostic Factors, and Surgical Outcome of Spheno-Orbital Meningioma	Germany	Retrospective	2000–2020	65	55	77%	I (52), II (13)	NA	NA	NA	NA	26 (40%)	15 (23%)	120
56	Dalle Ore [57], J Neurosurg, 2021	Hyperostosing Sphenoid Wing Meningiomas: Surgical Outcomes and Strategy for Bone Resection and Multidisciplinary Orbital Reconstruction	USA	Retrospective	NA	54	52 (30–79)	83%	I (45) e II (9)	28 (52%)	NA	40 (74%)	Visual field deficit, proptosis, diplopia	11 (20%)	18 (33%)	31
57	Gomes dos Santos [58], Surg Neurol Int, 2022	Spheno-Orbital Meningiomas: Is Orbit Reconstruction Mandatory? Long-Term Outcomes and Exophthalmos Improvement	Brazil	Retrospective	2008–2018	40	50 (NA)	88%	I (39) e II (1)	26 (65%)	8 (20%)	36 (90%)	Visual field deficit, headaches	26 (65%)	10 (25%)	39

Table 1. *Cont.*

	Study				Baseline Data					Presentation			Treatment	Mean Follow-Up Time (Months)
58	Locatelli [59], J Neurol Surg B Skull Base, 2022	The Role of the Trans-Orbital Superior Eyelid Approach in the Management of Selected Spheno-Orbital Meningiomas: In-Depth Analysis of Indications, Technique, and Outcomes from the Study of a Cohort of 35 Patients	Italy	Retrospective	2011–2021	35	57 (38–80)	77%	I (31), II (4)	11 (32%)	7 (20%)	22 (63%)	Visual field deficit, proptosis, diplopia, seizure	16 (46%)	NA	32
59	Wierzbowska [2], J Clin Med, 2023	Spheno-Orbital Meningioma and Vision Impairment—Case Report and Review of the Literature	Poland	Retrospective	NA	1	46	100%	I	Yes	No	Yes	NA	1 (100%)	NA	78

3.3. Efficacy Outcomes

Overall GTR rates were reported in 1542 patients. The overall rate of GTR following SOMs resection through any surgical approach was 57.3% (95%CI = 47.5–67.1%). Lesions treated through the MTA and anatomical class I lesions had the highest GTR rate at 59.8% (95%CI = 49.5–70.2%; $p = 0.001$) and 78.6% (95%CI = 60.1–97.1%; $p = 0.001$), while lesions treated through ETOA combined with EEA and WHO grade I lesions had the lowest GTR rate at 23.5% (95%CI = 0–52.5%; $p = 0.001$) and 43.1% (95%CI = 20.4–65.9%; $p = 0.001$). Overall recurrence rates were reported in 1409 patients. The overall rate of recurrence following SOMs resection through any surgical approach was 20.7% (95%CI = 16.6–24.8%). Figure 4 shows the forest plot of overall recurrence rates. Recurrence rates ranged from 4.4% (95%CI = 0–11.2%) for lesions treated through ETOA to 24.4% (95%CI = 19.4–29.4%) for lesions treated through MTA ($p = 0.014$). The overall rates of PFS 5-y and PFS 10-y were reported in 230 and 159 patients, and were 75.5% (95%CI = 70–81.1%) and 49.1% (95%CI = 41.3–56.8%), respectively. The overall rates of visual acuity and proptosis improvement were reported in 910 and 1132 patients and were 57.5% (95%CI = 51.7–63.3%) and 79.3% (95%CI = 73.7–84.8%), respectively. Figure 5 shows the forest plot of overall visual acuity improvement rates. Anatomical class I lesions had the highest visual acuity improvement rate at 71.5% (95%CI = 63.7–79.4%; $p = 0.003$). Lesions treated through the ETOA and anatomical class I lesions had the highest proptosis improvement rates at (60.1%, 95%CI = 38.0–82.2; $p = 0.001$) and 79.4% (95%CI = 57.3–100.0%; $p = 0.002$), respectively.

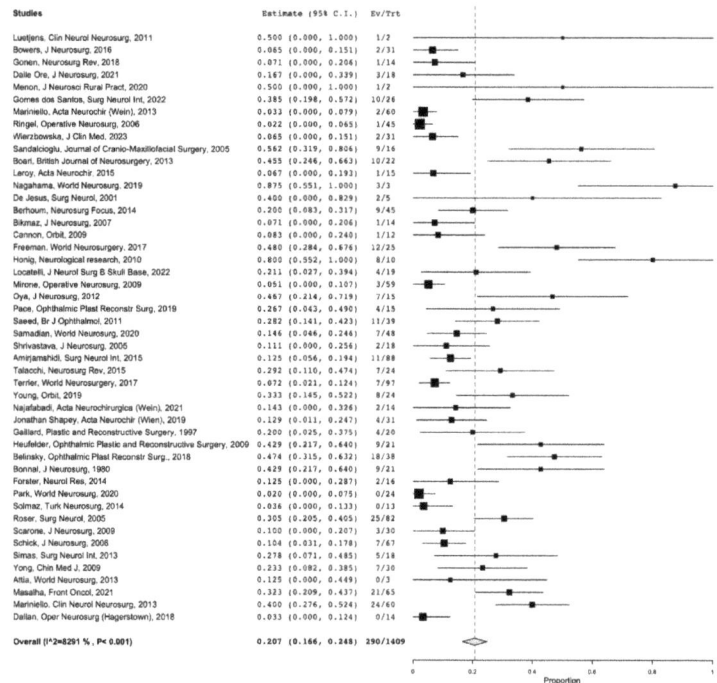

Figure 4. Forest plot of overall recurrence rates. (CIs = confidential intervals).

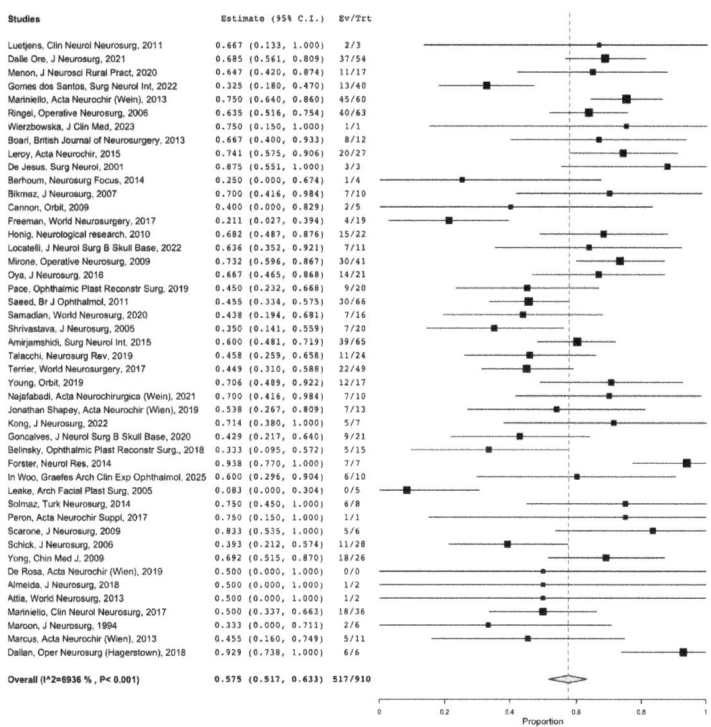

Figure 5. Forest plot of overall visual acuity improvement rates. (CIs = confidential intervals).

3.4. Safety Outcomes

Overall CN focal deficits and CSF leak rates were reported in 763 and 517 patients, respectively. The overall rate of CN focal deficits was 20.6% (95%CI = 14.9–26.3%). The lowest rate was reported for lesions treated through the ETOA (7.3%; 95%CI = 0–18.1%) and the highest rate was reported for lesions treated through the MTA (21.0%, 95%CI = 14.5–27.6%). The overall rate of CSF leak was 3.9% (95%CI = 2.3–5.5%). The CSF leak rate was highest for lesions treated through the combined ETOA and EEA (20.3%; 95%CI = 0–46.7%; $p = 0.551$) and was the lowest for lesions treated through the MTA (4.9%, 95%CI = 2.8–6.9%). Other complication rates were reported in 1181 patients. The overall rate was 13.9% (95%CI = 10.1–17.7%). The rate of other complications was the lowest for WHO grade I and II lesions (11.7%; 95%CI = 6.5–16.8%; $p = 0.001$). The efficacy and safety outcomes are summarized in Tables 2 and 3.

Table 2. Overall efficacy and safety outcomes.

	Overall % (95%CI)
GTR	57.3% (47.5–67.1)
Recurrence	20.7% (16.6–24.8)
PFS 5-y	75.5% (70.0–81.1)
PFS 10-y	49.1% (41.3–56.8)
Vision acuity improvement	57.5% (51.7–63.3)
Proptosis improvement	79.3% (73.7–84.8)
CN focal deficits	20.6% (14.9–26.3)
CSF leak	3.9% (2.3–5.5)
Other	13.9% (10.1–17.7)

Table 3. Subgroups efficacy and safety outcomes.

	MTA	ETOA	ETOA + EEA	p Value
	% (95%CI)	% (95%CI)	% (95%CI)	
GTR	59.8 (49.5–70.2)	41.3 (11.6–70.9)	23.5 (0–52.5)	0.001
Recurrence	24.4 (19.4–29.4)	4.4 (0–11.2)	NA	0.014
Vision acuity improvement	57.3 (51–63.5)	69.2 (41.5–96.9)	51.3 (16.7–85.9)	0.902
Proptosis improvement	60 (47.4–72.6)	79.4 (57.3–100)	69.8 (37.0–100)	0.002
CN focal deficits	21 (14.5–27.6)	7.3 (0–18.1)	20.3 (0–46.7)	0.411
CSF leak	4.9 (2.8–6.9)	5 (0–11.6)	20.3 (0–46.7)	0.551
Other	13.6 (9.5–17.7)	15.4 (1.6–29.2)	NA	0.866
	WHO Grade I	WHO Grades I + II	WHO Grades I + II + III	p Value
	% (95%CI)	% (95%CI)	% (95%CI)	
GTR	43.1 (20.4–65.9)	46.5 (26.8–66.1)	57.3 (47.5–67.1)	0.001
Recurrence	17.7 (1.6–33.9)	24.8 (14.9–34.7)	20.7 (16.6–24.8)	0.185
Vision acuity improvement	69.0 (47.6–90.4)	54.7 (41.1–68.3)	57.5 (51.7–63.3)	0.779
Proptosis improvement	77.3 (60.9–93.7)	74.0 (61.3–86.6)	79.3 (73.7–84.8)	0.013
CN focal deficits	12.4 (6.9–17.9)	15.4 (6.7–24.2)	20.6 (14.9–26.3)	0.224
CSF leak	5 (0–11.8)	5.2 (1.2–9.2)	3.9 (2.3–5.5)	0.983
Other	22.1 (5.1–39.2)	11.7 (6.5–16.8)	13.9 (10.1–17.7)	0.001
	Anatomical Class I	Anatomical Class I + II + III + IV		p Value
	% (95%CI)	% (95%CI)		
GTR	78.6 (60.1–97.1)	57.3 (47.5–67.1)		0.001
Recurrence	15.1 (6.5–23.7)	20.7 (16.6–24.8)		0.001
Vision acuity improvement	71.5 (63.7–79.4)	57.5 (51.7–63.3)		0.003
Proptosis improvement	60.1 (38–82.2)	79.3 (73.7–84.8)		0.001

3.5. Study Heterogeneity

The I2 values were >50%, indicating substantial heterogeneity for the following outcomes: GTR, recurrence, visual acuity improvement, proptosis improvement, CN focal deficits, and other complications. The I2 values were <50%, indicating a lack of substantial heterogeneity for the following outcomes: PFS 5-y, PFS 10-y, and CSF leak.

4. Discussion

As far as we know, this is the largest systematic literature review and meta-analysis available in the literature. Clinical and surgical outcomes of SOMs surgically treated have been analyzed. According to our findings, SOMs treated through the MTAs and anatomical class I lesions had the highest GTR rate, while ETOAs either as single or combined approach with EEAs offered the lowest GTR rate. On the other hand, MTAs presented the higher recurrence rates, and no statistically significant differences were detected between the different approaches regarding the PFS 5-y and PFS 10-y. Anatomical class I SOMs and SOMs treated with ETOA showed better rates of postoperative vision acuity and proptosis improvement. MTAs are more prone to postoperative CNs deficits, while combined ETOA and EEA have the highest rate of postoperative CSF leaks.

MTAs are commonly utilized for the surgical treatment of SOMs, with the pterional approach being the most frequently employed [60]. MTAs offer advantages such as wide exposure and the ability to achieve radical resection of hyperostotic bone. Recently, various EEAs and ETOAs, either as stand-alone options or in combination, have been described for SOMs removal [37,44,46,52,59]. EEAs are particularly effective for decompressing the medial part of the optic canal, while ETOAs enable further decompression of the hyperostotic bone and tumor removal, especially in lesions located more laterally [37]. Endoscopic approaches offer less invasive corridors and aesthetically pleasing results. However, due to the limitations in achieving GTR, these approaches should be reserved for selected patients with suspected benign SOMs exhibiting minimal intradural growth [14,60,61]. In such cases, the primary goal is symptom relief through decompression of the optic canal, with subsequent consideration of adjuvant radiotherapy (RT) for any residual tumor.

SOMs manifest as the expansion of the sphenoid bone, extending into the orbit and causing hyperostosis [42]. These tumors often spread to various adjacent areas, such as the sphenoid, orbital roof, middle fossa, superior orbital fissure (SOF), optic canal (OC), anterior clinoid, or cavernous sinus (CS). They can also invade the temporalis or lateral pterygoid muscles [62]. Due to their invasive nature, SOMs exhibit radiologic characteristics resembling malignancies [23]. However, in practical terms, most SOMs are classified as WHO-I tumors. The complete removal of SOMs through surgery is frequently limited by their infiltration into the SOF, CS, extraocular muscles, or cranial nerves [39]. The feasibility of performing aggressive resection has been a subject of debate. Reported rates of GTR in our series was 57.3% (95%CI = 47.5–67.1%). Simpson grade I resection with minimal morbidity is the main treatment goal. However, this often results in significant morbidity to the patient [4,56,63]. For this reason, over time the treatment paradigm has shifted from GTR to aggressive STR as respectful as possible of the healthy neurovascular structures surrounding the lesion [4]. Nowadays, the goal of surgery is, in fact, a symptomatic improvement compared to a GTR, for example, in the case of involvement of the optic canal with the aim of decompressing the optic nerve in order to maximize visual acuity outcomes. Accordingly, limited attempt at resection of meningioma within the cavernous sinus or with SOF involvement is performed given the risk of postoperative CN deficits [4]. This agrees with the data emerging from our study, which showed that anatomical class I lesions had the highest GTR rate, as the cavernous sinus, the orbital apex, and the intraorbital structures were not directly invaded [52,58]. Other examples of surgery aimed at improving the clinical outcome and respectful of the surrounding anatomical structures are reported in the literature. For example, Scarone et al. [20] published a series of 39 patients in which they excluded Simpson I resection in case of SOMs with SOF invasion. Ringel et al. [17] and Boari et al. [28], in a series of 63 and 40 patients, respectively, underline how the intraorbital and SOF extension prevents a GTR, as in the postoperative period there would be a considerable degree of morbidity such as not to justify the complete macroscopic removal of the lesion. Finally, Saeed et al. [29] have sanctified the concept of "symptom-oriented" resection rather than attempted GTR in a personal series of 66 patients [4,17].

According to the literature, proptosis is the most frequently observed preoperative finding and indication for surgery, with a reported occurrence rate of 45–100%. Postoperatively, proptosis improvement has been documented in 52–100% of patients [4,6,14,17,21,24,25,28,29,34,43,64]. Our study aligns with these findings, as we observed an overall clinical presentation of proptosis in 80% of cases. Additionally, the second most commonly reported preoperative finding in the literature is deteriorating visual function, which has been documented in 30–78% of cases [4,6,14,17,21,24,25,28,29,34,43,64]. Our study yielded similar results, with deteriorating visual function observed in 52% of cases. Postoperatively, visual function improvement has been reported in 21–87% of patients [4,6,14,17,21,24,25,28,29,33,34,43,64], consistent with our study's finding of 57.5% (95%CI = 51.7–63.3%). Furthermore, our study found that 79.3% (95%CI = 73.7–84.8%) of cases exhibited the specified characteristic. Ocular paresis is often the third most common presenting symptom associated with SOMs, in agreement with the data emerging from this review (13%) [3].

The patient's prognosis and quality of life heavily depend on visual acuity, rendering it a crucial clinical outcome for SOM patients [4]. To improve visual acuity, it is vital to optimize surgical interventions and postoperative follow-up [39]. According to this study, operating on patients, even those with minimal visual impairment or hyperostosis, appears to be beneficial in preventing the development of visual deficits [14,22,32,33,42,65]. The follow-up findings suggest that early surgery is predictive of favorable visual outcomes. Since SOMs tend to invade the bones near the cranial nerve foramina, early surgical intervention may help prevent extensive hyperostosis, narrowing of the foramina, and subsequent cranial nerve deficits [42]. Notably, involvement of the optic canal and intraorbital region has been identified as predictors of postoperative visual deficits. However, it should be noted that surgery itself carries the risk of new visual and cranial nerve deficits. In cases of very elderly patients, individuals with severe comorbidities, or those with extensive disease leading to complete blindness, the potential benefits of surgery may not always outweigh the risks of complications [14]. Nevertheless, in general, the risk of new complications is believed to be lower when patients undergo surgery early in their disease progression, as cranial nerves are less vulnerable when the degree of compression is less severe [54].

Complications following surgery for SOMs commonly include deficits in extraocular movements and trigeminal hypoesthesia [42]. Previous studies have indicated that postoperative deficits in extraocular movements involving CNs III, IV, and VI occur in approximately 7% to 68% of cases [17,25,42]. These findings are generally consistent with the results of this study, which reported a rate of 20.6% (95%CI = 14.9–26.3%). However, the latter figure is closer to the lower end of the range reported in existing literature. While cranial nerve palsies are often temporary, there are cases where they can be permanent. Diplopia, or double vision, tends to be more prevalent among patients who undergo resection of the periorbita [14]. Additionally, trigeminal hypoesthesia is a common comp li ca tion following surgery. Nevertheless, over the years, there has been a decrease in postoperative deficits affecting cranial nerves, likely attributable to a less aggressive surgical approach [3,4].

Over the past three decades, the surgical management of SOMs has undergone signif icant evolution, resulting in improved outcomes and reduced morbidity for patients. In the early 1990s, surgical approaches often involved extensive craniotomies and aggressive tumor resections, aiming to achieve complete tumor removal [66]. While this approach occasionally yielded favorable results, it was associated with considerable risks, such as visual impairment and injury to critical structures. As technological advancements and surgical expertise progressed, the trend shifted towards more conservative strategies in the late 1990s and early 2000s [17]. These techniques, including image-guided surgery and the use of endoscopes, prioritized functional preservation, especially vision, and resulted in reduced complications. By the 2010s, minimally invasive procedures, such as endoscopic endonasal surgery, gained prominence, offering excellent tumor control with minimal morbidity [56]. In 2023, a trend persists in favor of these less invasive techniques, showcasing their efficacy in achieving tumor control while preserving patient quality of life, particularly in terms of visual outcomes [59]. This gradual shift in surgical paradigms highlights the importance of not only eradicating the tumor but also ensuring the best possible functional outcomes for patients with spheno-orbital meningiomas.

Both recent studies and those conducted over 20 years ago provide evidence supporting the utilization of RT for subtotally resected meningiomas, demonstrating improved overall survival and PFS compared to surgery alone [9,17,20,28,64,67–70]. In cases of disease recurrence and residual tumor progression after primary microsurgery, secondary stereotactic radiosurgery (SRS) is frequently recommended [71]. SRS alone or in combination with hypo-fractionated radiotherapy offers particular advantages for treating SOMs located near the cavernous sinus and orbital apex, where surgical resection is limited, and preserving the neurovascular anatomy around the tumor is of utmost importance [9,17,20,28,64,67–70]. However, in situations where residual or recurrent lesions are in close proximity to CNs, a single dose of SRS may not be feasible [69]. Consequently, the systematic review highlights that fractionated SRS can serve as an effective approach, ensuring both appropriate aggressiveness towards the residual lesion and protection of the sur rounding neurovascular anatomy. This fractionated SRS approach achieves secondary tumor control while maintaining an acceptable adverse effect profile [71]. Nonetheless, advancements in dose reduction and treatment conformity strategies hold the potential to enhance the feasibility of this option in the future. Furthermore, other radiation modalities, such as external beam radiotherapy (EBRT), intensity-modulated radiotherapy (IMRT), and proton beam radiation therapy (PBRT), are being explored for their early applications in treating SOMs. These alternative radiation techniques offer additional options and potential benefits in the management of SOMs [50,72–74]. The role of RT in the treatment of SOMs remains a subject of ongoing debate. This systematic review highlights the lack of a standardized protocol among the authors regarding the use of RT for managing SOMs. According to the findings of this review, it is evident that residual WHO-I tumors do not typically receive secondary RT, regardless of the Simpson grade. However, in cases of recurrent WHO-I tumors, a combination of repeat surgery and postoperative radiotherapy appears to be the most commonly utilized and effective approach for disease control. Adjuvant RT is considered mandatory for WHO-II or WHO-III tumors.[75] Preliminary evidence suggests that RT may contribute to prolonged PFS, but the decision to administer RT should be carefully evaluated, considering factors such as age, tumor size, and pathology of the residual tumor [14,20].

Limitations

There are several limitations to the study. This meta-analysis was based primarily on single-center case series and, thus, has limitations inherent to single-center retrospective studies. While we were able to perform subgroup, analyses based on the surgical approach used, we were unable to perform more granular analyses stratifying outcomes by each WHO grade and anatomical class. Nonetheless, our study provides helpful information for providers who are considering surgery for the treatment of SOMs and provides guidance for future areas of investigation.

The limitations of this review stem from a dearth of high-quality studies and significant heterogeneity among those included, which may have constrained our ability to derive definitive conclusions. Moreover, we cannot disregard the possibility of publication bias, as studies reporting positive outcomes or statistically significant results tend to be more readily published. Such bias may have influenced the overall summary effect estimate, potentially leading to an overestimation of the treatment effect. Furthermore, our search strategy may have introduced limitations despite our comprehensive efforts; it is conceivable that some pertinent studies were inadvertently overlooked. Language restrictions and the exclusion of unpublished research may have also contributed to potential bias. Lastly, it is essential to consider the generalizability of our findings. The included studies may pertain to specific populations, interventions, or settings, thus potentially limiting the applicability of our results to other populations or clinical contexts.

5. Conclusions

Performing surgery for SOMs is intricate and challenging due to the tumor's diffuse nature and its proximity to critical structures. The goals of surgical treatment for SOMs have undergone an evolution. Presently, the primary objective of surgical intervention is to safeguard visual function and ameliorate proptosis, rather than pursuing complete tumor resection. When visual compromise is evident, surgery has the potential to enhance and stabilize visual function.

To optimize patient outcomes, a multidisciplinary approach involving a skull base team is essential. This team comprises neurosurgeons, ophthalmologists, otorhinolaryngologists, maxillofacial surgeons, and radiologists. Their collaborative efforts yield several advantages, including early detection of optic nerve compromise, preoperative and postoperative evidence-based management, and improved surgical resection and clinical outcomes facilitated by the combined expertise of the team members.

Author Contributions: Conceptualization, E.A., M.Z., L.D.M., M.M., T.I., M.M.F. and P.P.P.; methodology, E.A., M.Z., L.D.M., M.M., T.I., M.M.F. and P.P.P.; validation, E.A., M.Z., L.D.M., T.I., L.S., C.S., M.M.F. and P.P.P.; formal analysis, E.A. and L.D.M.; investigation, E.A. and L.D.M.; resources, L.S., C.S., A.T., F.F.A., M.M.F. and P.P.P.; data curation, E.A. and L.D.M.; writing—original draft preparation, E.A. and L.D.M.; writing—review and editing, E.A., M.Z. and L.D.M.; visualization, E.A., M.Z., L.D.M., M.M., A.R., T.I., L.S., C.S., A.T., A.P., S.P., F.F.A., M.M.F. and P.P.P.; supervision, M.Z.; project administration, L.S., C.S., A.T., F.F.A., M.M.F. and P.P.P. All authors have read and agreed to the published version of the manuscript.

Funding: This research received no external funding.

Institutional Review Board Statement: Not applicable.

Informed Consent Statement: Not applicable.

Data Availability Statement: Data available in a publicly accessible repository.

Conflicts of Interest: The authors declare no conflict of interest.

Abbreviations

Cerebro-spinal fluid (CSF), confidential intervals (CIs), cranial nerve (CN), endoscopic endonasal approaches (EEAs), endoscopic transorbital approaches (ETOAs), external beam radiotherapy (EBRT), gross total resection (GTR), intensity-modulated radiotherapy (IMRT), microsurgical transcranial (MTAs), spheno-orbital meningiomas (SOMs), Preferred Reporting Items for Systematic Reviews and Meta-Analysis (PRISMA), progression-free survival (PFS), stereotactic radiosurgery (SRS).

References

1. Shapey, J.; Jung, J.; Barkas, K.; Gullan, R.; Barazi, S.; Bentley, R.; Huppa, C.; Thomas, N.W. A single centre's experience of managing spheno-orbital meningiomas: Lessons for recurrent tumour surgery. *Acta Neurochir.* **2019**, *161*, 1657–1667. [CrossRef]
2. Wierzbowska, J.; Zegadło, A.; Patyk, M.; Rękas, M. Spheno-Orbital Meningioma and Vision Impairment-Case Report and Review of the Literature. *J. Clin. Med.* **2022**, *12*, 74. [CrossRef] [PubMed]
3. Nagahama, A.; Goto, T.; Nagm, A.; Tanoue, Y.; Watanabe, Y.; Arima, H.; Nakajo, K.; Morisako, H.; Uda, T.; Ichinose, T.; et al. Spheno-Orbital Meningioma: Surgical Outcomes and Management of Recurrence. *World Neurosurg.* **2019**, *126*, e679–e687. [CrossRef] [PubMed]
4. Freeman, J.L.; Davern, M.S.; Oushy, S.; Sillau, S.; Ormond, D.R.; Youssef, A.S.; Lillehei, K.O. Spheno-Orbital Meningiomas: A 16-Year Surgical Experience. *World Neurosurg.* **2017**, *99*, 369–380. [CrossRef]
5. Cannon, P.S.; Rutherford, S.A.; Richardson, P.L.; King, A.; Leatherbarrow, B. The surgical management and outcomes for spheno-orbital meningiomas: A 7-year review of multi-disciplinary practice. *Orbit* **2009**, *28*, 371–376. [CrossRef] [PubMed]
6. Young, J.; Mdanat, F.; Dharmasena, A.; Cannon, P.; Leatherbarrow, B.; Hammerbeck-Ward, C.; Rutherford, S.; Ataullah, S. Combined neurosurgical and orbital intervention for spheno-orbital meningiomas—The Manchester experience. *Orbit* **2020**, *39*, 251–257. [CrossRef] [PubMed]
7. Page, M.J.; McKenzie, J.E.; Bossuyt, P.M.; Boutron, I.; Hoffmann, T.C.; Mulrow, C.D.; Shamseer, L.; Tetzlaff, J.M.; Akl, E.A.; Brennan, S.E.; et al. The PRISMA 2020 statement: An updated guideline for reporting systematic reviews. *BMJ* **2021**, *372*, n71. [CrossRef] [PubMed]
8. Bonnal, J.; Thibaut, A.; Brotchi, J.; Born, J. Invading meningiomas of the sphenoid ridge. *J. Neurosurg.* **1980**, *53*, 587–599. [CrossRef]
9. Maroon, J.C.; Kennerdell, J.S.; Vidovich, D.V.; Abla, A.; Sternau, L. Recurrent spheno-orbital meningioma. *J. Neurosurg.* **1994**, *80*, 202–208. [CrossRef]
10. Gaillard, S.; Pellerin, P.; Dhellemmes, P.; Pertuzon, B.; Lejeune, J.P.; Christiaens, J.L. Strategy of craniofacial reconstruction after resection of spheno-orbital "en plaque" meningiomas. *Plast. Reconstr. Surg.* **1997**, *100*, 1113–1120. [CrossRef]
11. De Jesús, O.; Toledo, M.M. Surgical management of meningioma en plaque of the sphenoid ridge. *Surg. Neurol.* **2001**, *55*, 265–269. [CrossRef]
12. Leake, D.; Gunnlaugsson, C.; Urban, J.; Marentette, L. Reconstruction after resection of sphenoid wing meningiomas. *Arch. Facial Plast. Surg.* **2005**, *7*, 99–103. [CrossRef]
13. Roser, F.; Nakamura, M.; Jacobs, C.; Vorkapic, P.; Samii, M. Sphenoid wing meningiomas with osseous involvement. *Surg. Neurol.* **2005**, *64*, 37–43, discussion 43. [CrossRef]

4. Shrivastava, R.K.; Sen, C.; Costantino, P.D.; Della Rocca, R. Sphenoorbital meningiomas: Surgical limitations and lessons learned in their long-term management. *J. Neurosurg.* 2005, *103*, 491–497. [CrossRef] [PubMed]
5. Sandalcioglu, I.E.; Gasser, T.; Mohr, C.; Stolke, D.; Wiedemayer, H. Spheno-orbital meningiomas: Interdisciplinary surgical approach, resectability and long-term results. *J. Cranio-Maxillofac. Surg.* 2005, *33*, 260–266. [CrossRef] [PubMed]
6. Schick, U.; Bleyen, J.; Bani, A.; Hassler, W. Management of meningiomas en plaque of the sphenoid wing. *J. Neurosurg.* 2006, *104*, 208–214. [CrossRef]
7. Ringel, F.; Cedzich, C.; Schramm, J. Microsurgical technique and results of a series of 63 spheno-orbital meningiomas. *Neurosurgery* 2007, *60*, 214–221, discussion 221–222. [CrossRef] [PubMed]
8. Bikmaz, K.; Mrak, R.; Al-Mefty, O. Management of bone-invasive, hyperostotic sphenoid wing meningiomas. *J. Neurosurg.* 2007, *107*, 905–912. [CrossRef]
9. Li, Y.; Shi, J.; An, Y.; Zhang, T.; Fu, J.; Zhang, J.; Zhao, J. Sphenoid wing meningioma en plaque: Report of 37 cases. *Chin. Med. J.* 2009, *122*, 2423–2427.
10. Scarone, P.; Leclerq, D.; Héran, F.; Robert, G. Long-term results with exophthalmos in a surgical series of 30 sphenoorbital meningiomas. Clinical article. *J. Neurosurg.* 2009, *111*, 1069–1077. [CrossRef]
11. Heufelder, M.J.; Sterker, I.; Trantakis, C.; Schneider, J.-P.; Meixensberger, J.; Hemprich, A.; Frerich, B. Reconstructive and ophthalmologic outcomes following resection of spheno-orbital meningiomas. *Ophthal. Plast. Reconstr. Surg.* 2009, *25*, 223–226. [CrossRef] [PubMed]
12. Mirone, G.; Chibbaro, S.; Schiabello, L.; Tola, S.; George, B. En plaque sphenoid wing meningiomas: Recurrence factors and surgical strategy in a series of 71 patients. *Neurosurgery* 2009, *65*, 100–108, discussion 108–109. [CrossRef] [PubMed]
13. Civit, T.; Freppel, S. Sphenoorbital meningiomas. *Neurochirurgie* 2010, *56*, 124–131. [CrossRef] [PubMed]
14. Honig, S.; Trantakis, C.; Frerich, B.; Sterker, I.; Schober, R.; Meixensberger, J. Spheno-orbital meningiomas: Outcome after microsurgical treatment: A clinical review of 30 cases. *Neurol. Res.* 2010, *32*, 314–325. [CrossRef]
15. Oya, S.; Sade, B.; Lee, J.H. Sphenoorbital meningioma: Surgical technique and outcome. *J. Neurosurg.* 2011, *114*, 1241–1249. [CrossRef]
16. Luetjens, G.; Krauss, J.K.; Brandis, A.; Nakamura, M. Bilateral sphenoorbital hyperostotic meningiomas with proptosis and visual impairment: A therapeutic challenge. Report of three patients and review of the literature. *Clin. Neurol. Neurosurg.* 2011, *113*, 859–863. [CrossRef]
17. Mariniello, G.; de Divitiis, O.; Bonavolontà, G.; Maiuri, F. Surgical unroofing of the optic canal and visual outcome in basal meningiomas. *Acta Neurochir.* 2013, *155*, 77–84. [CrossRef]
18. Boari, N.; Gagliardi, F.; Spina, A.; Bailo, M.; Franzin, A.; Mortini, P. Management of spheno-orbital en plaque meningiomas: Clinical outcome in a consecutive series of 40 patients. *Br. J. Neurosurg.* 2013, *27*, 84–90. [CrossRef]
19. Saeed, P.; van Furth, W.R.; Tanck, M.; Freling, N.; van der Sprenkel, J.W.B.; Stalpers, L.J.A.; van Overbeeke, J.J.; Mourits, M.P. Surgical treatment of sphenoorbital meningiomas. *Br. J. Ophthalmol.* 2011, *95*, 996–1000. [CrossRef]
20. Simas, N.M.; Farias, J.P. Sphenoid Wing en plaque meningiomas: Surgical results and recurrence rates. *Surg. Neurol. Int.* 2013, *4*, 86. [CrossRef]
21. Attia, M.; Patel, K.S.; Kandasamy, J.; Stieg, P.E.; Spinelli, H.M.; Riina, H.A.; Anand, V.K.; Schwartz, T.H. Combined cranionasal surgery for spheno-orbital meningiomas invading the paranasal sinuses, pterygopalatine, and infratemporal fossa. *World Neurosurg.* 2013, *80*, e367–e373. [CrossRef] [PubMed]
22. Marcus, H.; Schwindack, C.; Santarius, T.; Mannion, R.; Kirollos, R. Image-guided resection of spheno-orbital skull-base meningiomas with predominant intraosseous component. *Acta Neurochir.* 2013, *155*, 981–988. [CrossRef] [PubMed]
23. Mariniello, G.; Bonavolontà, G.; Tranfa, F.; Maiuri, F. Management of the optic canal invasion and visual outcome in spheno-orbital meningiomas. *Clin. Neurol. Neurosurg.* 2013, *115*, 1615–1620. [CrossRef]
24. Forster, M.-T.; Daneshvar, K.; Senft, C.; Seifert, V.; Marquardt, G. Sphenoorbital meningiomas: Surgical management and outcome. *Neurol. Res.* 2014, *36*, 695–700. [CrossRef]
25. Solmaz, I.; Tehli, O.; Temiz, C.; Kural, C.; Hodaj, I.; Kutlay, M.; Gonul, E.; Daneyemez, M.K. Surgical strategies for the removal of sphenoorbital meningiomas. *Turk. Neurosurg.* 2014, *24*, 859–866. [CrossRef] [PubMed]
26. Talacchi, A.; De Carlo, A.; D'Agostino, A.; Nocini, P. Surgical management of ocular symptoms in spheno-orbital meningiomas. Is orbital reconstruction really necessary? *Neurosurg. Rev.* 2014, *37*, 301–309, discussion 309–310. [CrossRef]
27. Berhouma, M.; Jacquesson, T.; Abouaf, L.; Vighetto, A.; Jouanneau, E. Endoscopic endonasal optic nerve and orbital apex decompression for nontraumatic optic neuropathy: Surgical nuances and review of the literature. *Neurosurg. Focus* 2014, *37*, E19. [CrossRef]
28. Amirjamshidi, A.; Abbasioun, K.; Amiri, R.S.; Ardalan, A.; Hashemi, S.M.R. Lateral orbitotomy approach for removing hyperostosing en plaque sphenoid wing meningiomas. Description of surgical strategy and analysis of findings in a series of 88 patients with long-term follow up. *Surg. Neurol. Int.* 2015, *6*, 79. [CrossRef]
29. Leroy, H.-A.; Leroy-Ciocanea, C.I.; Baroncini, M.; Bourgeois, P.; Pellerin, P.; Labreuche, J.; Duhamel, A.; Lejeune, J.-P. Internal and external spheno-orbital meningioma varieties: Different outcomes and prognoses. *Acta Neurochir.* 2016, *158*, 1587–1596. [CrossRef]
30. Bowers, C.A.; Sorour, M.; Patel, B.C.; Couldwell, W.T. Outcomes after surgical treatment of meningioma-associated proptosis. *J. Neurosurg.* 2016, *125*, 544–550. [CrossRef]

41. Peron, S.; Cividini, A.; Santi, L.; Galante, N.; Castelnuovo, P.; Locatelli, D. Spheno-Orbital Meningiomas: When the Endoscopic Approach Is Better. *Acta Neurochir. Suppl.* **2017**, *124*, 123–128. [CrossRef]
42. Terrier, L.-M.; Bernard, F.; Fournier, H.-D.; Morandi, X.; Velut, S.; Hénaux, P.-L.; Amelot, A.; François, P. Spheno-Orbital Meningiomas Surgery: Multicenter Management Study for Complex Extensive Tumors. *World Neurosurg.* **2018**, *112*, e145–e156. [CrossRef]
43. Gonen, L.; Nov, E.; Shimony, N.; Shofty, B.; Margalit, N. Sphenoorbital meningioma: Surgical series and design of an intraoperative management algorithm. *Neurosurg. Rev.* **2018**, *41*, 291–301. [CrossRef]
44. Almeida, J.P.; Omay, S.B.; Shetty, S.R.; Chen, Y.-N.; Ruiz-Treviño, A.S.; Liang, B.; Anand, V.K.; Levine, B.; Schwartz, T.H. Transorbital endoscopic eyelid approach for resection of sphenoorbital meningiomas with predominant hyperostosis: Report of 2 cases. *J. Neurosurg.* **2018**, *128*, 1885–1895. [CrossRef]
45. Spheno-Orbital Meningiomas: An Analysis Based on World Health Organization Classification and Ki-67 Proliferative Index—PubMed. Available online: https://pubmed.ncbi.nlm.nih.gov/28350689/ (accessed on 19 July 2023).
46. Dallan, I.; Sellari-Franceschini, S.; Turri-Zanoni, M.; de Notaris, M.; Fiacchini, G.; Fiorini, F.R.; Battaglia, P.; Locatelli, D.; Castelnuovo, P. Endoscopic Transorbital Superior Eyelid Approach for the Management of Selected Spheno-orbital Meningiomas: Preliminary Experience. *Oper. Neurosurg.* **2018**, *14*, 243–251. [CrossRef] [PubMed]
47. Kong, D.-S.; Young, S.M.; Hong, C.-K.; Kim, Y.-D.; Hong, S.D.; Choi, J.W.; Seol, H.J.; Lee, J.-I.; Shin, H.J.; Nam, D.-H.; et al. Clinical and ophthalmological outcome of endoscopic transorbital surgery for cranioorbital tumors. *J. Neurosurg.* **2018**, *131*, 667–675. [CrossRef]
48. Pace, S.T.; Koreen, I.V.; Wilson, J.A.; Yeatts, R.P. Orbital Reconstruction via Deformable Titanium Mesh Following Spheno-Orbital Meningioma Resection: Ophthalmic Presentation and Outcomes. *Ophthal. Plast. Reconstr. Surg.* **2020**, *36*, 89–93. [CrossRef] [PubMed]
49. De Rosa, A.; Pineda, J.; Cavallo, L.M.; Di Somma, A.; Romano, A.; Topczewski, T.E.; Somma, T.; Solari, D.; Enseñat, J.; Cappabianca, P.; et al. Endoscopic endo- and extra-orbital corridors for spheno-orbital region: Anatomic study with illustrative case. *Acta Neurochir.* **2019**, *161*, 1633–1646. [CrossRef]
50. Menon, S.O.S.; Anand, D.; Menon, G. Spheno-Orbital Meningioma: Optimizing Visual Outcome. *J. Neurosci. Rural Pract.* **2020**, *11*, 385–394. [CrossRef] [PubMed]
51. Goncalves, N.; Lubbe, D.E. Transorbital Endoscopic Surgery for Sphenoid Wing Meningioma: Long-Term Outcomes and Surgical Technique. *J. Neurol. Surg. Part B Skull Base* **2020**, *81*, 357–368. [CrossRef]
52. Park, H.H.; Yoo, J.; Yun, I.-S.; Hong, C.-K. Comparative Analysis of Endoscopic Transorbital Approach and Extended Mini-Pterional Approach for Sphenoid Wing Meningiomas with Osseous Involvement: Preliminary Surgical Results. *World Neurosurg.* **2020**, *139*, e1–e12. [CrossRef] [PubMed]
53. Parish, J.M.; Shields, M.; Jones, M.; Wait, S.D.; Deshmukh, V.R. Proptosis, Orbital Pain, and Long-Standing Monocular Vision Loss Resolved by Surgical Resection of Intraosseous Spheno-Orbital Meningioma: A Case Report and Literature Review. *J. Neurol. Surg. Rep.* **2020**, *81*, e28–e32. [CrossRef] [PubMed]
54. Zamanipoor Najafabadi, A.H.; Genders, S.W.; van Furth, W.R. Visual outcomes endorse surgery of patients with spheno-orbital meningioma with minimal visual impairment or hyperostosis. *Acta Neurochir.* **2021**, *163*, 73–82. [CrossRef]
55. In Woo, K.; Kong, D.-S.; Park, J.W.; Kim, M.; Kim, Y.-D. Orbital decompressive effect of endoscopic transorbital surgery for sphenoorbital meningioma. *Graefe's Arch. Clin. Exp. Ophthalmol.* **2021**, *259*, 1015–1024. [CrossRef] [PubMed]
56. Masalha, W.; Heiland, D.H.; Steiert, C.; Krüger, M.T.; Schnell, D.; Scheiwe, C.; Schnell, O.; Grosu, A.-L.; Beck, J.; Grauvogel, J. Progression-Free Survival, Prognostic Factors, and Surgical Outcome of Spheno-Orbital Meningiomas. *Front. Oncol.* **2021**, *11*, 672228. [CrossRef] [PubMed]
57. Dalle Ore, C.L.; Magill, S.T.; Rodriguez Rubio, R.; Shahin, M.N.; Aghi, M.K.; Theodosopoulos, P.V.; Villanueva-Meyer, J.E.; Kersten, R.C.; Idowu, O.O.; Vagefi, M.R.; et al. Hyperostosing sphenoid wing meningiomas: Surgical outcomes and strategy for bone resection and multidisciplinary orbital reconstruction. *J. Neurosurg.* **2020**, *134*, 711–720. [CrossRef] [PubMed]
58. Dos Santos, A.G.; Paiva, W.S.; da Roz, L.M.; do Espirito Santo, M.P.; Teixeira, M.J.; Figueiredo, E.G.; da Silva, V.T.G. Spheno-orbital meningiomas: Is orbit reconstruction mandatory? Long-term outcomes and exophthalmos improvement. *Surg. Neurol. Int.* **2022**, *13*, 318. [CrossRef]
59. Locatelli, D.; Restelli, F.; Alfiero, T.; Campione, A.; Pozzi, F.; Balbi, S.; Arosio, A.; Castelnuovo, P. The Role of the Transorbital Superior Eyelid Approach in the Management of Selected Spheno-orbital Meningiomas: In-Depth Analysis of Indications, Technique, and Outcomes from the Study of a Cohort of 35 Patients. *J. Neurol. Surg. Part B Skull Base* **2022**, *83*, 145–158. [CrossRef]
60. Agosti, E.; Turri-Zanoni, M.; Saraceno, G.; Belotti, F.; Karligkiotis, A.; Rocca, G.; Buffoli, B.; Raffetti, E.; Hirtler, L.; Rezzani, R.; et al. Quantitative Anatomic Comparison of Microsurgical Transcranial, Endoscopic Endonasal, and Transorbital Approaches to the Spheno-Orbital Region. *Oper. Neurosurg.* **2021**, *21*, E494–E505. [CrossRef]
61. Agosti, E.; Saraceno, G.; Rampinelli, V.; Raffetti, E.; Veiceschi, P.; Buffoli, B.; Rezzani, R.; Giorgianni, A.; Hirtler, L.; Alexander, A.Y.; et al. Quantitative Anatomic Comparison of Endoscopic Transnasal and Microsurgical Transcranial Approaches to the Anterior Cranial Fossa. *Oper. Neurosurg.* **2022**, *23*, e256–e266. [CrossRef]
62. Mourits, M.P.; van der Sprenkel, J.W.B. Orbital meningioma, the Utrecht experience. *Orbit* **2001**, *20*, 25–33. [CrossRef] [PubMed]

53. Hsu, F.P.K.; Anderson, G.J.; Dogan, A.; Finizio, J.; Noguchi, A.; Liu, K.C.; McMenomey, S.O.; Delashaw, J.B. Extended middle fossa approach: Quantitative analysis of petroclival exposure and surgical freedom as a function of successive temporal bone removal by using frameless stereotaxy. *J. Neurosurg.* **2004**, *100*, 695–699. [CrossRef] [PubMed]
54. Honeybul, S.; Neil-Dwyer, G.; Lang, D.A.; Evans, B.T.; Ellison, D.W. Sphenoid wing meningioma en plaque: A clinical review. *Acta Neurochir.* **2001**, *143*, 749–757, discussion 758. [CrossRef] [PubMed]
55. Yannick, N.; Patrick, F.; Samuel, M.; Erwan, F.; Pierre-Jean, P.; Michel, J.; Stéphane, V. Predictive factors for visual outcome after resection of spheno-orbital meningiomas: A long-term review. *Acta Ophthalmol.* **2012**, *90*, e663–e665. [CrossRef]
56. Samii, M.; Tatagiba, M. Experience with 36 surgical cases of petroclival meningiomas. *Acta Neurochir.* **1992**, *118*, 27–32. [CrossRef]
57. Pompili, A.; Derome, P.J.; Visot, A.; Guiot, G. Hyperostosing meningiomas of the sphenoid ridge—Clinical features, surgical therapy, and long-term observations: Review of 49 cases. *Surg. Neurol.* **1982**, *17*, 411–416. [CrossRef]
58. Barbaro, N.M.; Gutin, P.H.; Wilson, C.B.; Sheline, G.E.; Boldrey, E.B.; Wara, W.M. Radiation therapy in the treatment of partially resected meningiomas. *Neurosurgery* **1987**, *20*, 525–528. [CrossRef]
59. Iwai, Y.; Yamanaka, K.; Ikeda, H. Gamma Knife radiosurgery for skull base meningioma: Long-term results of low-dose treatment. *J. Neurosurg.* **2008**, *109*, 804–810. [CrossRef]
70. Clark, B.G.; Candish, C.; Vollans, E.; Gete, E.; Lee, R.; Martin, M.; Ma, R.; McKenzie, M. Optimization of stereotactic radiotherapy treatment delivery technique for base-of-skull meningiomas. *Med. Dosim.* **2008**, *33*, 239–247. [CrossRef]
71. Gorman, L.; Ruben, J.; Myers, R.; Dally, M. Role of hypofractionated stereotactic radiotherapy in treatment of skull base meningiomas. *J. Clin. Neurosci.* **2008**, *15*, 856–862. [CrossRef]
72. Terpolilli, N.A.; Ueberschaer, M.; Niyazi, M.; Hintschich, C.; Egensperger, R.; Muacevic, A.; Thon, N.; Tonn, J.-C.; Schichor, C. Long-term outcome in orbital meningiomas: Progression-free survival after targeted resection combined with early or postponed postoperative radiotherapy. *J. Neurosurg.* **2019**, *133*, 302–312. [CrossRef] [PubMed]
73. Cohen-Inbar, O.; Tata, A.; Moosa, S.; Lee, C.-C.; Sheehan, J.P. Stereotactic radiosurgery in the treatment of parasellar meningiomas: Long-term volumetric evaluation. *J. Neurosurg.* **2018**, *128*, 362–372. [CrossRef] [PubMed]
74. El Shafie, R.A.; Czech, M.; Kessel, K.A.; Habermehl, D.; Weber, D.; Rieken, S.; Bougatf, N.; Jäkel, O.; Debus, J.; Combs, S.E. Clinical outcome after particle therapy for meningiomas of the skull base: Toxicity and local control in patients treated with active rasterscanning. *Radiat. Oncol.* **2018**, *13*, 54. [CrossRef] [PubMed]

Disclaimer/Publisher's Note: The statements, opinions and data contained in all publications are solely those of the individual author(s) and contributor(s) and not of MDPI and/or the editor(s). MDPI and/or the editor(s) disclaim responsibility for any injury to people or property resulting from any ideas, methods, instructions or products referred to in the content.

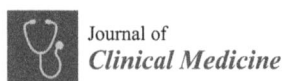 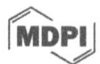

Brief Report

A Treatment Approach for Carotid Blowout Syndrome and Soft Tissue Reconstruction after Radiotherapy in Patients with Oral Cancer: A Report of 2 Cases

Tobias Moest [1,*], Marco Rainer Kesting [1], Maximilian Rohde [1], Werner Lang [2], Alexander Meyer [2], Manuel Weber [1] and Rainer Lutz [1]

1 Department of Oral and Maxillofacial Surgery, University Hospital Erlangen, Glückstraße 11, 91054 Erlangen, Germany
2 Department of Vascular Surgery, University Hospital Erlangen, Krankenhausstraße 12, 91054 Erlangen, Germany
* Correspondence: tobias.moest@uk-erlangen.de; Tel.: +49-9131-8533653; Fax: +49-9131-8534219

Abstract: Background: This retrospective case series study aims to demonstrate a salvage technique for the treatment of carotid blow-out syndrome (CBS) in irradiated head and neck cancer patients with a vessel-depleted neck. Methods: Between October 2017 and October 2021, two patients (N = 2) with CBS were treated at our institution in a multidisciplinary approach together with the Department of Vascular Surgery. Patients were characterized based on diagnoses, treatment procedures, and the subsequent postoperative course. Results: Surgical emergency intervention was performed in both cases. The transition zone from the common carotid artery (CCA) to the internal carotid artery (ICA) was resected and reconstructed with a xenogic (case 1) or autogenic (case 2) interposition (end-to-end anastomosis). To allow reconstruction of the vascular defect, an additional autologous vein graft was anastomosed to the interposition graft in an end-to-side technique, allowing arterial anastomosis for a free microvascular flap without re-clamping of the ICA. Because of the intraoperative ICA reconstruction, none of the patients suffered a neurological deficit. Conclusions: The techniques presented in the form of two case reports allow for acute bleeding control, cerebral perfusion, and the creation of a vascular anastomosis option in the vessel-depleted neck.

Keywords: carotid blow out syndrome; vessel graft; vessel-depleted neck; irradiation

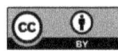

1. Introduction

Carotid blowout syndrome (CBS) is a rare and life-threatening complication in patients treated for head and neck cancer, most commonly with a history of prior surgery and radiotherapy. CBS is the result of vessel wall necrosis that can occur as a result of surgical and adjuvant tumor therapies, chronic inflammation, and fistula.

The general incidence of CBS in oncological procedures in the head and neck region is 3–4.5% [1,2], while the incidence in patients following previous radiotherapy varies from 4.5% to 21.1% [3,4]. According to Macdonald et al., the risk of CBS increases by a factor of 7.6 in patients with head and neck tumors [5].

Carotid artery rupture occurs mainly in the common carotid artery (CCA), near the bifurcation (60–70% of cases). A much smaller proportion also occurs in the internal carotid artery (ICA) [6–8]. In general, CBS is more common in atherosclerotic vessel segments with stenosis [9].

The main risk factor for the development of CBS is previous radiation therapy after tumor surgery [10]. Patients who have received more than 70 Gy have an up to 14-fold increased risk of developing CBS [11]. From a histopathological point of view, radiotherapy leads to the formation of free radicals, which in turn favor thrombosis, obliteration of the vasa vasorum of the vascular adventitia, and vascular fibrosis. The result is premature atherosclerotic change and significant vascular weakness. CBS is therefore the result of vascular weakness due to ischemia resulting from adventitial insufficiency [10].

Based on this, it is understandable that surgical procedures that result in damage to the adventitia increase the likelihood of CBS. Patients who underwent neck dissection surgery showed an eight-fold increased risk of CBS [11]. In particular, patients with recurrent tumors after previous surgical treatment with neck dissection and adjuvant radiotherapy, where additional radiotherapy is required if reoperation is not possible, are at particularly high risk of developing CBS.

The general incidence of CBS in re-irradiated patients with tumor recurrence is 0–17%. In these cases, tumor ingrowth into the CCA is an additional risk factor for CBS [12,13]. In general, the median cumulative dose of both radiotherapy modalities is between 110 and 130 Gy. Studies show an increased rate of CBS when the cumulative dose is >130 Gy [10].

Another risk factor is chronic inflammation in the sense of bacterial infection, which leads to thrombosis of the vasa vasorum of the arterial wall and has an increased susceptibility to the negative influence of inflammatory mediators in contaminated wound areas [6]. In addition to post-operative wound infections, oro- or pharyngocutaneous fistulae pose a high risk due to tryptic enzyme activity. Permanent contact with saliva leads to digestion of the arterial wall by tryptic enzymes, and bleeding may be provoked. Powitzky et al. showed in their study that 38% of CBS cases demonstrated inflammation, 40% fistula, and 55% tissue necrosis [6].

Due to the extremely high mortality rate of 76%, CBS is a feared complication [14]. In emergencies, CBS is treated by ligation of the CCA or ICA without consideration of collateral cerebral circulation, increasing the risk of neurological morbidity [15]. In the literature, mortality rates vary from 15–100%, with an average of 50% [10]. In addition to surgical treatment of CBS, endovascular interventions, including vascular plugging and covered stent repair, are considered feasible therapeutic options [11,16].

The aim of the present study was to present clinical examples of techniques that can be used for the surgical management of spontaneous and intraoperative CBS. The techniques presented in the form of two case reports allow acute hemorrhage control during permanent cerebral perfusion (intraluminal shunt) and the creation of a vascular anastomosis option in the avascular neck.

2. Patients, Materials and Methods

This interdisciplinary retrospective case series was performed at the Department of Oral and Maxillofacial Surgery in cooperation with the Department of Vascular Surgery (University Clinic Erlangen). Patients were identified by screening the digital clinic documentation system (MCC®, Meierhofer AG, Munich, Germany) and the digital patient files (Soarian Clinicals®, Cerner Health Services, Erlangen, Germany; Meona®, Meona GmbH, Freiburg, Germany).

Two patients with CBS were included in this retrospective analysis between October 2017 and October 2021. The Ethics Committee of the University Hospital Erlangen was consulted regarding the approval of the study. The committee decided that ethics approval was not required for retrospective case analyses.

3. Results

3.1. Case 1 (Spontaneous CBS)

In July 2017, a 76-year-old female Caucasian patient presented to our clinic with a recurrence of oral squamous cell carcinoma (OSCC) with infiltration of the mandible. She had previously undergone resection of an OSCC on the left cheek (2008, pT1 pN0 M0 G2 L0 V0 R0) and a second OSCC in the alveolar bone of the left mandible (2014, pT1 pN1 (1/1, perinodal) L0 V0 Pn0 G2 R0). Postoperative interstitial brachytherapy with up to 50 Gy in 2008/2009 and definitive concurrent radiotherapy (2014, total dose 64 Gy) and chemotherapy with 5-FU and cisplatin (10–12/2014) with maintenance chemotherapy with cisplatin (01/2015) were initially performed. In 10/2015, a recurrent tumor of the OSCC in the area of the anterior floor of the mouth and the alveolar crest of the left lower jaw (rpT4a pN0 (0/15) L0 V0 Pn0 G2 infiltration depth 0.5 cm, R0) was resected and reconstructed with a microvascular anastomosed upper arm graft.

The present recurrent tumor (rpT4a L0 V0 Pn0 G3 Rx), newly detected in July 2017, was treated with a partial mandibular resection (continuity resection). The mandible was reconstructed with a reconstruction plate (Stryker GmbH & Co. KG, Duisburg, Germany, 2.7 mm) and a free microvascular M. latissimus dorsi flap. The postoperative course was very complicated due to recurrent circulatory disturbances of the flap and cervical wound healing disorders, which were covered by a musculocutaneous anteriolateral thigh flap (ALT).

During the postoperative inpatient period, spontaneous erosive bleeding of the left CCA/ICA required emergency surgery. After systemic heparinization and clamping, the ruptured carotid bifurcation was resected, and the ICA was reconstructed with an on-table pericardial tube graft (bovine pericardium; PeriGuard Repair Patch® (Synovis, St. Paul, MN, USA), as autologous vessel grafts of adequate size were not available.

The tube graft was constructed with a linear stapler and anastomosed to the CCA and ICA by end-to-end anastomosis. As necrotic parts of the previous flap had to be removed, an approximately 3 cm-long arm vein graft (the cephalic vein of the right upper arm) was placed end-to-side on the pericardium to allow arterial anastomosis of a soft tissue graft. An upper arm flap was used to fill the cervical soft tissue defect resulting from the resection of the necrotic tissue mentioned above (Figures 1(D1) and 2).

The patient was discharged from the hospital on the 36th day after the operation. After discharge, the patient attended our six-weekly tumor follow-up in our outpatient clinic.

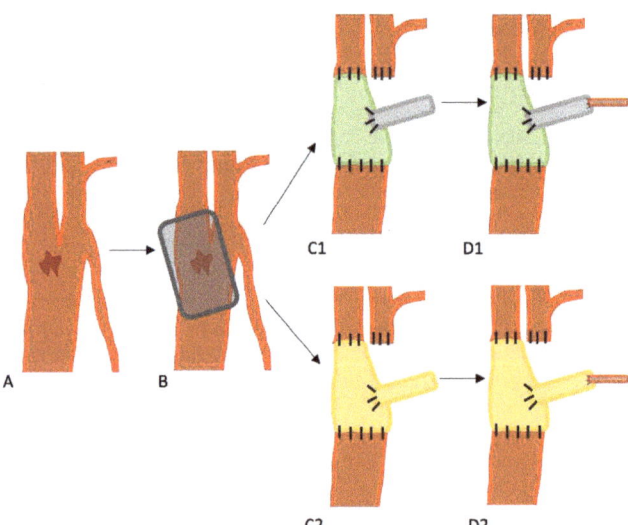

Figure 1. (**A**) Shows the typical location of carotid blow-out syndrome, which is often located at the junction of the CCA and ICA. (**B**) Shows the resected portions of the CCA, ICA, and ECA. (**C1,C2**) Illustrates the different reconstruction techniques: (**C1**) with a xenogenic graft (green) combined with an autologous second graft (grey); (**C2**) with an autologous graft (yellow) combined with an autologous second graft (yellow); (**D1,D2**) shows the anastomosis of the autologous graft (grey in (**D1**) and yellow in (**D2**)) with the arterial branch of the graft.

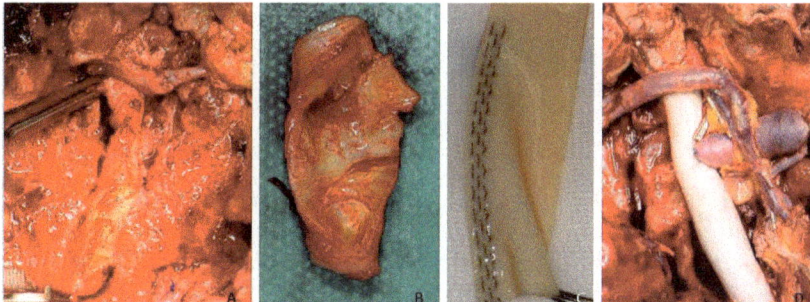

Figure 2. (**A**) Shows the intraoperative situation of the ruptured CCA near the bifurcation. (**B**) Resection of the CCA and the bifurcation to the ECA/ICA. (**C**) Individually table-made xenogenic interponate. (**D**) Anastomosed graft to the ICA/CCA with an additional graft for the microvascular free flap artery.

3.2. Case 2 (Intraoperative CBS)

A 65-year-old Caucasian male presented to our clinic in February 2021 with a suspected malignancy at the floor of the mouth, a significantly worsened general condition, and a weight loss of 10 kg within a few weeks. The staging CT scan showed a cT4a N2b OSCC on the right floor of the mouth. In March 2021, surgery was performed with a temporary tracheotomy, neck dissection of levels I-III on both sides, and resection of the floor of the mouth and the mandible from the left to right jaw angle. The mandible was reconstructed with a reconstruction plate (Stryker GmbH & Co. KG, Duisburg, Germany, 2.7 mm) in combination with a microvascular latissimus dorsi transplant, as osseous reconstruction was rejected by the patient.

Histopathological evaluation revealed a pT4a pN2c (2/43) L0 V0 Pn1 OSCC with bone infiltration of 1.4 cm, G2, R0. Due to the tumor size and lymph node involvement, the postoperative interdisciplinary tumor board recommended adjuvant radiochemotherapy to optimize tumor control. However, the planning CT showed signs of early recurrence, and definitive radiotherapy (increased final dose) and adjuvant chemotherapy were recommended, which were delivered from May 2021 to July 2021 with a total cumulative dose of 70 Gy to the oral floor and lymphatic drainage target volume. The recommended concurrent chemotherapy was rejected by the patient.

However, during the course of radiotherapy, a significant intraoral dehiscence with significant exposure of the reconstruction plate was observed, leading to severe aesthetic and functional impairment. Due to the risk of further complications, removal of the reconstruction plate was recommended. The patient has now requested osseous reconstruction of the mandible for future implant-prosthetic rehabilitation. Removal of the reconstruction plate alone, with the risk of permanent tracheostomy due to possible soft tissue collapse, was categorically rejected.

Because of the expected intraoperative soft tissue deficit due to previous radiotherapy, extraoral cervical soft tissue reconstruction with a microvascular ALT transplant in combination with a free fibula transplant was planned.

The procedure was performed using a "three-team approach". One team prepared the cervical vessels and removed the osteosynthesis material, while the second and third teams harvested the ALT and the free fibula transplant.

The preparation of the neck was extremely difficult due to extreme fibrosis of the soft tissues and significant scarring. Despite careful preparation, a wall weakness of the CCA was observed, leading to a wall defect with massive bleeding (CBS). As direct suture reconstruction was not possible, a vascular surgeon was consulted at once.

Systemic heparinization was initiated, followed by preparation of the carotid bifurcation and ligation of the external carotid artery (ECA). The area of perforation, which included parts of the ICA and parts of the CCA, was resected. To ensure cerebral perfusion, an intraluminal shunt system (FlexcelTM Carotid Shunt; Version 2020-05; LeMaitre Vascular; Burlington, MA, USA) was placed until an approximately 5 cm long venous segment of the greater saphenous vein was prepared and anastomosed to the ICA and CCA as an arterial interposition (end-to-end). To allow microvascular reconstruction of the cervical soft tissue dehiscence, an additional 2 cm-long vein graft was anastomosed to the interponate in an end-to-side technique, which could be used for arterial anastomosis of the ALT graft. This avoided further cross-clamping of the ICA during microsurgery. Due to the desolate cervical vascular status, the fibular graft was not completely harvested, transferred back to the lower leg, and replanted with osteosynthesis. The postoperative course was uneventful. No neurological deficit was noted. The patient was discharged on postoperative day 13 with a permanent tracheostomy tube. Postoperative angiography of the cervical vessels showed adequate perfusion (Figure 3). Postoperative care was provided in our outpatient clinic. After discharge, the patient attended our six-week tumor follow-up in our outpatient clinic.

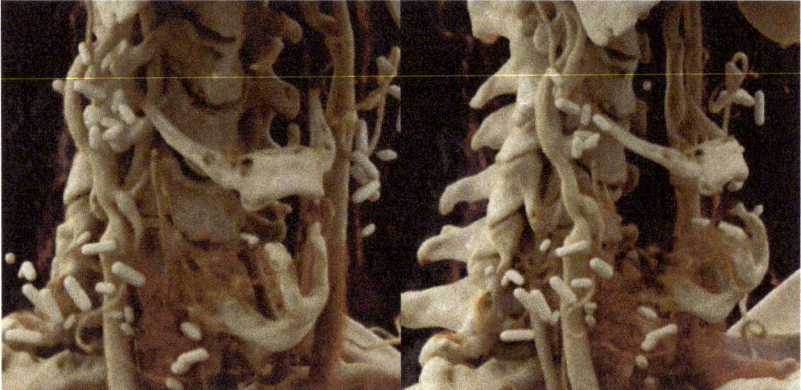

Figure 3. Three-dimensional reconstruction of the post-operative situation by angiography showing the interponate connecting the CCA to the ICA and the transition from the additional interponate to the arterial branch to the graft in case 2.

4. Discussion

The aim of this case series was to demonstrate techniques that allow for the management of CBS while at the same time enabling microvascular soft tissue reconstruction of cervical defects using free flaps. Two patient cases are presented.

The two cases have in common that the preoperative anatomical and soft tissue situations were extremely challenging. Both cases showed previous operations, wound infection/dehiscence, a previously irradiated neck (cases 1 + 2) and partial microvascular free flap necrosis (case 1). Both cases presented with CBS and cervical soft tissue defects too large for local management while at the same time presenting "vessel depleted necks" with no suitable vessels for microvascular anastomosis.

The literature describes different techniques for the handling of mass bleeding resulting from the erosion of the carotid bifurcation. The number of treatment techniques for acute CBS is more limited. Here, vascular ligation represents the ultima ratio, and a series of possible consequences should be considered. The direct neurologic consequences of ligation of the ICA are not predictable, and range from an asymptomatic course to a disabling major stroke [17].

Patients with a high risk for CBS often also show a "vessel depleted neck" due to multiple prior surgical and radiochemical interventions. In the same patient group, as is the case here, a microcvascular flap treatment may be necessary due to the size of the defect.

In order to make microvascular tissue transfer possible, individual solutions range from simple interposition grafts to extracorporeal perfusion devices [18–24].

As the standard vascular network defined by the ECA branches and the jugular vein is inaccessible in those cases, other recipient vessels for microvascular anastomoses have to be chosen.

For arterial anastomoses, branches of the subclavian (internal mammary artery and thyrocervical trunk) and axillary arteries (thoracoacromial artery) as well as the superficial temporal artery have been described in the literature [25–27].

For venous drainage, the accessory veins of the target artery can be prepared. Another option is to use the cephalic vein because of its reliable drainage, consistent anatomy, long pedicle, and high flow to the low-pressure system [18].

As mentioned above, CBS can occur under unfavorable conditions that require new strategies.

In addition to patient survival, the aim is to solve the acute bleeding problem, provide an anastomosis option for microsurgical defect treatment, and allow sufficient cerebral perfusion to prevent neurological damage. All these requirements were met with the two techniques described in this report.

In both cases, the choice of vascular graft depended on the presence/location of a suitable donor site, e.g., the presence of a microvascular donor site despite the "vessel depleted neck".

In case 1, a xenograft was used to manufacture a neo-ICA. In case 2, V. saphena magna was harvested by extending the surgical access to the ALT flap. The xenograft could be manufactured in length and diameter as required. The saphenous vein has nearly the same caliber as the ICA, and the length could be varied as required. This way, graft positioning was unproblematic, and no risk of kinking existed.

In case 2, a collateral circulation bridging the resected CCA/ICA gap was created using an intraluminal shunt. Installing the shunt takes about 5–8 min when performed by an experienced surgeon. During this period, the CCA as well as the ICA/ECA are clamped. The anastomosis of the additional lateral graft to the interposition graft for subsequent arterial flap anastomosis was performed before re-opening the clamps in order to avoid additional clamping of the interposition graft.

With the techniques described, simultaneous management of both acute bleeding (CBS) and soft tissue reconstruction was possible. In the treatment of the CBS, an almost optimal situation for microsurgical transplant anastomosis was constructed. Both patients experienced no further bleeding or neurological complications; cervical soft tissue reconstruction was successful.

5. Conclusions

ICA/CCA reconstruction with an autologous or xenogeneic vascular graft and an additional vascular branch for subsequent microvascular flap anastomosis is an effective method for the combined treatment of CBS and cervical soft tissue defects in patients with a "vessel depleted neck".

Author Contributions: Conceptualization, T.M.; Data curation, T.M.; Investigation, T.M., W.L., A.M., M.W. and R.L.; Supervision, M.R.K. and R.L.; Visualization, T.M. and M.R.; Writing—original draft, T.M. and M.R.; Writing—review and editing, M.R.K., M.R., W.L., A.M., M.W. and R.L. All authors have read and agreed to the published version of the manuscript.

Funding: This research received no external funding.

Institutional Review Board Statement: This retrospective chart review study involving human participants was in accordance with the ethical standards of the institutional and national research committee and with the 1964 Helsinki Declaration and its later amendments or comparable ethical standards. It did not require review by the IRB.

Informed Consent Statement: Informed consent was obtained from all subjects involved in the study.

Data Availability Statement: Additional chart data from all patients may be provided by contacting the corresponding author.

Conflicts of Interest: The authors declare no conflict of interest.

References

1. Leikensohn, J.; Milko, D.; Cotton, R. Carotid artery rupture. Management and prevention of delayed neurologic sequelae with low-dose heparin. *Arch. Otolaryngol.* **1978**, *104*, 307–310. [CrossRef]
2. Ketcham, A.S.; Hoye, R.C. Spontaneous carotid artery hemorrhage after head and neck surgery. *Am. J. Surg.* **1965**, *110*, 649–655. [CrossRef]
3. Joseph, D.L.; Shumrick, D.L. Risks of head and neck surgery in previously irradiated patients. *Arch. Otolaryngol.* **1973**, *97*, 381–384. [CrossRef] [PubMed]
4. Yim, D.; Rappaport, I.; Jose, L.; Kohut, R.; Shramek, J. Carotid artery and dermal graft. *Arch. Otolaryngol.* **1974**, *99*, 242–246. [CrossRef] [PubMed]
5. Macdonald, S.; Gan, J.; McKay, A.J.; Edwards, R.D. Endovascular treatment of acute carotid blow-out syndrome. *J. Vasc. Interv. Radiol.* **2000**, *11*, 1184–1188. [CrossRef] [PubMed]
6. Powitzky, R.; Vasan, N.; Krempl, G.; Medina, J. Carotid blowout in patients with head and neck cancer. *Ann. Otol. Rhinol. Laryngol.* **2010**, *119*, 476–484. [CrossRef]
7. Razack, M.S.; Sako, K. Carotid artery hemorrhage and ligation in head and neck cancer. *J. Surg. Oncol.* **1982**, *19*, 189–192. [CrossRef]
8. Liang, N.L.; Guedes, B.D.; Duvvuri, U.; Singh, M.J.; Chaer, R.A.; Makaroun, M.S.; Sachdev, U. Outcomes of interventions for carotid blowout syndrome in patients with head and neck cancer. *J. Vasc. Surg.* **2016**, *63*, 1525–1530. [CrossRef]
9. Luo, C.B.; Teng, M.M.; Chang, F.C.; Chang, C.Y.; Guo, W.Y. Radiation carotid blowout syndrome in nasopharyngeal carcinoma: Angiographic features and endovascular management. *Otolaryngol. Head Neck Surg.* **2008**, *138*, 86–91. [CrossRef]
10. Suárez, C.; Fernández-Alvarez, V.; Hamoir, M.; Mendenhall, W.M.; Strojan, P.; Quer, M.; Silver, C.E.; Rodrigo, J.P.; Rinaldo, A.; Ferlito, A. Carotid blowout syndrome: Modern trends in management. *Cancer Manag. Res.* **2018**, *10*, 5617–5628. [CrossRef]
11. Chen, Y.J.; Wang, C.P.; Wang, C.C.; Jiang, R.S.; Lin, J.C.; Liu, S.A. Carotid blowout in patients with head and neck cancer: Associated factors and treatment outcomes. *Head Neck* **2015**, *37*, 265–272. [CrossRef] [PubMed]
12. Kasperts, N.; Slotman, B.J.; Leemans, C.R.; de Bree, R.; Doornaert, P.; Langendijk, J.A. Results of postoperative reirradiation for recurrent or second primary head and neck carcinoma. *Cancer* **2006**, *106*, 1536–1547. [CrossRef] [PubMed]
13. Cengiz, M.; Özyiğit, G.; Yazici, G.; Doğan, A.; Yildiz, F.; Zorlu, F.; Gürkaynak, M.; Gullu, I.H.; Hosal, S.; Akyol, F. Salvage reirradiaton with stereotactic body radiotherapy for locally recurrent head-and-neck tumors. *Int. J. Radiat. Oncol. Biol. Phys.* **2011**, *81*, 104–109. [CrossRef] [PubMed]
14. McDonald, M.W.; Moore, M.G.; Johnstone, P.A. Risk of carotid blowout after reirradiation of the head and neck: A systematic review. *Int. J. Radiat. Oncol. Biol. Phys.* **2012**, *82*, 1083–1089. [CrossRef]
15. Lu, H.J.; Chen, K.-W.; Chen, M.-H.; Chu, P.-Y.; Tai, S.-K.; Wang, L.-W.; Chang, P.M.-H.; Yang, M.-H. Predisposing factors, management, and prognostic evaluation of acute carotid blowout syndrome. *J. Vasc. Surg.* **2013**, *58*, 1226–1235. [CrossRef] [PubMed]
16. Brinjikji, W.; Cloft, H.J. Outcomes of endovascular occlusion and stenting in the treatment of carotid blowout. *Interv. Neuroradiol.* **2015**, *21*, 543–547. [CrossRef] [PubMed]
17. Moore, O.S.; Karlan, M.; Sigler, L. Factors influencing the safety of carotid ligation. *Am. J. Surg.* **1969**, *118*, 666–668. [CrossRef] [PubMed]
18. Horng, S.Y.; Chen, M.T. Reversed cephalic vein: A lifeboat in head and neck free-flap reconstruction. *Plast. Reconstr. Surg.* **1993**, *92*, 752–753. [CrossRef]
19. Havlik, R.; Ariyan, S. Repeated use of the same myocutaneous flap in difficult second operations of the head and neck. *Plast. Reconstr. Surg.* **1994**, *93*, 481–488. [CrossRef]
20. Fichter, A.M.; Ritschl, L.M.; Rau, A.; Schwarzer, C.; von Bomhard, A.; Wagenpfeil, S.; Wolff, K.-D.; Mücke, T. Free flap rescue using an extracorporeal perfusion device. *J. Cranio-Maxillofac. Surg.* **2016**, *44*, 1889–1895. [CrossRef]
21. Wolff, K.D.; Ervens, J.; Herzog, K.; Hoffmeister, B. Experience with the osteocutaneous fibula flap: An analysis of 24 consecutive reconstructions of composite mandibular defects. *J. Cranio-Maxillofac. Surg.* **1996**, *24*, 330–338. [CrossRef] [PubMed]
22. Cheng, H.T.; Lin, F.Y.; Chang, S.C. Evidence-based analysis of vein graft interposition in head and neck free flap reconstruction. *Plast. Reconstr. Surg.* **2012**, *129*, 853e–854e. [CrossRef]
23. Moubayed, S.P.; Giot, J.P.; Odobescu, A.; Guertin, L.; Harris, P.G.; Danino, M.A. Arteriovenous fistulas for microvascular head and neck reconstruction. *Plast. Surg.* **2015**, *23*, 167–170. [CrossRef]
24. Ethunandan, M.; Cole, R.; Flood, T.R. Corlett loop for microvascular reconstruction in a neck depleted of vessels. *Br. J. Oral. Maxillofac. Surg.* **2007**, *45*, 493–495. [CrossRef] [PubMed]
25. Roche, N.A.; Houtmeyers, P.; Vermeersch, H.F.; Stillaert, F.B.; Blondeel, P.N. The role of the internal mammary vessels as recipient vessels in secondary and tertiary head and neck reconstruction. *J. Plast. Reconstr. Aesthet. Surg.* **2012**, *65*, 885–892. [CrossRef] [PubMed]

26. Urken, M.L.; Vickery, C.; Weinberg, H.; Buchbinder, D.; Biller, H.F. Geometry of the vascular pedicle in free tissue transfers to the head and neck. *Arch. Otolaryngol. Head Neck Surg.* **1989**, *115*, 954–960. [CrossRef]
27. Frohwitter, G.; Rau, A.; Kesting, M.R.; Fichter, A. Microvascular reconstruction in the vessel depleted neck—A systematic review. *J. Cranio-Maxillofac. Surg.* **2018**, *46*, 1652–1658. [CrossRef]

Disclaimer/Publisher's Note: The statements, opinions and data contained in all publications are solely those of the individual author(s) and contributor(s) and not of MDPI and/or the editor(s). MDPI and/or the editor(s) disclaim responsibility for any injury to people or property resulting from any ideas, methods, instructions or products referred to in the content.

MDPI
St. Alban-Anlage 66
4052 Basel
Switzerland
www.mdpi.com

Journal of Clinical Medicine Editorial Office
E-mail: jcm@mdpi.com
www.mdpi.com/journal/jcm

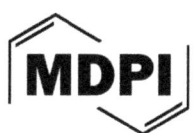

Disclaimer/Publisher's Note: The statements, opinions and data contained in all publications are solely those of the individual author(s) and contributor(s) and not of MDPI and/or the editor(s). MDPI and/or the editor(s) disclaim responsibility for any injury to people or property resulting from any ideas, methods, instructions or products referred to in the content.

www.ingramcontent.com/pod-product-compliance
Lightning Source LLC
LaVergne TN
LVHW070155120526
838202LV00013BA/1141